Resources for People

with

Disabilities and Chronic Conditions

Resources for Rehabilitation
Lexington, Massachusetts

Resources for Rehabilitation
22 Bonad Road
Winchester, MA 01890
(781) 368-9094   FAX (781) 368-9096
e-mail: info@rfr.org   www.rfr.org

Resources for People with Disabilities and Chronic Conditions, 4th edition

ISBN 0-929718-30-5

Resources for Rehabilitation is a nonprofit organization dedicated to providing training and information to professionals and the public about the needs of individuals with disabilities and the resources available to meet those needs.

Library of Congress Cataloging-in-Publication Data

Resources for People with Disabilities and Chronic Conditions
5th ed.
  p.   cm.

      Includes bibliographical references and index
      ISBN 0-929718-30-5 (alk.paper)
1. Handicapped--Rehabilitation--United States--Directories.
2. Handicapped--Services for--United States--Directories.
3. Chronically ill--Rehabilitation--United States--Directories.
4. Chronically ill--Services for--United States--Directories.
I. Resources for Rehabilitation (Organization)
HV1553.R482
362.4'048'02573--dc21   2002001030

For a complete listing of publications available from Resources for Rehabilitation, see pages 324-328.

TABLE OF CONTENTS

HOW TO USE THIS BOOK **7**

Chapter 1
LIVING WITH A DISABILITY OR CHRONIC CONDITION **9**
   Responses to disability and chronic conditions **10**
   How disabilities and chronic conditions affect the family **11**
   Where to find local services **13**
   Rehabilitation **14**
   Computers and disabilities **15**
   Self-help groups **16**
   Conclusion **17**
   Organizations **19**
   Publications and tapes **32**

Chapter 2
LAWS THAT AFFECT PEOPLE WITH DISABILITIES **43**
   Organizations **50**
   Publications and tapes **57**

Chapter 3
CHILDREN AND YOUTHS **63**
   Family and peer relationships **65**
   Laws that affect children and youths **66**
   Organizations **71**
   Publications and tapes **78**
   Financial aid for postsecondary education **88**

Chapter 4
MAKING EVERYDAY LIVING EASIER **89**
   Environmental adaptations and assistive devices **89**
   Organizations **91**
   Publications and tapes **93**
   Travel and recreation **96**
   Travel and transportation organizations **98**
   Adaptive sports and recreation organizations **102**
   Publications and tapes **107**
   Resources for assistive devices **111**

Chapter 5
COMMUNICATION DISORDERS 113

HEARING DISORDERS 113
Causes and types of hearing impairment and deafness 113
Hearing loss in children 115
Hearing loss in elders 117
Psychological aspects of hearing loss 118
Professional service providers 119
Where to find services 120
Environmental adaptations 121
Assistive devices 122
Organizations 126
Publications and tapes 134
Resources for assistive devices 143

SPEECH DISORDERS 147
Causes and types of speech impairments 147
Psychological aspects of speech impairments 148
Professional service providers 148
Where to find services 149
Assistive devices 149
Organizations 151
Publications and tapes 156
Resources for assistive devices 161

Chapter 6
DIABETES 164
Types of diabetes 165
Diabetes in children 168
Diabetes in elders 170
Psychological aspects of diabetes 170
Professional service providers 172
Where to find services 172
Assistive devices 172
How to recognize an insulin reaction and give first aid 173
Organizations 176
Publications and tapes 181
Special equipment for people with visual impairment 191

Chapter 7
EPILEPSY 193
Types of seizures 193
Treatment of epilepsy 194
Epilepsy in children 197
Epilepsy in elders 198
Psychological aspects of epilepsy 199
Professional service providers 200
Where to find services 201
How to recognize a seizure and give first aid 201
Organizations 205
Publications and tapes 208

Chapter 8
LOW BACK PAIN 218
The back 218
Nonspecific low back pain 219
Other types of back pain 220
Psychological aspects of low back pain 222
Professional service providers 223
Where to find services 223
Modifications in daily living 224
Organizations 227
Publications and tapes 231

Chapter 9
MULTIPLE SCLEROSIS 235
Diagnosis of multiple sclerosis 235
Types of multiple sclerosis 236
Treatment of multiple sclerosis 236
Psychological aspects of multiple sclerosis 239
Professional service providers 240
Where to find services 241
Environmental adaptations 241
Organizations 245
Publications and tapes 249

Chapter 10
SPINAL CORD INJURY 259
The spinal cord 260
Treatment and complications of spinal cord injury 260
Spinal cord injury in youths 262
Aging and spinal cord injury 263
Psychological aspects of spinal cord injury 263
Professional service providers 265
Where to find services 266
Modifications in everyday living 267
Organizations 271
Publications and tapes 277

Chapter 11
VISUAL IMPAIRMENT AND BLINDNESS 285
Major types and causes of visual impairment and blindness 285
Visual impairment and blindness in children 287
Visual impairment and blindness in elders 288
Psychological aspects of vision loss 288
Professional service providers 289
Where to find services 290
Environmental adaptations 290
Assistive devices 293
Organizations 295
Publications and tapes 303
Resources for assistive devices 312

INDEX TO ORGANIZATIONS 314

PUBLICATIONS FROM RESOURCES FOR REHABILITATION . 324

HOW TO USE THIS BOOK

The services available for people with disabilities and chronic conditions have increased in recent years to meet the needs of this growing population. The vast array of services and the eligibility criteria for these services may be confusing to individuals and service providers alike. Furthermore, many individuals and service providers are unaware of these services.

This book is designed to help individuals with disabilities and chronic conditions, their family members, and service providers find services and products that contribute to achieving the maximum level of independence possible. It provides information on a wide variety of organizations, publications, and assistive devices. Because individuals have different lifestyles, needs, and degrees of impairment, this book is organized so that readers may select the resources that are most appropriate to their specific needs.

Each chapter includes an introductory narrative, information about national organizations that provide services to people with disabilities and chronic conditions, and information about relevant publications and tapes. Chapters 1, 2, and 4, "Living with a Disability or Chronic Condition," "Laws That Affect People with Disabilities," and "Making Everyday Living Easier," provide information that is useful no matter what disability or condition the reader is interested in. Similarly, Chapter 3, "Children and Youths," although aimed at a specific age group, is relevant to this group regardless of the specific disability or condition.

Beginning with Chapter 5, each chapter has introductory material describing causes and effects of the condition or impairment; special information concerning the needs of children and elders, when appropriate; psychological aspects; information on professional service providers and where to find services; assistive devices; major organizations serving people with the condition or disability; and publications and tapes. Descriptions of organizations, publications and tapes, and resources for assistive devices are alphabetical within sections. Although many of the publications described are available in libraries or bookstores, for those who wish to purchase the books by mail or phone, the addresses and phone numbers of publishers and distributors are included. Only directories that have timely information and those that are updated regularly are included. Publications that are out of print may be located at libraries or bookstores that specialize in locating out of print books.

Developments in computer technology, such as the Internet and e-mail, have greatly increased access to information for the general population as well as people with disabilities and chronic conditions. E-mail and Internet addresses are provided for organizations when available.

The use of "TTY" in the listings indicates a teletypewriter, a special telephone system for individuals who are deaf or have hearing impairments and those who have speech impairments (also known as a "TDD," telecommunication device for the deaf or "TT," text telephone). The use of "V/TTY" indicates that the same telephone number is used for both voice and TTY. Toll-free numbers may begin with "800," "888," "877," or "866."

The use of the phrase "alternate formats" in the listings indicates that, in addition to standard print, publications may also be available in large print, audiocassette, braille, or computer disk.

All of the material in this book is up-to-date, and prices were accurate at the time of publication. However, it is always advisable to contact publishers and manufacturers to inquire about availability and current prices.

Chapter 1

LIVING WITH A DISABILITY OR CHRONIC CONDITION

The number of individuals who live with a disability or chronic condition constitutes a significant proportion of the population. A recent survey estimates that in 1997, 52.6 million Americans, or 19.7% of the population, lived with a disability that limits their functional or socially defined activities (McNeil: 2001). This figure does not include those Americans who live in institutions.

The large portion of Americans with disabilities is attributable to several factors. Advances in medical technology have increased the survival rates of individuals who have experienced severe trauma and babies who are born with diseases that formerly were life-threatening. Similarly, advances in technology have enabled the general population to live longer. An increase in the prevalence of disabilities and chronic conditions has accompanied this increased longevity.

A wide variety of services exists for this population in both the private and the public sectors. Federal laws have mandated a variety of programs that provide rehabilitation services and independent living programs. Such programs exist at the regional, state, and local levels. Special programs and services are available at hospitals, libraries, senior centers, independent living centers, and in educational institutions at all levels, from preschool through postsecondary education.

Although the services that exist are both numerous and varied, it is commonplace to discover that people who need these services have not received information about them or about the implications of their own condition. Individuals interviewed by William Roth (1981) repeatedly made this point. For example, one individual who was paralyzed said the following about his hospital stay:

> I hardly ever saw or talked with my doctor. An aide used to come by and check me. I think it would have been a lot more helpful for me to talk to the doctor and have him explain all the aspects of my disability and how I could function in my daily life with it. Maybe the doctors didn't know about independent living. But even if they didn't, they should have tried to get me off the catheter and give a lot of counseling to me and my family.
> ... They should have classes for people who are disabled to inform them about their disability and what it means....I probably learned more from other people in wheelchairs than I did from any of the doctors... (pp. 42-43)

Researchers have found that physicians often lack knowledge about rehabilitation services or have a negative attitude toward rehabilitation. Greenblatt (1989) found that ophthalmologists are themselves unaware of many of the services that exist to help people who are visually impaired or blind. Her study (1991) of people who had recently been diagnosed with irreversible vision loss found that these individuals are often given a diagnosis with no explanation of the available services or devices that would enable them to function independently and to continue working.

Researchers in the field of aphasia noted:

> ...many physicians dismiss aphasia rehabilitation as an irrelevant endeavor...As the 20th century progressed, however, physicians became less involved with aphasia rehabilitation and seemed to adopt the pessimistic attitude of hopelessness" (Albert and Helm-Estabrooks: 1988, 1206)

A negative attitude on the part of some physicians and inadequate information about rehabilitation leave people with disabilities and chronic conditions in a position where they are marginal to both the fields of medicine and rehabilitation. Physicians, who are attuned more to the needs of patients with acute conditions than those with chronic conditions, in essence often write off many of these patients. Rehabilitation professionals are not aware of these individuals and therefore are unable to provide services to them. In many instances, individuals never receive rehabilitation services or else years elapse before they do.

RESPONSES TO DISABILITY AND CHRONIC CONDITIONS

The diagnosis of a disability or chronic condition changes a person's life dramatically. To many members of society, people with physical impairments bear a stigma; their social status has decreased and they become the objects of others' curiosity. People with disabilities are aware of the way in which society views them. As a result, some people try to "pass" or to hide their disabilities. Many individuals who experience their first physical impairment in later life once held the same stereotypes that they now fear will be applied to them.

It is normal for people who have recently learned that they have a disability or chronic condition to go through a series of emotions including depression, denial, bargaining, anger, and acceptance. These reactions are similar to those that occur after other losses, such as the death of a loved one. Not every individual experiences all of these reactions. Some people may be chronically depressed; some may deny the permanency or severity of their loss; others may accept the loss and move on to acceptance of rehabilitation services and assistive devices.

Knowledge of the person's reactions to previous stressful situations may provide insight into his or her responses to a disability or chronic condition. It is common to rely on coping mechanisms that have been developed over a course of a lifetime. Religious faith, family, and friends may help some individuals to face disability and cope with it in a positive manner. An individual's reactions may be shaped by the severity of the disability or condition and whether it occurs suddenly or gradually. When the onset of disability is gradual and early intervention measures are taken, the individual may be motivated to learn new ways of accomplishing ordinary tasks. In addition, the individual may be better able to handle depression; retain a positive self-image; and strive to be independent. Both the individual and family members have time to plan for necessary changes, although anxiety over the future course of the condition may be severe.

When a disability or chronic condition has a sudden onset, the individual may be in a state of shock. Depression, the most common response to loss, often follows shock. Both shock and depression are normal precedents to emotional recovery. Depression is not always recognized, because it may be masked by weakness, apathy, irritability, and passivity (Hollander: 1982). Denial of the presence of the disability is also a common reaction. Service

10

providers and family members must not encourage the belief that the condition will be reversed. Individuals must fully accept their condition before emotional recovery can occur. Individuals who deny their conditions should be referred for counseling; otherwise, it is unlikely that rehabilitation will be effective.

It is especially difficult to cope with those chronic conditions that fluctuate in their severity and impact. Conditions such as multiple sclerosis and diabetes can leave people relatively free of symptoms for a period of time and then cause devastating problems, such as loss of vision. Adjusting to the current situation is difficult enough; add to this the fear that the condition may worsen and it is easy to understand why people in these circumstances have great emotional burdens.

Brooks and Matson (1987) have described the broad array of coping mechanisms and skills that individuals with multiple sclerosis must develop in order to feel that they have a sense of control over their condition and their lives. They must make decisions about medications and treatment; search for information about their disease; adapt their environment to accommodate their current situation; and take measures to relieve anxiety. All of these factors affect employment, family life, and relationships outside the family.

The knowledge that there are services available to help cope with what may at first seem overwhelming can make the difference in maintaining the ability to continue functioning independently. Learning about new technology that enables people with disabilities and chronic conditions to function in their everyday activities may prove to be the factor that enables these individuals to come to grips with the new dimension of their lives.

The roles of professional service providers may be crucial in shaping individuals' responses to a disability or a chronic condition. Professionals can help people with disabilities to continue functioning in socially productive roles and to avoid the feeling that they need to "pass." Combating negative attitudes among professionals toward people with disabilities is an essential first step in serving this growing population.

HOW DISABILITIES AND CHRONIC CONDITIONS AFFECT THE FAMILY

Diagnosis of a disability or chronic condition in a family member can cause disruption in the healthiest of families. Coping with a crisis situation puts strain on any relationship; coping with the inevitability of a permanent change causes strain between marital partners, parents and offspring, and between members of the nuclear and extended families. Stress may be related to providing adequate health care, financial concerns, disruption of familiar patterns of everyday living and work, and sexual relations.

It is crucial that family members understand the nature of the condition and its effects on daily functioning. Holding realistic expectations for what the affected family member can and cannot do contributes to the individual's ability to cope with the situation. Being overly protective and trying to do everything for the affected family member may result in diminished self-esteem and independence. On the other hand, expecting the individual to carry out activities that are unrealistic or implying that the limitations are "only in the head" creates a great deal of additional stress. People with disabilities and chronic conditions often express the fear of being a burden on family members; when their relatives suggest that they can accomplish tasks that are physically impossible for them, the affected individuals will be reluctant to ask for assistance at any time.

Individuals who are part of well adjusted marriages and families are likely to cope better with their newly diagnosed conditions than individuals in strained relationships. Just as individual coping patterns are developed over a lifetime of experience, family responses to crises are similar to those that they have exhibited in the past. Individuals with supportive marital partners find their marriages to be a source of support, while individuals in weaker relationships may tend to use their condition as an excuse for the strain in their marriages (Rodgers and Calder: 1990).

With increasing lifespans for people with disabilities and chronic conditions, the responsibilities of caregivers have increased. For children with disabilities, parents must help decide appropriate courses of education, training, and care that will enable the children to become as independent as possible once they reach adulthood. Spouses of individuals with recently acquired disabilities or chronic conditions must often take on new roles within the family and the household, while at the same time helping the partner whose health has changed to adapt to the new situation. For elders who are expected to live for years with a disability or chronic condition, family members must help decide the best options for long term care and housing.

With family structures changing and more women in the work force, it is essential that society develop policies and programs that enable family members to meet the needs of their relatives and continue to have healthy relationships with other members of their family. Often the help of a social worker or a psychologist is necessary to help the family restructuring that takes place following the development of a disability or chronic condition. The emotional needs of the spouse or partner must also be considered. Since the spouse or partner has the additional role of providing emotional and physical support for the individual who has developed a disability or chronic condition, he or she will likely need support also. Self-help groups of other spouses or partners in similar situations may prove helpful. Hulnick and Hulnick (1989) suggest that counselors can help family members "reframe" the context of the situation so that they respond positively, learn and grow from the new situation, and empower themselves to make choices.

Local and state governments, private agencies that provide case management services, and voluntary organizations that are dedicated to one disease or disability often have programs to help family members as well as the individuals with disabilities and chronic conditions. Short term respite programs that enable caregivers to have time to themselves, adult day care programs, provision of personal attendants or home health aides, and special programs for children and elders have been developed as a way for caregivers to give adequate care and also tend to their own personal needs. Meeting the financial needs of dependent family members often requires the help of an attorney who specializes in family law.

Parents of children with disabilities and chronic conditions worry about what will happen to the children when the parents are no longer alive. Group homes enable adults who are not capable of living on their own to live in a setting with different levels of supervision. An alternative is for adult siblings to care for their sister or brother. Individuals who take on the responsibility of caring for a brother or sister with a disability or chronic condition must understand the major commitment that they are making in terms of both time and emotions.

These adults must learn how to navigate service systems and how to advocate effectively. Often they must help make decisions regarding medical treatment and other important services; evaluate assistive devices; and provide services such as transportation that help their brother or sister carry out everyday activities.

Locating the appropriate service providers and self-help groups is often a challenge for family members and may prove frustrating at first. Persevering until the goals of health care, rehabilitation, and maximum levels of independence have been achieved is not only rewarding but enables the family to develop new patterns of living that become familiar and normal for all members.

WHERE TO FIND LOCAL SERVICES

A good place to start the search for services is the information and referral office of the local United Way. Other sources of information are local directories of service agencies available in the reference collection of many public libraries. Libraries often have their own special programs for people with disabilities, and some have special needs centers or special reading equipment for people with visual impairments.

State and municipal offices established to serve people with disabilities are other sources of referrals. A study of major cities in the United States (Groch: 1991) found that over half had established special offices to deal with disability issues. The remainder had designated an individual to deal with these issues, and the overwhelming majority (86%) had appointed a person to coordinate the requirements of Section 504 of the Rehabilitation Act (see Chapter 2, "Laws That Affect People with Disabilities" for a discussion of this section). It is likely that these cities have now appointed individuals to coordinate the cities' efforts to meet the requirements of the Americans with Disabilities Act, which was passed about one and a half years after the survey was completed. At the time of the survey, the cities responded that they provided a wide variety of services, including accessible housing, transportation, public education about disability, job placement, referrals, and special recreational activities.

Rehabilitation agencies, described below, are a major source of assistance for people with disabilities and chronic conditions. Some departments of rehabilitation, human or health services, aging, and education may provide respite care to families of individuals with disabilities. Respite care is temporary help designed to relieve caretakers of the need to be "on call" for 24 hours a day. It relieves the caretaker's emotional burden and allows time to tend to personal needs.

Veterans are eligible for special benefits and rehabilitation services. The U.S. Department of Veterans Affairs (VA) has established a number of special services, including the provision of prosthetics for veterans with service related disabilities. Visual Impairment Services Teams (VIST) help veterans with vision problems. The VA will specially adapt the homes of veterans with disabilities.

REHABILITATION

In fiscal year 1995, approximately 1.3 million adults received services from state vocational rehabilitation programs. Over 200,000 were considered to be successfully rehabilitated, meaning that they had been suitably employed for at least 60 days. This figure represents nearly half (46.1%) of those exiting the rehabilitation system (Kaye: 1998).

The rehabilitation process helps individuals who have irreversible impairments or chronic conditions to continue functioning in society. Rehabilitation is appropriate when medical and surgical interventions are incapable of restoring functioning to normal. Rehabilitation services may include any or all of the following:

- rehabilitation counseling
- job placement
- provision of assistive equipment, prostheses, and medical supplies
- vocational training to remain in one's current position or to learn a new skill
- adapting the home or work environment
- training in activities of daily living and homemaking
- transportation services

Rehabilitation services are provided by both public and private agencies. In the United States, each state is required by law to have a public agency that is responsible for providing vocational rehabilitation services. In many states, there are separate agencies to serve people who are visually impaired or blind. In the remaining states, services for people who are visually impaired or blind are provided within the general vocational rehabilitation agency. Many states offer special rehabilitation services for children and elders. The federal government provides financial support for rehabilitation services and sets standards for service delivery, as required by the Rehabilitation Act of 1973 and its amendments (see Chapter 2, "Laws That Affect People with Disabilities") and administered by the Rehabilitation Services Administration, U.S. Department of Education.

Some rehabilitation professionals provide services independently on a fee-for-service basis. (Rehabilitation counselors are certified by the Commission on Rehabilitation Counselor Certification, listed in "ORGANIZATIONS" section below.) Rehabilitation services are offered in group settings, in residential settings, or at home.

There is no one rehabilitation plan that will work for all individuals. Individuals must work jointly with rehabilitation counselors to set their goals and establish an appropriate rehabilitation plan to meet those goals. The federal government requires that individuals sign an Individual Written Rehabilitation Program that indicates they approve of the rehabilitation strategy developed jointly with counselors in state rehabilitation agencies. It is also important to involve family members in the rehabilitation process so that they will support, not undermine, the person's attempts to remain independent.

The Client Assistance Program is a federally mandated program that requires states to provide information to all clients and potential clients about the benefits available under the Rehabilitation Act (see Chapter 2, "Laws That Affect People with Disabilities") and to assist clients in obtaining these benefits.

Individuals with severe disabilities often require assistance with personal care, transportation, and special equipment. Independent living programs enable people with disabilities to continue functioning within the community with a minimal amount of assistance. A crucial element of the independent living movement is that consumers have control over the types of services provided. For some, this means living at home, with or without attendant care, and maintaining employment. Attendants assist people with disabilities in activities such as bathing, grooming, dressing, food preparation, and household tasks. Provisions of both Social Security and Medicaid laws have been used to finance the services of attendants. People with disabilities or chronic conditions may opt to live in group residences, where individuals live under supervision but maintain a degree of responsibility for their own care and maintenance. Independent living programs or centers are sometimes administered by state vocational rehabilitation agencies and sometimes are free-standing organizations administered by individuals with disabilities themselves.

Ideally, the approach to medical treatment and rehabilitation planning should be carried out jointly by health professionals and rehabilitation professionals. Because the medical profession is largely oriented toward cure rather than rehabilitation, such a collaborative approach is often a difficult goal to attain.

COMPUTERS AND DISABILITIES

Personal computers (PCs) have opened up a wide variety of opportunities for people who have disabilities or chronic conditions. Used alone, adapted computers enable individuals to perform tasks that would be otherwise inaccessible to them; retaining a job is just one major opportunity that computers offer to people with disabilities. Using computers with online subscription services and the Internet, it is possible to communicate with people all over the world. This instant communication provides up-to-the-minute information about new developments and the opportunity to "chat" with individuals in similar situations. Many of these services are free, with the exception of telephone charges or subscription fees for online services. World Wide Web pages provide access to information from service agencies, professional societies, educational institutions, and commercial organizations, as well as individuals who have established their own pages. Web sites listed throughout this book provide links to a wide variety of disability resources.

A variety of formats is available to receive and exchange information. When you join a usenet group, you may read messages and respond to them as well as submit your own information and questions. In order to join a usenet group, your host computer must provide access. When you subscribe to a usenet group, you will automatically receive all new messages whenever you log on. If you decide to exchange messages with just one member, you may send mail directly to that individual's e-mail address.

Listserv enables you to receive information by sending a message to an e-mail address stating you would like to subscribe. You may add your own messages which may in turn generate responses from other members of a group. Protocol requires that you then summarize your responses and mail them to all other members of the listserv group.

PubMed, a web site that provides access to MEDLINE, a medical database that enables the user to perform searches of the medical literature by topic and author, is available at most libraries. PubMED is also available over the Internet at no charge, directly from the National Library of Medicine, as are several other online databases. MEDLINE performs searches of major medical journals and provides both citations and abstracts of articles. After searching MEDLINE and reading abstracts of the articles on the web site, it is possible to order the articles through the organization that provides the service. You may also find the articles at local libraries. If your library does not have the articles you want, ask the reference librarians to obtain them from other libraries. Be certain to ask the charge, as it may be less expensive for you to visit the other libraries yourself.

SELF-HELP GROUPS

Self-help groups enable individuals with similar problems or conditions to discuss their problems and offer mutual assistance. Self-help groups offer a number of benefits to participants, including learning to develop coping strategies; acquiring a sense of control over life; combating isolation and alienation; and developing information networks. In addition, members of self-help groups often express a sense of increased self-esteem, because they have offered help to other members of the group.

Self-help group members often believe that their peers are more understanding and patient than professional counselors, health care providers, or even family members, because they have had similar experiences. The person who needs help may feel weak or incompetent, no matter what his or her profession or background. Receiving help from a peer tends to minimize these feelings.

Professional service providers are ideally suited to identify and bring together individuals with common problems, and they often are able to offer a site where meetings may be held. However, professionals must understand the new role that they play in helping to create a self-help group. Madara (no date) recommends that professionals assume the role of consultants, providing advice and counsel but not assuming any responsibility for leadership, decision making, or group tasks. A professional who is the catalyst for the formation of a group must disengage from this initial role to allow the group to develop autonomously. Since professionals often tend to encourage dependent client relationships, they must guard against this type of relationship if a group is to offer true mutual support.

Identifying a group facilitator or coordinator is the first step in developing self-help groups for individuals with disabilities and chronic conditions, their spouses or partners, their parents, or their siblings. One method is to identify someone who has had group experience. Former patients or clients who have had experience in coping with disabilities are likely candidates for starting a group. Another method is to identify an organized, articulate person who has experienced a disability and has some background in a club or other organization. Announcements in publications, at meetings, and on hospital and agency bulletin boards are also good recruitment techniques. Once the group is established, it is up to the members to decide how frequently to meet; the types of discussions or programs to have; and how to recruit members.

It is sometimes necessary to be creative in establishing self-help groups for people with disabilities. Individuals who have difficulty traveling because of mobility impairments may

16

have difficulty arranging for transportation to the meeting site. One solution to this problem is to hold meetings by having telephone conference calls (Romness et al.: 1992). While this system may have the disadvantage of not providing face-to-face contact, it does provide the participants with the opportunity to discuss common problems with peers and may eliminate some of the feelings of isolation. For individuals with hearing impairments who are not fluent in sign language, interpreters may be employed in order to conduct a self-help meeting.

Interpreted captioning is a system that enables people with hearing loss who are not fluent in sign language or speechreading to understand the conversation at group meetings (Grant and Walsh: 1990). There are several methods of interpreted captioning, including visual recording, where a volunteer uses large sheets of paper to record the meeting in words, symbols, and graphics, and real time captioning, where an operator types the dialogue from a meeting into a computer. The computer display may be presented in enlarged form by projection onto a screen or wall; alternatively, large print software may be sufficient to enable members of the group to read the proceedings.

The most recent form of self-help group has evolved as a result of the technological advances in personal computing. Individuals with a computer and modem may now join a usenet group, where they may exchange information with others who experience the same disabilities or conditions. Individuals have the opportunity to discuss their insights, offer advice, and ask questions; other individuals respond to their questions and comments.

While exchanging information over computer lines is significantly different in character from meeting face-to-face with a group, it provides information and helps to combat social isolation for those in rural areas and those who are unable to leave their homes. It may also serve as a first step in meeting someone with a similar experience who lives in the same geographic area.

CONCLUSION

Rehabilitation, independent living programs, and self-help groups are some of the options available to help individuals with disabilities and chronic conditions. When these local services are used in conjunction with the resources described in this book, people with disabilities and chronic conditions may overcome depression and function to the maximum level of independence possible. The ability to function independently will have great consequences on the individual's self-esteem, on relationships with family members and significant others, and on employment.

References

Albert, Martin and Nancy Helm-Estabrooks
1988 "Diagnosis and Treatment of Aphasia, Part II" JAMA 259:8(February 26): 1205-1210
Brooks, Nancy A. and Ronald R. Matson
1987 "Managing Multiple Sclerosis" Volume 6, pp. 73-106 in Julius A. Roth and Peter Conrad (eds.) Research in the Sociology of Health Care Greenwich, CT: JAI Press Inc.

Grant, Nancy C. and Birrell Walsh
1990 "Interpreted Captioning: Facilitating Interactive Discussion Among Hearing Impaired Adults" International Journal of Technology and Aging 3:2(Fall/Winter):133-144

Greenblatt, Susan L.
1991 "What People with Vision Loss Need to Know" pp. 7-20 in Susan L. Greenblatt (ed.) Meeting the Needs of People with Vision Loss: A Multidisciplinary Perspective Lexington, MA: Resources for Rehabilitation
1989 "The Need for Coordinated Care" pp. 25-38 in Susan L. Greenblatt (ed.) Providing Services for People with Vision Loss: A Multidisciplinary Perspective Lexington, MA: Resources for Rehabilitation

Groch, Sharon
1991 "Public Services Available to Persons with Disabilities in Major U.S. Cities" Journal of Rehabilitation July/August/September 23-26

Hollander, Laura-Lee
1982 "Normal Aging" pp. 1-39 in Martha Logigian (ed.) Adult Rehabilitation: A Team Approach for Therapists Boston, MA: Little Brown & Co.

Hulnick, Mary R. and H. Ronald Hulnick
1989 "Life's Challenges: Curse or Opportunity? Counseling Families of Persons with Disabilities" Journal of Counseling and Development 68(November/December):166-170

Kaye, H. Stephen
1998 "Vocational Rehabilitation in the United States" Disability Statistics Abstract Number 20, March

Madara, Edward
no Developing Self-Help Groups - General Steps and Guidelines for Professionals
date Denville, NJ: New Jersey Self-Help Clearinghouse

McNeil, John M.
2001 Americans With Disabilities 1997, Washington, DC: U.S. Bureau of the Census Current Population Reports P70-73

Rodgers, Jennifer and Peter Calder
1990 "Marital Adjustment: A Valuable Resource for the Emotional Health of Individuals with Multiple Sclerosis" Rehabilitation Counseling Bulletin 34:1(September):24-32

Romness, Sharon, Vicki Bruce, and Catherine Smith-Wilson
1992 "Multiple Sclerosis Telephone Self-Help Support Groups" pp. 220-223 in Alfred H. Katz et al. (eds.) Self-Help: Concepts and Applications Philadelphia, PA: The Charles Press, Publishers

Roth, William
1981 The Handicapped Speak Jefferson, NC: McFarland

ORGANIZATIONS

<u>Agency for Healthcare Research and Quality</u> (AHRQ)
2101 East Jefferson Street, Suite 501
Rockville, MD 20852
(301) 594-1364   e-mail: info@ahrq.gov   www.ahrq.gov

A federal agency that funds research studies on effectiveness of medical treatments, economic aspects of health care policy, and quality of care. Publishes monthly newsletter, "Research Activities." Free. Newsletter and reports also available on the web site.

<u>American Disabled for Attendant Programs Today</u> (ADAPT)
PO Box 9598
Denver, CO 80209
(303) 333-6698

or

ADAPT/Incitement
1339 Lamar SE Drive, Suite 101
Austin, TX 78704
(512) 442-0252   FAX (512) 442-0522
e-mail: adapt@adapt.org   www.adapt.org

An organization dedicated to changing the structure of long term care and helping people with disabilities live in the community with supports instead of being sent to nursing homes and other institutions. Publishes "INCITEMENT," a newsletter describing ADAPT activities, three or four times a year (available in standard print and on audiocassette), free. ADAPT has supported federal legislation, the Community Attendant Services Act (CASA), to provide personal attendants to individuals with disabilities. No membership fees, but a willingness to participate in ADAPT's activities is required.

<u>American Indian Rehabilitation Research and Training Center</u>
Northern Arizona University
PO Box 5630
Flagstaff, AZ 86011-5630
(928) 523-4791   FAX (928) 523-9127
www.nau.edu/ihd/airrtc

Conducts research and training to improve vocational rehabilitation services for American Indians with disabilities. Publishes resource and training manuals, directories, research reports, and newsletter, "American Indian Rehabilitation," biannually. Free

American Self-Help Clearinghouse
100 Hanover Avenue, Suite 202
Cedar Knolls, NJ 07927
(973) 326-6789   FAX (973) 326-9467   www.selfhelpgroups.org

Provides information and contacts for national self-help groups, information on model groups and individuals who are starting new networks, and state or local self-help clearinghouses.

Beach Center on Disability
c/o Life Span Institute
University of Kansas
3136 Haworth Hall
1200 Sunnyside Avenue
Lawrence, KS 66045
(785) 864-7600 (V/TTY)   FAX (785) 864-7605
e-mail: beach@dole.lsi.ukans.edu   www.beachcenter.org

A federally funded center that conducts research and training in the factors that contribute to the successful functioning of families with members who have disabilities. A catalogue of publications describes monographs and tapes related to family coping, professional roles, and service delivery. Free

ClinicalTrials.gov
clinicaltrials.gov

This confidential web site has information on more than 4,000 Federal and private medical studies. Lists location of clinical trials, design and purpose, criteria for participation, information about the disease and treatment being studied, and links to personnel who are recruiting participants. Also available at www.nlm.nih.gov

Combined Health Information Database (CHID)
Ovid Technologies, Attn: CHID Database
333 7th Avenue
New York, NY 10001
(800) 950-2035   (212) 563-3006
e-mail: chid@aerie.com   chid.nih.gov

A federally sponsored database that includes bibliographic citations and abstracts from journals, reports, books, and patient education brochures.

Commission on Accreditation of Rehabilitation Facilities (CARF)
4891 East Grant Road
Tucson, AZ 85712
(520) 325-1044 (V/TTY)   FAX (520) 318-1129
e-mail: webmaster@carf.org   www.carf.org

Conducts site evaluations and accredits organizations that provide rehabilitation, pain management, adult day services, and assisted living. Provides a free list of accredited organizations in a specific state.

Commission on Rehabilitation Counselor Certification
1835 Rohlwing Road, Suite E
Rolling Meadows, IL 60008
(847) 394-2104
www.crccertification.com

Provides certification to rehabilitation counselors.

Disability.gov
www.disability.gov

This web site provides links to a wide variety of information and resources of the federal government that are related to disability.

DisabilityResources.org
Disability Resources, Inc.
Dept. IN
4 Glatter Lane
Centereach, NY 11720
(631) 585-0290 (V/FAX)   e-mail: pubs@disabilityresources.org
www.disabilityresources.org

The web site provides information about resources for independent living, including "The DRM Regional Resource Directory." Publishes "Disability Resources Monthly," $33.00. Available in standard print and audiocassette. Free sample available on the web site.

Disability Statistics Center
3333 California Street, Suite 340
San Francisco, CA 94118
(415) 502-5210   (415) 502-5205 (TTY)
FAX (415) 502-5208   e-mail distats@itsa.ucsf.edu
www.dsc.ucsf.edu

A federally funded research center that monitors the status of people with disabilities, including the cost of having a disability, access to health care, and employment. Produces "Disability Statistics Reports" and "Disability Statistics Abstracts." Free. Also available on the web site.

Genetic Alliance
4301 Connecticut Avenue, NW, Suite 404
Washington, DC 20008
(800) 336-4363   (202) 966-5557   FAX (202) 966-8553
e-mail: info@geneticalliance.org   www.geneticalliance.org

This coalition of individuals, professionals, and genetic support groups provides education and services to families and individuals affected by genetic disorders. Membership, individuals, $35.00; genetic support groups, $55.00; other organizations, $75.00; includes monthly newsletter, "ALERT." Publishes "Alliance Directory of National Genetic Support Organizations and Related Resources;" members, $15.00; nonmembers, $35.00. Also available as a searchable database on the web site.

Healthfinder
e-mail: healthfinder@health.org   www.healthfinder.gov

Sponsored by the federal government, this web site provides information about government agencies that are related to health, as well as online publications such as a medical dictionary.

The Healthpages
www.thehealthpages.com

Provides articles on a wide variety of diseases and conditions. Also provides information on physicians and facilities that treat specific disorders in specified metropolitan areas.

HealthWeb
www.healthweb.org

This web site is operated by a consortium of university libraries. The site provides links to a variety of noncommercial health sites that have been evaluated by the librarians.

Independent Living Research Utilization (ILRU)
2323 South Shepherd, Suite 1000
Houston, TX 77019
(713) 520-0232   (713) 520-5136 (TTY)   FAX (713) 520-5785
e-mail: ilru@bcm.tmc.edu   www.ilru.org

Develops and disseminates information; conducts training programs; sponsors conferences; and produces a wide variety of publications for people who administer independent living centers.

Maintains ILRU National Database on Independent Living Programs; available on web site.

International Association of Rehabilitation Professionals (IARP)
3540 Soquel Avenue, Suite A
Santa Cruz, CA 95062
(800) 240-9059   (831) 464-4892
FAX (831) 464-4881   e-mail: iarpwebhelp@yahoo.com
www.rehabpro.org

A professional membership organization for rehabilitation professionals who work as case managers, in long term disability, and consulting on disability management, life care planning, and ADA compliance. Holds annual meeting. Membership, $107.00 plus local chapter fee; includes journal "RehabPro." "IARP National Directory," printed annually, is available on the web site.

Librarians' Index to the Internet
lii.org

This searchable, annotated subject directory on Internet resources includes subjects such as disabilities, health, medicine, and seniors.

Medicinenet
www.medicinenet.com

Sponsored by physicians, this web site provides information on diseases, procedures and tests, drugs, a medical dictionary, and links to other health sites.

National Association on Alcohol, Drugs, and Disability, Inc. (NAADD)
2165 Bunker Hill Drive
San Mateo, CA 94402
(650) 578-8047 (V/TTY)   FAX (650) 286-9205
e-mail: jdem@aimnet.com   www.naadd.org

Promotes awareness and education about substance abuse in individuals with disabilities. Newsletters and other publications are available on the web site.

National Center for Medical Rehabilitation Research (NCMRR)
Building 61E, Room 2A03
6100 Executive Boulevard, MSC 7510
Bethesda, MD 20892
(301) 402-2242   FAX (301) 402-0832
e-mail: tuels@box-t.nih.gov   www.nichd.nih.gov

Part of the National Institute on Child Health and Human Development, this federal agency conducts and supports research to develop ways of improving the lives of individuals with disabilities, including research to develop technology and assistive devices.

National Center for the Dissemination of Disability Research (NCDDR)
Southwest Educational Development Laboratory
211 East Seventh Street, Suite 400
Austin, TX 78701
(800) 266-1832   (512) 476-6861   FAX (512) 476-2286
e-mail: NCDDR@sedl.org   www.ncddr.org

This federally funded organization conducts surveys related to disability, provides a structure for the dissemination of disability research funded by the National Institute on Disability and Rehabilitation Research, conducts demonstrations of successful strategies, and provides technical assistance.

National Council on Disability (NCD)
1331 F Street, NW, Suite 850
Washington, DC 20004
(202) 272-2004   (202) 272-2074 (TTY)   FAX (202) 272-2022
e-mail: mquigley@ncd.gov   www.ncd.gov

An independent federal agency mandated to study and make recommendations about public policy for people with disabilities. Holds regular meetings and hearings in various locations around the country. Publishes monthly newsletter, "NCD Bulletin," available in standard print, alternate formats, and on the web site. Free

National Family Caregivers Association (NFCA)
10400 Connecticut Avenue, Suite 500
Kensington, MD 20895
(800) 896-3650   FAX (301) 942-2302
e-mail: info@nfcacares.org   www.nfcacares.org

A membership organization for individuals who provide care for others at any stage of their lives or with any disease or disability. Maintains an information clearinghouse. Membership, U.S. family caregivers, free; other individuals, $20.00; professionals, $40.00; nonprofit organizations, $60.00; and group medical practices, home health agencies, etc., $100.00. Membership includes quarterly newsletter, "Take Care!" which provides information and resources for family caregivers.

National Health Information Center (NHIC)
Office of Disease Prevention and Health Promotion
PO Box 1133
Washington, DC 20013-1133
(800) 336-4797   In MD, (301) 565-4167   FAX (301) 984-4256
FAXBACK (301) 468-1204   e-mail: nhicinfo@health.org   nhic-nt.health.org
www.health.gov/nhic/pubs/default.htm

Maintains a database of health-related organizations and a library. Provides referrals related to health issues for both professionals and consumers. Publications enable individuals to locate information and resources in the federal government. Free publications list; also available on the web site. Publications on the web site include "Federal Health Information Centers and Clearinghouses" with telephone numbers and web sites for federal health information and referral services by topic.

National Institutes of Health Information
www.nih.gov/health

Provides a single access point to the National Institutes of Health, including their individual clearinghouses, publications, and the Combined Health Information Database. Provides information on hotlines, PubMed, clinical trials and drug information.

National Institute on Disability and Rehabilitation Research (NIDRR)
U.S. Department of Education
400 Maryland Avenue, SW
Washington, DC 20202
(202) 205-8134   (202) 205-4475 (TTY)   FAX (202) 205-8515
www.ed.gov/offices/OSERS/NIDRR

A federal agency that supports research into various aspects of disability and rehabilitation, including demographic analyses, social science research, and the development of assistive devices.

National Library of Medicine (NLM)
8600 Rockville Pike
Building 38, Room 2S-10
Bethesda, MD 20894
(888) 346-3656   (301) 594-5983
www.ncbi.nlm.nih.gov/PubMed

Operates PubMed, a web site which provides access to MEDLINE, a computerized database that provides access to articles in major medical journals from around the world. Users may search for a specific health related topic and receive citations and abstracts of articles.

Available directly through NLM, the Internet, and at most medical, public, and university libraries.

National Organization for Rare Disorders (NORD)
PO Box 8923
New Fairfield, CT 06812-8923
(800) 999-6673   (203) 746-6518   (203) 746-6927 (TTY)
FAX (203) 746-6481   e-mail: orphan@rarediseases.org
www.rarediseases.org

Federation of voluntary health organizations that serve individuals with rare or "orphan" diseases. Maintains a confidential patient networking program for individuals and family members who have been diagnosed with a rare disorder. Membership, $30.00. Reprints of articles on rare diseases available from the NORD Rare Disease Database for $7.50 per copy; abstracts available free on web site. Publishes newsletter, "Orphan Disease Update," three times a year; free.

National Organization on Disability (NOD)
910 16th Street, NW, Suite 600
Washington, DC 20006
(202) 293-5960   (202) 293-5968 (TTY)   FAX (202) 293-7999
e-mail: ability@nod.org   www.nod.org

An organization dedicated to achieving the full participation of people with disabilities in all aspects of community life. Works with a network of local agencies to achieve this goal. Provides technical assistance and maintains an informational database. Offers an electronic newsletter on disability issues. Free

National Rehabilitation Association (NRA)
633 South Washington Street
Alexandria, VA 22314
(703) 836-0850   (703) 836-0849 (TTY)
FAX (703) 836-0848   e-mail: info@nationalrehab.org
www.nationalrehab.org

A membership organization for rehabilitation professionals and independent living center affiliates. Includes special divisions for independent living, counseling, job placement, etc. Legislative alerts appear on NRA's web site. Regular membership, $91.00, includes "Journal of Rehabilitation" and newsletter, "Contemporary Rehab;" student membership, $20.00.

National Rehabilitation Information Center (NARIC)
1010 Wayne Avenue, Suite 800
Silver Spring, MD 20910
(800) 346-2742   (301) 562-2400   (301) 495-5626 (TTY)
FAX (301) 562-2401   e-mail: naricinfo@kra.com   www.naric.com

A federally funded center that responds to telephone and mail inquiries about disabilities and support services. Maintains REHABDATA, a database with publications and research references. Some NARIC publications are available on the web site.

National Resource Center for Parents with Disabilities
Through the Looking Glass
2198 Sixth Street, Suite 100
Berkeley, CA 94710-2204
(800) 644-2666   (800) 804-1616 (TTY)   (510) 848-1112
FAX (510) 848-4445   e-mail: tlg@lookingglass.org
www.lookingglass.org

A federally funded center that conducts research on the needs of parents with disabilities. Conducts research on special equipment and techniques of caring for babies. Maintains a national network of parents with disabilities, their families, researchers, and service providers. Publishes quarterly newsletter, "Parenting with a Disability," which provides information about the center's activities, publications in the field, and practical suggestions for parents. Available in standard print and alternate formats. Free. Also publishes "Adaptive Babycare Equipment: Guidelines, Prototypes, and Resources," a book that describes products to help individuals with disabilities diaper, bathe, dress, feed, and play with their babies; $30.00; parents on fixed incomes, $15.00. Also available with a 12 minute video that demonstrates the use of adaptive babycare equipment; $79.00 for the set.

National Self-Help Clearinghouse
Graduate School and University Center of the City University of New York
365 5th Avenue, Suite 3300
New York, NY 10016
(212) 817-1822   e-mail: info@selfhelpweb.org   www.selfhelpweb.org

Makes referrals to local self-help groups.

Native American Research and Training Center (NARTC)
University of Arizona
1642 East Helen Street
Tucson, AZ 85719
(520) 621-5075 (V/TTY)   FAX (520) 621-9802
e-mail: lclore@u.arizona.edu   www.ahsc.arizona.edu/nartc

A federally funded center that conducts research to develop model rehabilitation programs for Native Americans with disabilities or chronic illnesses. Conducts training programs for service providers, managers, and consumers.

Rehabilitation Engineering and Assistive Technology Society of North America/RESNA
1700 North Moore Street, Suite 1540
Arlington, VA 22209
(703) 524-6686   (703) 524-6639 (TTY)   FAX (703) 524-6630
e-mail: info@resna.org   www.resna.org

Multidisciplinary professional membership organization for people involved with improving technology for people with disabilities. Conducts a variety of projects, including research in the area of assistive technology and rehabilitation technology service delivery and technical assistance to statewide programs to develop technology. Membership, regular, $150.00; institutional, $500.00; corporate, $525.00; includes semi-annual journal, "Assistive Technology" and quarterly newsletter, "RESNA News." Special membership rates for consumers and for students, $50.00 without journal; $80.00 with journal.

Research and Training Center on Independent Living (RTC/IL)
University of Kansas
4089 Dole Life Span Institute
1000 Sunnyside Avenue
Lawrence, KS 66045
(785) 864-4095 (V/TTY)   FAX (785) 864-5063
www.lsi.ukans.edu/rtcil/rtcil.htm

A federally funded center that conducts research and training on the variables that affect independent living. Publications catalogue, free.

Research and Training Center on Rural Rehabilitation
52 Corbin Hall
University of Montana
Missoula, MT 59812
(800) 732-0323 (V/TTY)   (406) 243-5467 (V/TTY)
FAX (406) 243-4730   e-mail muarid@selway.umt.edu   ruralinstitute.umt.edu

A federally funded center that conducts research and training on issues that affect service delivery of rehabilitation in rural areas. Maintains a directory of rural disability services throughout the country. Publishes a newsletter, "The Rural Exchange," free. Available in alternative formats and on the web site.

Resources for Rehabilitation
22 Bonad Road
Winchester, MA 01890
(781) 368-9094   FAX (781) 368-9096
e-mail: orders@rfr.org   www.rfr.org

Provides training and information to professionals who serve people with disabilities and to the public. Publications, custom designed training programs, program evaluations, and needs assessments.

Sibling Support Project
Children's Hospital and Medical Center
PO Box 5371
Seattle, WA 98105
(206) 527-5712   FAX (206) 527-5705
e-mail: dmeyer@chmc.org   www.seattlechildrensorg/sibsupp

Maintains a database of sibling programs across the U.S. Includes programs for young siblings of children with developmental disabilities, chronic illness, or for adult siblings.

Society for Disability Studies (SDS)
Department of Disability and Human Development
University of Illinois at Chicago
1640 West Roosevelt Road, # 236
Chicago, IL 60608
(312) 996-4664 (V/TTY)   FAX (312) 413-2918   e-mail: cg16@uic.edu
www.uic.edu/orgs/sds

Membership organization of practitioners, clinicians, and social scientists interested in the study of issues related to disability. Holds an annual meeting. Membership, $95.00; low income, $30.00.

Substance Abuse Resources & Disability Issues (SARDI)
Rehabilitation Research and Training Center on Drugs and Disability
School of Medicine, Wright State University
PO Box 927
Dayton, OH 45401-0927
(937) 775-1484 (V/TTY)   FAX (937) 775-1495
www.med.wright.edu/som/sardi

A federally funded research center that investigates the relationship between drug use and disabilities. Free newsletter, "SARDI Online."

TASH: The Association for Persons with Severe Handicaps
29 West Susquehanna Avenue, Suite 210
Baltimore, MD 21204
(410) 828-8274   (410) 828-1306 (TTY)   FAX (410) 828-6706
e-mail: info@tash.org   www.tash.org

A national advocacy organization that disseminates information to improve the education and increase the independence of individuals with severe disabilities. Holds an annual conference. Publishes a quarterly journal, "Journal of the Association for Persons with Severe Handicaps" and the "TASH Newsletter" (both included with membership). Regular membership, $88.00; associate membership, $45.00.

United Way of America (UWA)
701 North Fairfax Street
Alexandria, VA 22314
(800) 411-8929 to obtain telephone number of closest United Way office
(703) 836-7100   FAX (703) 683-7840
www.unitedway.org

An umbrella organization of local human service organizations. National office will direct callers to the local United Way, which in turn will provide referral to a specific local service agency.

Untangling the Web
West Virginia Rehabilitation Research and Training Center
806 Allen Hall, PO Box 6122
Morgantown, WV 26506
(304) 293-5314 (V/TTY)   e-mail: walls@rtc1.icdi.wvu.edu
www.icdi.wvu.edu

This web site provides links to a wide variety of other web sites, organized by disability.

U.S. Department of Veterans Affairs (VA)
(800) 827-1000   www.va.gov

This nationwide toll-free number connects veterans with the VA regional office in their vicinity.

Vocational Rehabilitation and Employment
Veterans Benefits Administration
U.S. Department of Veterans Affairs (VA)
(800) 827-1000 (connects with regional office)
www.vba.va.gov/bln/vre/index.htm

Provides education and rehabilitation assistance and independent living services to veterans with service related disabilities through offices located in every state as well as regional centers, medical centers, and insurance centers. Medical services are provided at VA Medical Centers, Outpatient Clinics, Domiciliaries, and Nursing Homes. VONAPP (VA Online Application) enables veterans to apply for benefits on the Internet.

Well Spouse Foundation
30 East 40th Street, Suite PH
New York, NY 10016
(800) 838-0879   (212) 685-8815   FAX (212) 685-8676
e-mail: wellspouse@aol.com   www.wellspouse.org

A network of support groups that provide emotional support to husbands, wives, and partners of people who are chronically ill. Membership, individuals, $25.00; professionals, $50.00; includes bimonthly newsletter, "Mainstay." Publishes pamphlets discussing "Guilt," "Anger," "Isolation," and "Looking Ahead." $1.50 each; $5.00 per set.

World Institute on Disability (WID)
510 16th Street, Suite 100
Oakland, CA 94612
(510) 763-4100   (510) 208-9496 (TTY)   FAX (510) 763-4109
e-mail: webpoobah@wid.org   www.wid.org

A public policy center founded and operated by individuals with disabilities, WID conducts research, public education, and training. It also develops model programs related to disability. It deals with issues such as personal assistance, public transportation, employment, and access to health care. WID's Research and Training Centers are federally funded centers that study personal assistance services, federal independent living initiatives, and community integration issues.

After the Diagnosis
by JoAnn LeMaistre
Alpine Guild
PO Box 4846
Dillon, CO 80435
(800) 869-9559   FAX (970) 269-9378
e-mail: information@alpineguild.com
www.alpineguild.com

Written by a woman with multiple sclerosis, this book describes the emotional responses to health changes due to physical disabilities, chronic illness, and aging. $12.95 plus $3.00 shipping and handling

Alcohol, Disabilities, and Rehabilitation
by Susan A. Storti
Thomson Learning, Florence, KY

This book discusses alcohol abuse in individuals with disabilities and chronic conditions. Includes treatment and rehabilitation strategies. Out of print

American Rehabilitation
Superintendent of Documents
PO Box 371954
Pittsburgh, PA 15250-7954
(866) 512-1800   (202) 512-1800   FAX (202) 512-2250
e-mail: gpoaccess@gpo.gov   www.access.gpo.gov

Published by the Rehabilitation Services Administration, this quarterly magazine provides information on rehabilitation programs, services, and publications. $18.75

Building Community: A Manual Exploring Issues of Women and Disability
Educational Equity Concepts
100 Fifth Avenue, Second Floor
New York, NY 10011
(212) 243-1110 (V/TTY)   FAX (212) 627-0407
e-mail: info@edequity.org   www.edequity.org

A collection of readings and activities that explore the relationship between gender and disability bias. $24.95 plus 15% shipping and handling

Chronic Illness: The Constant Companion
United Learning
1560 Sherman Avenue, Suite 100
Evanston, IL 60201
(800) 421-2363   (847) 328-6700   FAX (847) 328-6706
e-mail: agc@mcs.net   www.agcmedia.com

This videotape relates the stories of individuals who cope with a chronic illness. Includes discussion of changes in lifestyle and relationships as well as emotional issues. 32 minutes $95.00 plus $3.00 shipping and handling

Clinical Trials: What You Should Know before Volunteering to Be a Research Subject
by J. Joseph Giffels
Demos Medical Publications
386 Park Avenue South, Suite 201
New York, NY 10016
(800) 532-8663   (212) 683-0072   FAX (212) 683-0118
e-mail: info@demospub.com   www.demosmedpub.com

This book provides answers to questions concerning the rights of individuals who choose to participate in clinical trials. $9.95 plus $4.00 shipping and handling. Orders made on the Demos web site receive a 15% discount.

The Comfort of Home: An Illustrated Step-by-Step Guide for Caregivers
by Maria M. Meyer with Paula Derr
Demos Medical Publications
386 Park Avenue South, Suite 201
New York, NY 10016
(800) 532-8663   (212) 683-0072   FAX (212) 683-0118
e-mail: info@demospub.com   www.demosmedpub.com

This book is a practical guide to the safety considerations of home care, nutrition, communicating with health care professionals, end of life decisions, and everyday activities. $23.00 plus $4.00 shipping and handling. Orders made on the Demos web site receive a 15% discount.

Computer and Web Resources for People with Disabilities
Alliance for Technology Access
2173 East Francisco Boulevard, Suite L
San Rafael, CA 94901
(800) 455-7970   (415) 455-4575   (415) 455-0491 (TTY)
FAX (415) 455-0654   e-mail: atainfo@atacess.org
www.ataccess.org

This book guides readers in making decisions based on personal goals and resources related to assistive technology. Includes resource list of organizations and vendors. Softcover, $20.95; spiral bound, $27.95; disk, $27.95; plus $3.00 shipping and handling.

A Delicate Balance: Living Successfully with Chronic Illness
by Susan Milstrey Wells
Harper Collins
PO Box 588
Dunmore, PA 18512
(800) 242-7737   www.harpercollins.com

In this book, the author, and 20 other individuals with chronic illness relate their experiences in searching for a diagnosis, finding compassionate health care, and learning to live with chronic illness. $17.50

Dictionary of Rehabilitation
by Myron G. Eisenberg
Springer Publishing Company
536 Broadway
New York, NY 10012
(212) 431-4370   FAX (212) 941-7842
e-mail: springer@springerpub.com springerpub.com

This book defines the core terms used in the rehabilitation field. $43.95 plus $4.75 shipping and handling

Disability Funding News
CD Publications
8204 Fenton Street
Silver Spring, MD 20910
(800) 666-6380   FAX (301) 588-6385   www.cdpublications.com

This semimonthly publication contains information about funding opportunities from the federal government and private foundations. $329.00

Disability in America: Toward a National Agenda for Prevention
by Andrew M. Pope and Alvin R. Tarlow (eds.)
National Academy Press
2101 Constitution Avenue, NW
Lockbox 285
Washington, DC 20055
(888) 624-8373   (202) 334-3313   FAX (202) 334-2451
e-mail: zjones@nas.edu   www.nap.edu

The report of a panel of experts, this book examines the magnitude of disability in the U.S., recommends a model to prevent disabilities, and makes a series of policy recommendations. $71.50 plus $4.00 shipping and handling. A 20% discount is offered to individuals who purchase books through the National Academy's Web Bookstore. May be read on the web site, free.

Disability in the United States: A Portrait from National Data
by Susan Thompson-Hoffman and Inez Fitzgerald-Storck (eds.)
Springer Publishing Company, New York, NY

This book is a collection of articles based on data collected from a variety of federal agencies. Analyzes the relationship between a wide variety of demographic characteristics and disability with implications for future policy and research. Out of print

Disability Studies Quarterly
David Pfeiffer
University of Hawaii Center for Disability Studies
University of Hawaii at Manoa
1776 University Avenue, UA 4-6
Honolulu, HI 96822
www.cds.hawaii.edu/DSQ

A quarterly electronic journal with reports on recent research findings, upcoming meetings, and grant solicitations. Reviews of books and audio-visual materials. Free. Available in standard print and alternate formats. Contact Carol Gill [(312) 996-4664 (V/TTY); e-mail: cgl@uic.edu].

Enabling America: Assessing the Role of Rehabilitation Science and Engineering
by Edward N. Brandt, Jr. and Andrew Pope (eds.)
National Academy Press
2101 Constitution Avenue, NW
Lockbox 285
Washington, DC 20055
(888) 624-8373   (202) 334-3313   FAX (202) 334-2451
e-mail: zjones@nas.edu   www.nap.edu

Written by a multidisciplinary group of experts, this book assesses the practical implications of current knowledge in rehabilitation science as well as the costs of disability and rehabilitation. It reviews technology transfer, education and training of rehabilitation science personnel, and the status of federal research policy. It recommends a course for administering rehabilitation programs and research. $54.95 plus $4.00 shipping and handling. A 20% discount is offered to individuals who purchase books through the National Academy's Web Bookstore. May be read on the web site, free.

Enabling Romance: A Guide to Love, Sex, and Relationships for People with Disabilities
by Ken Kroll and Erica Levy Klein
Nine Lives Press
PO Box 220
Horsham, PA 19044
(888) 850-0344, extension 109   (215) 675-9133, extension 109
FAX (215) 675-9376   e-mail: kim@leonardmediagroup.com
www.newmobility.com

Written by a man who has a disability and his wife who does not, this book provides examples of how people with a variety of disabilities have established fulfilling relationships. $15.95 plus $3.00 shipping and handling

Encyclopedia of Disability and Rehabilitation
by Arthur E. Dell Orto and Robert P. Marinelli (eds.)
Macmillan Library Reference, New York, NY

Written by a variety of experts in the field of disability, this reference book includes articles ranging from AIDS to stroke, advocacy to wheelchairs, and aging to work. Out of print

Family Challenges: Parenting with a Disability
Aquarius Health Care Videos
5 Powderhouse Lane
PO Box 1159
Sherborn, MA 01770
(508) 651-2963   FAX (508) 650-4216
e-mail: aqvideos@tiac.net   www.aquariusproductions.com

In this videotape, the children and spouses of parents with disabilities describe their relationships and coping strategies. 25 minutes. $195.00 plus $9.00 shipping and handling

Federal Register
New Orders, Superintendent of Documents
PO Box 371954
Pittsburgh, PA 15250-7954
(866) 512-1800   (202) 512-1530
FAX (202) 512-2250   e-mail: gpoaccess@gpo.gov
www.access.gpo.gov/su_docs/aces/aces140.html

A federal publication printed every weekday with notices of all regulations and legal notices issued by federal agencies. Domestic subscriptions, $764.00 annually for second class mailing of paper format; $264.00 annually for microfiche. Access to the Federal Register is available through the Internet at the address listed above at no charge.

Foundations of the Vocational Rehabilitation Process
by Stanford E. Rubin and Richard T. Roessler
Pro-Ed
8700 Shoal Creek Boulevard
Austin, TX 78757
(800) 897-3202   FAX (800) 397-7633   www.proedinc.com
A textbook with complete coverage of the development of vocational rehabilitation programs in the U.S., legislative history, and procedures used by professionals to conduct client assessments and deliver services. $46.00 plus 10% shipping and handling

Grants for Organizations Serving People with Disabilities
Research Grant Guides, Inc.
PO Box 1214
Loxahatchee, FL 33470
(561) 795-6129   FAX (561) 795-7794
www.researchgrant.com

This book provides profiles of foundations and federal sources of funding, including areas of interest and eligibility requirements. Includes chapters with advice on proposal writing. $69.00 plus $10.00 handling fee.

Helping Yourself Help Others: A Book for Caregivers
by Rosalynn Carter with Susan K. Golant
Random House, Order Department
400 Hahn Road, PO Box 100
Westminster, MD 21157
(800) 733-3000   (410) 848-1900   FAX (410) 386-7013
www.randomhouse.com

This book focuses on family caregivers, offering suggestions for everyday problems such as physical and emotional needs, isolation, burnout, and dealing with professional caregivers. Lists of organizations, books, and resources included. $14.00

How to Help Children Through a Parent's Serious Illness
by Kathleen McCue with Ron Bonn
St. Martin's Griffin
c/o VHPS
16365 James Madison Highway
Gordonville, VA 22942
(800) 321-9299   www.stmartins.com

This book presents practical guidelines to help parents explain their illness to children of different ages, how to understand the children's reactions, and how to seek professional help. Includes a chapter on chronic illness. $12.95 plus $4.50 shipping and handling

Journal of Disability Policy Studies
Pro-Ed
8700 Shoal Creek Boulevard
Austin, TX 78757
(800) 897-3202   FAX (800) 397-7633   www.proedinc.com
A journal, published twice a year, with articles related to legislative policy and regulatory matters as well as articles from a range of academic disciplines. Individuals, $39.00; institutions, $95.00.

Journal of Rehabilitation Research and Development (JRRD)
Scientific and Technical Publications Section
Rehabilitation Research and Development Service
103 South Gay Street, 5th floor
Baltimore, MD 21202
(410) 962-1800   FAX (410) 962-9670   e-mail: pubs@vard.org
www.vard.org

A journal that includes articles on disability, rehabilitation, sensory aids, gerontology, and disabling conditions. Annual supplements provide research progress reports. Clinical supplements report on specific topics. Published six times a year. Available in standard print and on the web site. Free

Life Services Planning for the Elderly and Persons with Disabilities
Commission on Mental and Physical Disability Law
American Bar Association
740 15th Street, NW, 9th Floor
Washington, DC 20005
(202) 662-1570   (202) 662-1012   FAX (202) 662-1032
e-mail: hammillj@staff.abanet.org   www.abanet.org

This three book series provides guidance for individuals, families, and service providers about estates, financial issues, health care, and government benefits. $20.00 plus $5.00 shipping and handling

Living a Healthy Life with Chronic Conditions
by Kate Lorig, Halsted Holman, David Sobel, Diana Laurent, Virginia Gonzalez, and Marian Minor
Bull Publishing Company
PO Box 208
Palo Alto, CA 94302
(800) 676-2855   FAX (650) 327-3300   www.bullpub.com

This book recommends strategies for dealing with chronic illnesses, carrying out normal activities, and managing emotional issues. Includes chapters on exercise, communication, nutrition, intimacy, and advance directives. $18.95 plus $3.00 shipping and handling

Mainstay: For the Well Spouse of the Chronically Ill
by Maggie Strong
Bradford Books
45 Lyman Road
Northampton, MA 01060
(413) 586-5207

Written by a woman whose husband was diagnosed with multiple sclerosis at age 46, this book provides her personal account and others' stories, practical suggestions, and advice from health care professionals. $15.00 plus $3.00 shipping and handling; prepayment by check required.

Making Disability
by Paul Higgins
Charles C. Thomas, Publisher
2600 South First Street
Springfield, IL 62704
(800) 258-8980   (217) 789-8980   FAX (217) 789-9130
e-mail: books@ccthomas.com   www.ccthomas.com

Written by a sociologist, this book examines disability as a social phenomenon rather than a defect. It discusses the depiction of disability, experiencing disability, serving individuals with disabilities, and developing disability policy. Hardcover, $57.95; softcover, $39.95; plus $5.95 shipping and handling.

Making Wise Medical Decisions: How to Get the Information You Need
22 Bonad Road
Winchester, MA 01890
(781) 368-9094   FAX (781) 368-9096
e-mail: orders@rfr.org   www.rfr.org

This book includes information about where to go and what to read in order to make informed, rational, medical decisions. It describes how to obtain relevant health information and evaluate medical tests and procedures, health care providers, and health facilities. Includes chapters on protecting the health of children who are ill; special issues facing elders; and people with chronic illnesses and disabilities and the health care system. $42.95 plus $5.00 shipping and handling (See last page of this book for order form.)

No Pity: People with Disabilities Forging a New Civil Rights Movement
by Joseph P. Shapiro
Random House, Order Department
400 Hahn Road, PO Box 100
Westminster, MD 21157
(800) 733-3000   (410) 848-1900   FAX (410) 386-7013
www.randomhouse.com

This book describes the evolution of the disability rights movement and profiles its leaders.
$15.00 plus $4.00 shipping and handling

NORD Resource Guide
National Organization for Rare Disorders (NORD)
100 Route 37, PO Box 8923
New Fairfield, CT 06812-8923
(800) 999-6673   (203) 746-6518   (203) 746-6927 (TTY)
FAX (203) 746-6481   e-mail: orphan@rarediseases.org
www.rarediseases.org

This directory lists organizations that support individuals with rare diseases and disabilities.
$45.00 plus $5.00 shipping and handling

Ragged Edge
Advocado Press Inc.
Box 145
Louisville, KY 40201
e-mail: editor@ragged-edge-mag.com
www.ragged-edge-mag.com

This bimonthly magazine reports on disability issues from the perspective of disability rights
activists. Individuals, $17.50; institutions, $35.00. Available free on the web site.

Report on Disability Programs
Business Publishers
8737 Colesville Road, Suite 1100
Silver Spring, MD 20910-3928
(800) 274-6737   (301) 589-5103   FAX (301) 589-8493
e-mail: bpinews@bpinews.com   www.bpinews.com

A biweekly newsletter with information on policies promulgated by federal agencies, laws, and
funding sources. $327.00

The Self-Help Sourcebook Online
American Self-Help Clearinghouse
100 Hanover Avenue, Suite 202
Cedar Knolls, NJ 07927
(973) 326-6789   FAX (973) 326-9467   www.selfhelpgroups.org

This online database provides information on national and model self-help groups, online mutual help groups and networks, and self-help clearinghouses. Includes ideas on starting self-help groups and opportunities to link with others to develop new groups.

Silent Storm
c/o United Cerebral Palsy of America/New Jersey
354 South Broad Street
Trenton, NJ 08608
(888) 322-1918   (609) 392-4004   (609) 392-7044 (TTY)

This videotape explores substance abuse among individuals with disabilities and describes programs designed to meet their needs. Open or closed captioned. 10 minutes. Accompanying brochure available in English and Spanish. $45.00 plus $5.00 shipping and handling

Staring Back: The Disability Experience from the Inside Out
by Kenny Fries (ed.)
Penguin Putnam, Inc.
(800) 788-6262   www.penguinputnam.com

This anthology includes essays, poems, and works of fiction written by individuals who have a broad range of disabilities. $17.00

Surviving Your Spouse's Chronic Illness
by Chris McGonigle
Von Holtzbrinck Publishing Services, Gordonsville, VA

Building on her own background as the well spouse of a man with multiple sclerosis, the author interviewed more than 40 spouses of women and men with chronic conditions and describes the emotional and psychological aspects of their experiences. Out of print

That All May Worship
National Organization on Disability (NOD)
910 16th Street, NW, Suite 600
Washington, DC 20006
(202) 293-5960   (202) 293-5968 (TTY)   FAX (202) 293-7999
e-mail: ability@nod.org   www.nod.org

An interfaith guide to help congregations make their facilities accessible to people with disabilities. $10.00.

To Everything There is a Season: A Guide for Caregivers of Farmers and Ranchers with Disabilities
Breaking New Ground Resource Center
Purdue University
1146 ABE Building
West Lafayette, IN 47907
(800) 825-4264   (765) 494-5088 (V/TTY)   FAX (765) 496-1356
e-mail: bng@ecn.purdue.edu   www.agrability.org

This resource kit is targeted to rural caregivers. Includes a videotape, brochure, and written resources. $85.00

Us and Them
by Fred Simon and Janet Kam
Fanlight Productions
4196 Washington Street, Suite 2
Boston, MA 02131
(800) 937-4113   (617) 469-4999   FAX (617) 469-3379
e-mail: fanlight@fanlight.com   www.fanlight.com

This videotape is about relationships between people who have disabilities and those who do not. 32 minutes, black and white. $69.00 plus $9.00 shipping and handling

What Psychotherapists Should Know about Disability
by Rhoda Olkin
Guilford Publications
72 Spring Street
New York, NY 10012
(800) 365-7006   (212) 431-9800   FAX (212) 966-6708
e-mail: info@guilford.com   www.guilford.com

Written by a clinician who has a disability, this book examines a minority model of disability and describes the disability experience of stereotypes and attitudes, affect and everyday experiences. Includes chapters on laws and social history, families, etiquette with individuals with disabilities, special issues in therapy, and assistive technology. Hardcover, $42.00; softcover, $22.00; plus $4.50 shipping and handling.

Chapter 2

LAWS THAT AFFECT PEOPLE WITH DISABILITIES

(For laws specifically related to children and education, see Chapter 3, "Children and Youths")

Laws affecting people with disabilities cover a wide range of issues, including health care, financial benefits, housing, rehabilitation, civil rights, transportation, access to public buildings, and employment. For those who are not specialists in the law, it is sometimes difficult to keep abreast of the laws and their amendments. At the same time, people with disabilities may be able to continue living independently if they are aware of their rights and know how to locate the proper equipment and professional services. In many instances, government programs provide financial assistance for their needs.

In 1990, the *Americans with Disabilities Act* (ADA) was passed. The ADA (P.L. 101-336) increased the steps employers must take to accommodate employees with disabilities and required that new buses and rail vehicles, facilities, and public accommodations be accessible. The ADA defines disability as "a physical or mental impairment that substantially limits one or more of the major life activities..." [such as speaking, hearing, seeing, or walking]; "a record of such impairment;" or "being regarded as having such an impairment." Thus individuals who have been cured of cancer or mental illness may still be regarded by others as having a disability and may experience discrimination. Others may have a physical condition that does not limit activity, such as disfiguring scars from injuries incurred in an automobile accident, but are regarded as disabled. Individuals in these situations are covered by the law.

The major provisions of the ADA are as follows:

• Title I prohibits discrimination against individuals with disabilities who are otherwise qualified for employment and requires that employers make "reasonable accommodations." "Reasonable accommodations" include making existing facilities accessible and job restructuring (e.g., reassignment to a vacant position, modification of equipment, training, provision of interpreters and readers). Employers are protected from "undue hardship" in complying with this provision; the financial situation of the employer and the size and type of business are considered when determining whether an accommodation would constitute "undue hardship." The provisions of this section apply to employers with 15 or more employees. (For a more detailed discussion of the employment aspects of the ADA, see "Meeting the Needs of Employees with Disabilities," described in "PUBLICATIONS" section below).

• Title II prohibits discrimination by public entities (i.e., local and state governments) and requires that individuals with disabilities be entitled to the same rights and benefits of public programs as other individuals. For example, local programs for elders may not discriminate against those elders who have low vision or other disabilities; they are entitled to receive the same benefits of the programs as elders who do not have disabilities.

• Title III requires that public accommodations, businesses, and services be accessible to individuals with disabilities. Public accommodations are broadly defined to include places such as hotels and motels, theatres, museums, schools, shopping centers and stores, banks, restaurants, and professional service providers' offices. Effective January 26, 1993, most new construction for public accommodations must be accessible to individuals with disabilities.

• Requires that bus and railroad transportation systems address the needs of individuals with disabilities by purchasing adapted equipment, modifying facilities, and providing special transportation services that are comparable to regular transportation services.

• Title IV mandates that telephone companies provide relay services 24 hours a day, 7 days a week for individuals with hearing or speech impairments. Relay services enable individuals who have teletypewriters (TTYs) or another computer device that is capable of communicating across telephone lines to communicate with individuals who do not have such devices.

Copies of the ADA and all federal laws are available from Senators and Representatives. Agencies charged with formulating regulations and standards include the Architectural and Transportation Barriers Compliance Board, the U.S. Department of Transportation, the Equal Employment Opportunity Commission, the Federal Communications Commission, and the Attorney General. Regulations for enforcing individual sections of the ADA are available from the federal agencies charged with promulgating them and in the "Federal Register" (see "PUBLICATIONS" section below). In addition, many private agencies that work with individuals with disabilities have copies of the ADA available for distribution to the public.

In 1999, the Supreme Court ruled in Olmstead, Commissioner, Georgia Department of Human Resources, et al. v. L.C. et al. that the ADA requires community placement instead of institutionalization whenever possible. The case was brought by two women who were both mentally retarded and mentally ill. Both had lived in state mental institutions for many years. Now their mental health professionals were recommending that they be placed in community-based treatment, but the state refused, saying it was more cost effective to keep the women hospitalized. The Supreme Court rejected the state's argument, citing Congress's intent that isolation and segregation were discrimination per se, and returned the case to the lower level court to determine appropriate relief. As a result of the Olmstead ruling, governments must place individuals in the community rather than in institutions whenever possible. This includes elders, who are often placed in nursing homes when supplemental in-home services could allow them to remain in their own homes.

In 2002, the Supreme Court unanimously ruled that the ADA does not protect individuals with impairments that prevent them from carrying out manual tasks related to their jobs. In the case of Toyota Motor Manufacturing of Kentucky v. Williams, the Court said that workers must show that an impairment has substantial effect beyond the workplace in order to be covered by the ADA.

Other major laws affecting people with disabilities include the *Rehabilitation Act of 1973* (P.L. 93-112) and its amendments, which are the centerpieces of federal law related to rehabilitation. States must submit a vocational rehabilitation plan to the Rehabilitation Services Administration indicating how the designated state agency will provide vocational training, counseling, and diagnostic and evaluation services required by the law. Subsequent reauthorizations of and amendments to the Rehabilitation Act expanded the services provided under this law. For example, the "Client Assistance Program" authorizes states to inform clients and other persons with disabilities about all available benefits under the Act and to assist them in obtaining all remedies due under the law (P.L. 98-221). "Comprehensive Services for Independent Living" (P.L. 95-602) expands rehabilitation services to individuals with severe disabilities, regardless of their vocational potential, making services available to many people who are no longer in the work force. The Act broadly defines services as any "service that will enhance the ability of a handicapped individual to live independently or function within his family and community..." These services may include counseling, job placement, housing, funds to make the home accessible, funds for prosthetic devices, attendant care, and recreational activities. The Rehabilitation Act Amendments of 1992 (P.L. 102-569) establish state rehabilitation advisory councils composed of representatives of independent living councils, parents of children with disabilities, vocational rehabilitation professionals, and business; the role of these councils is to advise state vocational rehabilitation agencies and to prepare an annual report for the governor. Each state agency was required to establish performance and evaluation standards by September 30, 1994. The amendments also establish a National Commission on Rehabilitation Services to study the quality and adequacy of rehabilitation services provided by the states. The Rehabilitation Act Amendments of 1998 (P.L. 105-220, part of the Workforce Investment Partnership Act) aim to bring more Americans with disabilities into the mainstream workforce and requires federal agencies to adopt accessible electronic information systems, so that individuals with disabilities have comparable access as those without disabilities. Section 508 of the Workforce Investment Partnership Act of 1998 (which includes the Rehabilitation Act Amendments of 1998) requires that the federal government provide access to electronic and information technology for all individuals with disabilities who are federal employees or who are members of the public seeking information or services from federal agencies. If a federal agency claims that procurement of accessible technology poses an "undue burden," it must ensure that access to information is provided through alternative means.

Section 503 of the Rehabilitation Act requires any contractor that receives more than $10,000 in contracts from the federal government to take affirmative action to employ individuals with disabilities. The Office of Federal Contract Compliance Programs within the U.S. Department of Labor is responsible for enforcing this provision (see "ORGANIZATIONS" section below). *Section 504* prohibits any program that receives federal financial assistance from discriminating against individuals with disabilities who are otherwise eligible to benefit from their programs. Virtually all educational institutions are affected by this law, including private postsecondary institutions which receive federal financial assistance under a wide variety of programs. Programs must be physically accessible to individuals with disabilities, and construction begun after implementation of the regulations (June 3, 1977) must be designed so that it is in compliance with standard specifications for accessibility. Federal agencies must have an affirmative action plan for hiring, placing, and promoting individuals with disabilities and for making their facilities accessible. The Civil Rights Division of the U.S. Department of Justice is responsible for enforcing this section.

The *Ticket to Work and Work Incentives Improvement Act of 1999* (P.L. 106-170) increases the choices for rehabilitation and vocational services, creates new options and incentives for states to offer a Medicaid buy-in for workers with disabilities, and extends Medicare coverage for an additional four and one-half years for people on disability who return to work.

Supplementary Security Income (SSI) is a federal minimum income maintenance program for elders and individuals who are blind or disabled and who meet a test of financial need. Monthly *Social Security Disability Insurance* (SSDI) benefits are available to individuals who are disabled and their dependents. To be eligible, individuals must have paid Social Security taxes for a specified number of years (dependent upon the applicant's age); must not be working; and must be declared medically disabled by the state disability determination service or through an appeals process. The disability must be expected to last at least 12 months or to result in death. Individuals who are blind and age 55 to 65 may receive monthly benefits if they are unable to carry out the work (or similar work) that they did before age 55 or becoming blind, whichever is later. Individuals who apply for disability insurance from the Social Security Administration must undergo an evaluation carried out by a state disability evaluation team, composed of physicians, psychologists, and other health care professionals. Social Security disability benefits are not retroactive, so it is important to apply for them immediately after becoming disabled.

Individuals who have received SSDI for two consecutive years are eligible for *Medicare*, a federal health insurance program, which may cover some of the necessary outpatient therapy or supplies discussed in this book. However, Medicare does not cover eyeglasses (except for recipients who have undergone cataract surgery), low vision aids, or hearing aids. *Medicaid* is a health insurance plan for individuals who are considered financially needy (i.e., recipients of financial benefits from governmental assistance programs such as Temporary Assistance to Needy Families, formerly called Aid to Families with Dependent Children, or Supplemental Security Income).

Medicaid is a joint federal/state program. While federal law requires that each state cover hospital services, skilled nursing facility services, physician and home health care services, and diagnostic and screening services, states have great discretion in other areas. Payments for prosthetics and rehabilitation equipment vary greatly from state to state.

The *Health Insurance Portability and Accountability Act of 1996* (P.L. 104-191), also known as the Kennedy-Kassebaum law, protects individuals from being denied health insurance due to a pre-existing medical condition when they move from one job to another or if they become unemployed. "Portability" means that once individuals have been covered by health insurance, they are credited with having medical coverage when they enter a new plan. Group health plans, health insurance plans such as HMOs, Medicare, Medicaid, military health plans, Indian Health Service medical care, and public, state or federal health benefits are considered creditable coverage (Fuch et al.: 1997). Coverage of a pre-existing medical condition may not be limited for more than 12 months for individuals who enroll in the health plan as soon as they are eligible (18 months for those who delay enrollment). Although the Act creates federal standards, the states have considerable flexibility in their requirements for insurers. The U.S. Departments of Treasury, Health and Human Services, and Labor are responsible for enforcing the provisions of the Act.

The medical and social service benefits available from organizations receiving federal assistance are guaranteed by federal laws and protected by the Office for Civil Rights of the

U.S. Department of Health and Human Services (HHS). When an individual feels that his or her rights have been violated, a complaint should be filed with the regional office of HHS (see "ORGANIZATIONS" section below).

The *Family and Medical Leave Act of 1993* (P.L.103-3) requires employers with 50 or more employees at a worksite or within 75 miles of a worksite to permit eligible employees 12 workweeks of unpaid leave during a 12 month period in order to care for themselves, a spouse, son or daughter, or parent who has a serious health condition. During this period of leave, the employer must continue to provide group health benefits for the employee under the same conditions as the employee would have received while working. Upon return from leave, the employee must be restored to the same position he or she had prior to the leave or to a position with equivalent pay, benefits, and conditions of employment. Special regulations apply to employees of school systems and private schools and employees of the federal civil service.

The *Telecommunications Act of 1996* (P.L. 104-104) has several sections that apply to individuals with disabilities. Section 254 redefines "universal service" to include schools, health facilities, and libraries, and requires that the Federal Communications Commission (FCC) work with state governments to determine what services must be made universally available and what is considered "affordable." Section 255 requires that telecommunication equipment manufacturers and service providers be accessible to all individuals with disabilities, "if readily achievable." Section 713 requires that video services be accessible to individuals with hearing impairments via closed captioning and to individuals with visual impairments via descriptive video services. Section 706 requires that the FCC encourage the development of advanced telecommunications technology that provides equal access for individuals with disabilities, especially school children. The FCC is authorized to establish regulations and time tables for implementing these sections.

The *Technology-Related Assistance for Individuals with Disabilities Act Amendments of 1994* (P.L. 103-218) strengthens the original Act, passed in 1988. The Act mandates state-wide programs for technology-related assistance to determine needs and resources; to provide technical assistance and information; and to develop demonstration and innovation projects, training programs, and public awareness programs. The amendments set priorities for consumer responsiveness, advocacy, systems change, and outreach to underrepresented populations such as the poor, individuals in rural areas, and minorities.

The *Fair Housing Amendments Act of 1988* (P.L. 100-430) requires that multifamily dwellings of four or more units first occupied after March 13, 1991 be accessible to individuals with disabilities. Tenants with disabilities have the legal right to make modifications to rental housing at their own expense in order to meet their needs. However, the residence must be restored to its original condition "within reason" when the tenant moves. In addition, HUD has established programs to house individuals with disabilities who are homeless.

Section 202 of the *Housing and Community Development Act of 1987,* Direct Loan Program for Housing for the Elderly or Handicapped, provides loans to nonprofit organizations to sponsor development of housing for elders and persons with disabilities, including units eligible for Section 8 rent subsidies. Under amendments to the *Housing and Community Development Act of 1987* (P.L. 100-242), the U.S. Department of Housing and Urban

Development (HUD) provides direct loans for the development of projects for elders and individuals with disabilities. These developments may consist of apartments or group homes for up to 15 residents. In 2000, HUD released the final rule that allows individuals and families to use Section 8 vouchers for home ownership. Public housing authorities who participate in the Homeownership Program can allow individuals and families to convert current Section 8 vouchers from rental to mortgage supplements and allow individuals and families who are eligible in the future to choose between mortgage and rental subsidies.

The Rural Housing Service of the U.S. Department of Agriculture offers a variety of homeownership programs for individuals who are elderly, disabled, or low-income and who live in rural areas, including direct loan and loan guarantee programs, home repair loan and grant programs, and rental assistance (see "ORGANIZATIONS" section below). Fannie Mae, a private company, offers HomeChoice, Community Living, and Retrofitting mortgages that make homeownership and home modifications possible for individuals with disabilities or who have family members with disabilities living with them (see "ORGANIZATIONS" section below).

Section 811 of the National Affordable Housing Act of 1990, Supportive Housing for People with Disabilities, enables nonprofit organizations to develop group homes, independent living facilities, and intermediate care facilities licensed by state Medicaid agencies. Applications are available from the U.S. Department of Housing and Urban Development field offices.

Individuals who feel that they have experienced discrimination in housing may file complaints with HUD or a state or local fair housing agency, or they may file a civil suit.

The federal government allows special tax credits for people who are totally disabled and additional standard deductions for those who are legally blind. Legal blindness is defined as acuity of 20/200 or less in the better eye with the best possible correction or a field of 20 degrees or less diameter in the better eye. Tax deductions for business expenses include disability related expenditures, and deductions for medical expenses include special equipment, such as wheelchairs, TTYs, also called telecommunications devices for the deaf (TDDs) and text telephones (TTs), and the like. Contact the Internal Revenue Service (see "ORGANI-ZATIONS" section below) to obtain publications that explain these benefits, including Publication 501, "Exemptions, Standard Deduction, and Filing Information," and Publication 524, "Credit for the Elderly or the Disabled."

All states and many local governments have adopted their own laws regarding accessibility. Information about these laws may be obtained from the state or local office serving people with disabilities. In many areas, special legal services for people with disabilities are available, often with fees on a sliding scale. Check with the local bar association or with a law school. Some lawyers specialize in the legal needs of people with disabilities.

It is possible to locate the text of federal laws and information about federal programs on many sites on the Internet. The Library of Congress provides information on the status of proposed legislation, Congressional reports, and how to contact members of Congress at thomas.loc.gov.

Reference

Fuch, Beth C. et al.
1997 The Health Insurance Portability and Accountability Act of 1996: Guidance Washington DC: Library of Congress, Congressional Research Service

Architectural and Transportation Barriers Compliance Board (ATBCB)
1331 F Street, NW, Suite 1000
Washington, DC 20004
(800) 872-2253   (800) 993-2822 (TTY)   (202) 272-5434
(202) 272-5449 (TTY)   FAX (202) 272-5447
e-mail: info@access-board.gov   www.access-board.gov

A federal agency charged with developing standards for accessibility in federal facilities, public accommodations, and transportation facilities as required by the Americans with Disabilities Act and other federal laws. Publishes the "Uniform Federal Accessibility Standards," which describes accessibility standards for buildings and dwelling units developed for four federal agencies. Provides technical assistance, sponsors research, and distributes publications. Publishes a free bimonthly newsletter, "Access Currents." Publications available in standard print, alternate formats, and on the web site. Complaint forms may be downloaded from the web site.

Clearinghouse on Disability Information
Office of Special Education and Rehabilitative Services (OSERS)
U.S. Department of Education
400 Maryland Avenue, SW
Washington, DC 20202
(800) 872-5327   (800) 437-0833 (TTY)   (202) 205-8241
FAX (202)) 401-0689   e-mail: customerservice@inet.ed.gov
www.ed.gov/offices/OSERS

Responds to inquiries about federal legislation and programs for people with disabilities and makes referrals.

Client Assistance Program (CAP)
Rehabilitation Services Administration
U.S. Department of Education
330 C Street, SW, Switzer Building, Room 3223
Washington, DC 20202
(202) 205-9315

Established by the Rehabilitation Act of 1973, as amended, CAP provides information and advocacy for individuals with disabilities served under the Act and Title I of the Americans with Disabilities Act. Assistance is also provided to facilitate employment.

Commission on Mental and Physical Disability Law
American Bar Association
740 15th Street, NW, 9th Floor
Washington, DC 20005
(202) 662-1570   (202) 662-1012 (TTY)   FAX (202) 662-1032
e-mail: hammillj@staff.abanet.org   www.abanet.org

Operates a Disability Legal Support Center, which provides searches of databases of laws, legal cases, and recent developments in the field of disability. Provides technical consultations on rights, enforcement, and other issues related to the Americans with Disabilities Act.

Disability.gov
www.disability.gov

This web site provides links to a wide variety of information and resources of the federal government that are related to disability.

Disability Rights Education and Defense Fund (DREDF)
2212 6th Street
Berkeley, CA 94710
(510) 644-2555 (V/TTY)   FAX (510) 841-8645
e-mail: dredf@dredf.org   www.dredf.org

Provides technical assistance, information, and referrals on laws and rights; provides legal representation to people with disabilities in both individual and class action cases; trains law students, parents, and legislators. ADA Hotline [(800)-466-4232 (V/TTY)] provides information on the Americans with Disabilities Act. Quarterly newsletter, "Disability Rights News," available in standard print, alternate formats, and on the web site. Free

Disability Rights Section
U.S. Department of Justice, Civil Rights Division
950 Pennsylvania Avenue, NW
Washington, DC 20530
(800) 514-0301   (800) 514-0383 (TTY)
FAX (202) 307-1198   www.usdoj.gov/crt/ada/adahom1.htm

Responsible for enforcing Titles II and III of the Americans with Disabilities Act. Copies of its regulations are available in standard print, alternate formats, and on the web site. Callers may request publications, obtain technical assistance, and speak to an ADA specialist.

Equal Employment Opportunity Commission (EEOC)
1801 L Street, NW, 10th floor
Washington, DC 20507
(800) 669-3362 to order publications
(800) 669-4000 to speak to an investigator
(800) 669-6820 (TTY)
In the Washington, DC metropolitan area, (202) 663-4900
(202) 663-4494 (TTY)   www.eeoc.gov

Responsible for promulgating and enforcing regulations for the employment section of the ADA. Copies of its regulations are available in standard print, alternate formats, and on the web site.

Fannie Mae
(800) 732-6643
www.fanniemae.com

This private company offers mortgage products designed to help individuals with disabilities attain home ownership. Publishes "A Home of Your Own Guide," for housing educators and counselors who work with individuals with disabilities. Standard print edition available through the Fannie Mae Distribution Center, (800) 471-5554. Free. Also available on the web site.

Federal Communications Commission (FCC)
445 12th Street, SW
Washington, DC 20554
(888) 225-5322   (888) 835-5322 (TTY)   (202) 418-0190
(202) 418-2555 (TTY)   e-mail: fccinfo@fcc.gov   www.fcc.gov/cib/dro

Responsible for developing regulations for telecommunication issues related to federal laws, including the ADA and the Telecommunications Act of 1996. The Consumer Information Bureau (CIB) provides a free e-mail subscription with new information related to disabilities.

Internal Revenue Service (IRS)
(800) 829-1040   (800) 829-4059 (TTY)
www.irs.gov

The IRS provides technical assistance about tax credits and deductions related to accommodations for disabilities. To receive Publication 554, "Older Americans Tax Guide," Publication 501, "Exemptions, Standard Deduction, and Filing Information;" Publication 907, "Tax Highlights for Persons with Disabilities;" and Publication 524, "Credit for the Elderly or the Disabled," call (800) 829-3676; (800) 829-4059 (TTY). These publications are available on the web site.

National Council of State Housing Agencies (NCSHA)
444 North Capitol Street, NW, Suite 438
Washington, DC 20001
(202) 624-7710   FAX (202) 624-5899   www.ncsha.org

Membership organization of state housing agencies. Web site offers a "State Housing Finance Agency Directory" that lists assistance available for home modifications and home ownership programs.

National Council on Disability (NCD)
1331 F Street, NW, Suite 850
Washington, DC 20004
(202) 272-2004   (202) 272-2074 (TTY)
FAX (202) 272-2022   e-mail: mquigley@ncd.gov   www.ncd.gov

An independent federal agency mandated to study and make recommendations about public policy for people with disabilities. Holds regular meetings and hearings in various locations around the country. Publishes monthly newsletter, "NCD Bulletin," available in standard print, alternate formats, and on the web site. Free

National Home of Your Own Alliance
Center for Housing and New Community Economics
Institute on Disability
University of New Hampshire
7 Leavitt Lane, Suite 101
Durham, NH 03824
(800) 220-8770   alliance.unh.edu

The web site provides extensive information about housing for individuals with disabilities, including the Section 8 Homeownership Rule; "A Home of Your Own Guide" for prospective home owners; and information about state housing coalitions, funding sources, and other resources.

Nolo Law for All
Nolo Press
950 Parker Street
Berkeley, CA 94710
(800) 992-6656   (510) 549-1976
FAX (800) 645-0895   e-mail: order@nolo.com   www.nolo.com

This web site provides information on legal topics, updates legislation and court decisions, and features articles from "Nolo News." Free publications catalogue.

Office for Civil Rights, U.S. Department of Health and Human Services
200 Independence Avenue, SW
Washington, DC 20201
(877) 696-6775   (202) 619-0700   (202) 863-0101 (TTY)
FAX (202) 619-3818   www.hhs.gov

Responsible for enforcing laws and regulations that protect the rights of individuals seeking medical and social services in institutions that receive federal financial assistance. Individuals who feel their rights have been violated may file a complaint with one of the ten regional offices located throughout the country. Calling (800) 368-1019 connects you with the regional office closed to you. A special phone number has been established for the office that enforces the health privacy regulations, (866) 827-7748 or e-mail to ocrprivacy@os.dhhs.gov

Office of Civil Rights, U.S. Department of Education
330 C Street, SW
Washington, DC 20202
(800) 421-3481   (877) 521-2172 (TTY)   (202) 205-5413
FAX (202) 205-9862   e-mail: OCR@ed.gov
www.ed.gov/offices/OCR

Responsible for enforcing laws and regulations designed to protect the rights of individuals in educational institutions that receive federal financial assistance. Individuals who feel their rights have been violated may file a complaint with one of the ten regional offices located throughout the country.

Office of Civil Rights, Federal Transit Administration
400 7th Street, SW, Room 9102
Washington, DC 20590
(202) 366-3472   FAX (202) 366-3475
e-mail: ada.assistance@fta.dot.gov   www.fta.dot.gov

Responsible for investigating complaints covered by regulations set forth in the Americans with Disabilities Act regarding the transportation of individuals with disabilities. Call the ADA Assistance Line, (888) 446-4511, to request a complaint form.

Office of Fair Housing and Equal Opportunity
U.S. Department of Housing and Urban Development (HUD)
451 7th Street, SW, Room 5204
Washington DC 20140
(800) 669-9777   (800) 927-9275 (TTY)   (202) 927-9275 (TTY)e
mail: fheo_webmanager@hud.gov
www.hud.gov/fheo.html

This agency enforces the Fair Housing Act and will inform callers how to file a complaint with one of the ten regional HUD offices. Information about the Fair Housing Act and a complaint form are available on the web site.

Office of Federal Contract Compliance Programs (OFCCP)
U.S. Department of Labor, Employment Standards Administration
200 Constitution Avenue, NW, Room C-3325
Washington, DC 20210
(888) 378-3227   (202) 219-9475
FAX (202) 219-6195
www.dol.gov/dol/esa/public/ofcp_org.htm

Reviews contractors' affirmative action plans; provides technical assistance to contractors; investigates complaints; and resolves issues between contractors and employees. Ten regional offices throughout the country serve as liaisons with the national office and with district offices under their jurisdiction.

Office of General Counsel, U.S. Department of Transportation
400 7th Street, SW
Washington, DC 20590
(202) 366-9306   (202) 755-7687 (TTY)   FAX (202) 366-9313
www.dot.gov

Responsible for providing information and interpretation of the regulations for transportation of individuals with disabilities required by the Rehabilitation Act and the Americans with Disabilities Act. Regulations available in standard print and audiocassette.

Rural Housing Service National Office
U.S. Department of Agriculture
Room 5037, South Building
14th Street and Independence Avenue, SW
Washington, DC 20250
(202) 720-4323   www.rurdev.usda.gov/rhs

Provides home ownership, renovation, and repair programs for individuals with disabilities who live in rural areas.

Social Security Administration
6401 Security Boulevard
Baltimore, MD 21235
(800) 772-1213   (800) 325-0778 (TTY)   www.ssa.gov

To apply for Social Security benefits based on disability, phone the number above to set up an appointment with a Social Security representative, or visit the local Social Security office.

Thomas
Library of Congress
thomas.loc.gov

This web site provides a database of recent laws and pending legislation, as well as information about the committees of Congress and the text of the "Congressional Record." Searches for legislation and laws may be done by topic or public law number. Since changes are expected in Social Security, Medicare, Medicaid, and other government programs, this database is a good resource for the status of pending legislation.

U.S. Department of Housing and Urban Development (HUD)
451 7th Street, SW, Room 5240
Washington, DC 20410
(202) 708-0404   FAX (202) 708-1251   www.hud.gov
HUD Discrimination Hotline: (800) 669-9777; (800) 927-9275 (TTY)

Operates programs to make housing accessible, including loans for developers of independent living and group homes and loan and mortgage insurance for rehabilitation of single or multifamily units. Individuals who feel their rights have been violated may file a complaint with one of the ten regional offices located throughout the country.

<u>Americans with Disabilities Act: Questions and Answers</u>
Equal Employment Opportunity Commission (EEOC)
Publications Distribution Center
PO Box 12549
Cincinnati, OH 45212-0549
(800) 669-3362   (800) 800-3302 (TTY)   FAX (513) 489-8692
www.eeoc.gov

This booklet's question and answer format provides explanations of the ADA's effects on employment, state and local governments, and public accommodations. Available in standard print, alternate formats, and on the web site. Free. Also available at www.pueblo.gsa.gov. Click on "Federal Programs."

<u>The Appeals Process</u>
<u>Disability Benefits</u>
<u>How We Decide if You Are Still Disabled</u>
<u>Social Security Disability Programs Can Help</u>
<u>Social Security: What You Need to Know When You Get Disability Benefits</u>
<u>Ticket to Work and Work Incentives Improvement Act of 1999</u>
<u>Working While Disabled... How We Can Help</u>
<u>Your Right to Question the Decision to Stop Your Disability Payments</u>
Social Security Administration (see "ORGANIZATIONS" section above)
(800) 772-1213   (800) 325-0778 (TTY)   www.ssa.gov

These booklets provide basic information about Social Security programs for individuals with disabilities. The Social Security Administration distributes many other titles, including many that are available in standard print, alternate formats, and the web site and at local Social Security offices. Free

<u>Directory of Legal Aid and Defender Offices</u>
National Legal Aid and Defender Association
1625 K Street, NW, 8th Floor
Washington, DC 20006
(202) 452-0620   FAX (202) 872-1031   www.nlads.org

A directory of legal aid offices throughout the U.S. Includes chapters on disability protection/advocacy, health law, and senior citizens. Updated biennially. $70.00

Federal Benefits for Veterans and Dependents
Federal Consumer Information Center
PO Box 100
Pueblo, CO 81002
(888) 878-3256
e-mail: catalog.pueblo.gsa.gov   www.pueblo.gsa.gov

Describes the benefits available under federal laws. $5.00. Also available on the web site.
Click on "Federal Programs."

Federal Register
New Orders, Superintendent of Documents
PO Box 371954
Pittsburgh, PA 15250-7954
(866) 512-1800   (202) 512-1530
FAX (202) 512-2250   e-mail: gpoaccess@gpo.gov
www.access.gpo.gov/su_docs/aces/aces140.html

A federal publication printed every weekday with notices of all regulations and legal notices
issued by federal agencies. Domestic subscriptions, $764.00 annually for second class mailing
of paper format; $264.00 annually for microfiche. Access to the Federal Register is available
through the Internet at the address listed above at no charge.

A Guide to Disability Rights Laws
Federal Consumer Information Center
PO Box 100
Pueblo, CO 81002
(888) 878-3256   e-mail: catalog.pueblo@gsa.gov www.pueblo.gsa.gov

This brochure summarizes federal laws that are applicable to individuals with disabilities and
lists the agencies that enforce them. Free. Also available on the web site.

A Guide to Legal Rights for People with Disabilities
by Marc D. Stolman
Demos Medical Publishing
386 Park Avenue South, Suite 201
New York, NY 10016
(800) 532-8663   (212) 683-0072   FAX (212) 683-0118
e-mail: info@demospub.com   www.demosmedpub.com

This book discusses civil rights, insurance, benefits, and legal issues faced by individuals with
disabilities. $24.95 plus $4.00 shipping and handling. Orders made on the Demos web site
receive a 15% discount.

Guide to Using the Family and Medical Leave Act: Questions and Answers
National Partnership for Women and Families
1875 Connecticut Avenue, NW, Suite 710
Washington, DC 20009
(202) 986-2600   FAX (202) 986-2539
www.nationalpartnership.org

This booklet answers the most frequently asked questions about the law. Available in English and Spanish. Free. Also available on the web site.

Insurance Solutions--Plan Well, Live Better: A Workbook for People with Chronic Illnesses or Disabilities
by Laura D. Cooper
Demos Medical Publishing
386 Park Avenue South, Suite 201
New York, NY 10016
(800) 532-8663   (212) 683-0072   FAX (212) 683-0118
e-mail: info@demospub.com   www.demosmedpub.com

This book enables readers to find and evaluate insurance options. Includes checklists, worksheets, and exercises. $24.95 plus $4.00 shipping and handling. Orders made on the Demos web site receive a 15% discount.

Know Your Rights
National Technical Information Service (NTIS)
5285 Port Royal Road
Springfield, VA 22161
(800) 553-6847   (703) 605-4600   FAX (703) 605-6900
e-mail: orders@ntis.fedworld.gov   www.ntis.gov

This videotape explains the legal rights of residents in nursing homes, using actual examples. Available in English and Spanish. 9 minutes. $50.00 plus $5.00 shipping and handling

Laws Enforced by the U.S. Equal Employment Opportunity Commission
Equal Employment Opportunity Commission (EEOC)
Publications Distribution Center
PO Box 12549
Cincinnati, OH 45212-0549
(800) 669-3362   (800) 800-3302 (TTY)   FAX (513) 489-8692
www.eeoc.gov

Included in this booklet are Title VII of the Civil Rights Act of 1964, Equal Pay Act, Age Discrimination in Employment Act, Rehabilitation Act of 1973, Title I of the Americans with Disabilities, and the Civil Rights Act of 1991. Free

Medicare & You
Centers for Medicare and Medicaid Services (CMS)
formerly Health Care Financing Administration (HCFA)
7500 Security Boulevard
Baltimore, MD 21244
(800) 633-4227   (877) 486-2048   (410) 786-3000
www.hcfa.gov   www.medicare.gov

This booklet provides basic information about Medicare including eligibility, enrollment, coverage, and options. Available in English and Spanish in standard print and alternate formats. Free. Also available on the web site.

Meeting the Needs of Employees with Disabilities
Resources for Rehabilitation
22 Bonad Road
Winchester, MA 01890
(781) 368-9094   FAX (781) 368-9096
e-mail: orders@rfr.org   www.rfr.org

This book provides information to help people with disabilities retain or obtain employment. Information on government programs and laws, supported employment, training programs, environmental adaptations, and the transition from school to work are included. Chapters on mobility, vision, and hearing and speech impairments include information on organizations, products, and services that enable employers to accommodate the needs of employees with disabilities. $44.95 plus $5.00 shipping and handling. (See order form on last page of this book.)

Mental and Physical Disability Law Reporter
Commission on Mental and Physical Disability Law
American Bar Association
740 15th Street, NW, 9th Floor
Washington, DC 20005
(202) 662-1570   (202) 662-1012 (TTY)   FAX (202) 662-1032
e-mail: hammillj@staff.abanet.org   www.abanet.org

A bimonthly journal with court decisions, legislative and regulatory news, and articles on treatment, accessibility, employment, education, federal programs, etc. Individuals, $289.00; organizations, $349.00. Reprints of articles from back issues available.

Removing Barriers to Health Care: A Guide for Health Professionals
Center for Universal Design
North Carolina State University
219 Oberlin Road
Raleigh, NC 27695
(800) 647-6777   (919) 515-3082 (V/TTY)   FAX (919) 515-3023
e-mail: cud@ncsu.edu   www.design.ncsu.edu/cud

This booklet provides guidelines for access to health care facilities. Reviews the design standards of the Americans with Disabilities Act and suggests methods for courteous interactions with individuals with disabilities. Free

Report on Disability Programs
Business Publishers
8737 Colesville Road, Suite 1100
Silver Spring, MD 20910-3928
(800) 274-6737   (301) 589-5103   FAX (301) 589-8493
e-mail: bpinews@bpinews.com   www.bpinews.com

A biweekly newsletter with information on policies promulgated by federal agencies, laws, and funding sources. $327.00

Social Security, Medicare & Pensions: A Source Book
by Joseph Matthews and Dorothy Matthews Berman
Nolo Press
950 Parker Street
Berkeley, CA 94710
(800) 992-6656   (510) 549-1976   FAX (800) 645-0895
e-mail: order@nolo.com   www.nolo.com

This book provides information on Social Security, Medicare and Medicaid, Supplemental Security Income, veterans' benefits, and civil service benefits. It also discusses a variety of Internet sites related to these topics. $29.95 plus $5.00 shipping and handling

A Summary of Department of Veterans Affairs Benefits
(800) 827-1000   www.va.gov

This booklet is available from any VA regional office. Free

<u>Tax Options and Strategies for People with Disabilities</u>
by Steven Mendelsohn
Demos Medical Publishing
386 Park Avenue South, Suite 201
New York, NY 10016
(800) 532-8663   (212) 683-0072   FAX (212) 683-0118
e-mail: info@demospub.com   www.demosmedpub.com

This book describes provisions in the tax laws that affect individuals with disabilities, including access to retirement funds to defray disability related expenses, deductions available for assistive technology, incentives for employers to hire individuals with disabilities, and dependent care. $29.95 plus $4.00 shipping and handling. Orders made on the Demos web site receive a 15% discount.

Chapter 3

CHILDREN AND YOUTHS

Approximately four million children under age 18 have a disability, defined as limitations in activities due to a chronic health problem or impairment (Wenger et al.: 1996). In the 1993-94 school year, 12.2% of all students were designated as having a disability. Nearly 600,000 children under age six participated in preschool programs, and 4.7 million children age six or over participated in elementary or secondary school programs for children with disabilities supported by the federal government (Kaye: 1997).

When parents learn that their child has a disability or chronic condition, they are often overwhelmed by their own emotional responses and the pressure to provide the child with the best possible medical and rehabilitation services. At a time when they often feel guilty, frightened about their child's future, and depressed, they must learn about a new system of services and how to integrate these services into their family life.

Parents are rarely prepared for this situation, unless by chance they have friends or family members who have dealt with a similar condition in their own family. How families cope with a child with a disability or chronic condition is influenced by a variety of factors, including educational level of parents, financial status, personality characteristics of family members, and the availability of services to help the child. Although some families may break up as a result of the stress caused by having a child with a disability or chronic condition, others become closer (Shapiro: 1983).

Because parents experience such intense emotional reactions to a child's disability or illness, counseling to help them cope with their own emotions will contribute to their ability to help the child. Such counseling may be available from medical professionals, social workers or psychologists, rehabilitation counselors, and other parents in similar situations. Talking with other parents either in private or at a parent support group helps parents to learn that their emotional responses are normal. Parent groups also serve as a mechanism for parents to channel energy into productive ways of helping their child. Support groups, which in many cases are focused on a specific disability, help parents to learn about the services available for their child and how to interact effectively with a variety of professionals. In addition to providing information and referrals, parent groups may also have a system of providing respite care.

The professional's responsibility to the family goes far beyond initial discussions of a disability or chronic condition. One study found that parents expressed dissatisfaction with the behavior of physicians and other health care professionals who had not provided the assistance and information needed for making informed decisions about their children's care (Davis, H.: 1991). Parents expressed the need to be treated with respect, to be spoken to in an unpatronizing manner, to have their expertise as parents acknowledged, and to have their family as a whole considered.

Gill (1991) observed that traditional medical training focuses on the physical aspects of disability and ignores the social realities of living with a disability. She recommends that physicians and other health professionals go beyond traditional medical training and get to know individuals with disabilities who live and work independently and successfully. This knowledge should enable professionals to refer individuals with recently diagnosed disabilities and their families to other individuals with disabilities; these relationships may contribute to the development or renewal of self-esteem and independence.

Teplin recommends that professionals discuss the parents' questions and concerns; recognize that early intervention and parent education are important for normal development; and recognize that the physician must take the initiative in making referrals to supportive agencies and resources. Failure to make referrals may cause the family to "flounder needlessly, while the infant misses valuable opportunities for cognitive, motor, and emotional development" (Teplin: 1988, 302).

Noting that several studies have documented that pediatricians have been lacking in their role as case managers for children who are chronically ill, McInerny (1984) makes numerous recommendations to improve the situation. Included are the need to understand the family's strengths and weaknesses in order to help them build upon their strengths; to discuss with the parents how to inform the child about his or her condition; and to make referrals to service providers such as nurse practitioners and social workers as well as parent support groups.

Fowler and colleagues (1985) found that a fifth of the teachers they studied were unaware of the health problems of children in their classrooms, including epilepsy, diabetes, and asthma. Education of classroom teachers regarding the needs of children who have disabilities or chronic conditions is especially important, as teachers may be called upon to respond to such emergencies as epileptic seizures and insulin reactions. They need to know the types of activities that are permissible and those that must be restricted to protect the children's health. On the other hand, they must not be overprotective, unnecessarily limiting the children's activities, or they will be contributing to a sense of inadequacy. Parents and teachers must cooperate to ensure that children with disabilities and chronic conditions strive for a maximum amount of independence in order to prevent the inability to mature. The child's primary care physician, usually a pediatrician, may play an important role in the child's adjustment to the school setting. Walker (1984) suggests that pediatricians educate classroom teachers about the special needs of children they treat. These include effects of medication, special dietary requirements, toileting assistance, use of special equipment, and any limitations on activities.

An investigation by the National Council on Disability (1990) found that there are numerous aspects of education for children with disabilities that must be improved. Noting that fewer students with disabilities complete high school or attend postsecondary institutions than students who do not have disabilities, the report found that parents often view their relations with school personnel as adversarial; that services are often difficult to obtain, especially in rural areas, for minority students, and for students with low incidence disabilities; that schools have low expectations for students with disabilities, resulting in passing them through the schools without providing an adequate education; and that many parents are uninformed about their rights under the law.

Although numerous professionals may be involved in helping children with disabilities and chronic conditions, ultimately it is the parents' responsibility to ensure that their child receives optimal medical care, rehabilitation, and education. Gliedman and Roth make several suggestions to help parents achieve this goal, including:

- Monitor your child's progress closely and keep copies of your child's records.
- Keep records of visits with professionals, including dates, who was present, and what was said.
- If you do not understand any terms that are used, ask for a translation into "lay" language.
- Learn as much as you can about your child's condition.
- Stay in touch with your child's teacher.
- Listen to your child when he or she expresses individual needs.

(1980: 184-185)

Just as teachers and other professionals need to understand the family's needs and dynamics, so too must parents understand that professionals have their own perspectives and organizational structures. Greenberg (1994) points out that professionals must follow organizational policies and meet deadlines which may not seem important to parents. When working together, both parents and professionals must communicate their perspectives to meet the needs of the child.

FAMILY AND PEER RELATIONSHIPS

Stress factors which affect the families of children with disabilities or chronic conditions include financial problems, often caused by limitations of health insurance coverage; lack of information about medical and community services available; and the need to restructure the family itself to accommodate the needs of the child. Parents who share the responsibility of caring for the child may alleviate some of the stress in family dynamics. For example, it may be wise to schedule visits to physicians' and other service providers' offices so that parents can both attend and share the responsibility for the child's care. Patterson (1991) noted that in cases where one parent takes the major responsibility for the child (most frequently the mother), he or she often forms a strong dyad with the child, disrupting the parents' own dyad. Sabbeth (1984) reported that while parents of children with disabilities often do not have much time to spend alone together and may unconsciously or consciously blame each other for the child's condition, research indicates that the divorce rate is not higher among these couples than in a control group.

When other children are in the family, the situation is compounded by the need to preserve a sense of normalcy and at the same time help the child who has a disability or chronic condition. Siblings may be jealous of the attention paid to their brother or sister. They may feel embarrassed to have a sibling whose physical appearance or behavior is abnormal, and they may fear rejection by their peers. Siblings as well as the affected children need information about the disability or condition in order to be comfortable and to quell their anxieties.

As the child develops and enters different environments, it is important for his or her peers to be educated about the disability or condition. Parents who tell their children to keep their condition a secret are giving them the message that there is something to be ashamed of (Weitzman: 1984). Their peers must learn that individuals who are different should not be viewed negatively. Children who do not have disabilities should be encouraged to ask adults questions about disabilities. They should be told that teasing will hurt the other child's feelings. Weiserbs and Gottlieb (1992) found that younger children expressed more positive attitudes toward children with disabilities than older children, reflecting a less powerful influence of peer groups on the younger group. They suggest that teachers employ a rotating "partner" system for all students rather than assigning responsibility for a student with a disability to one or two classmates. The stigma of association with a peer who is disabled is avoided when all students work with partners.

Disability awareness programs in schools, religious organizations, and youth groups offer an opportunity to educate children about a specific disability or a range of conditions. The "Kids on the Block" (see "ORGANIZATIONS" section below) puppets and programs enable children to simulate an experience with a disability, thereby encouraging understanding and acceptance.

Disabilities and chronic conditions may be especially difficult to cope with during adolescence and teenage years. It is during this stage that body image receives a great deal of emphasis and that relationships with the opposite sex begin. Youths with disabilities may wonder about their ability to have normal sexual relationships and to have children but may find it difficult to discuss this matter with their parents. Unfortunately, health care providers and professional counselors also neglect the subject of sexuality when working with youths with disabilities and chronic conditions (Davis, S. et al.: 1991).

Children with disabilities or chronic conditions often benefit from participation in programs which match them with adult role models. The adults share their life experiences and provide a sounding board for questions about school, recreation, employment, social life, and many other issues. Working with these youngsters gives the adults an opportunity to share their life experience, provide inspiration, and give something back to the community.

Children and youths with disabilities and chronic conditions use a wide variety of assistive devices at home, in the classroom, and in recreation. Many special aids have been developed to make independent learning and living safe and comfortable. Often family members, teachers, or other professionals create assistive devices to meet a particular need.

LAWS THAT AFFECT CHILDREN AND YOUTHS

(This section covers laws that are specific to children and education. For laws that affect individuals of all ages who have disabilities, including children, see Chapter 2, "Laws That Affect People with Disabilities.")

The enactment of the *Education of the Handicapped Act* (P.L. 94-142) in 1975 broke ground for the expansion of educational services for children with disabilities and established legal rights for these children to obtain an appropriate education from the public school system. The law requires that states provide all children with disabilities an appropriate public education in the least restrictive setting. Special education services provided in public school classrooms, at home, and in hospitals and institutions are included. Related services that states must provide include transportation; physical, occupational, audiological, and speech therapy; and psychological services. In addition, the U.S. Department of Education is mandated to provide funding for a variety of programs that train special educators and other professional personnel to serve children with special needs.

In order for states to receive federal funding for programs for children with disabilities, the state department of education must establish a plan and procedures for providing these services and require that local educational agencies maintain Individualized Education Programs (IEPs) for each child served. Federal funds are allocated to states based on the number of children with disabilities served.

In addition, the federal law mandates that regional resource centers be established to provide technical assistance to professional educators who provide services for children and youths with disabilities. These centers may be operated by a college or university, state or local education agency, or private nonprofit organization that has received a federal grant for this purpose. The state educational agency is required to publish a listing of the resource centers in the state. Parent Training and Information Centers, also mandated by federal law, assist parents with IEP meetings, publish newsletters, and provide training on topics such as technology, transition, and other related issues (Ziegler: 1992).

The *Education of the Handicapped Act Amendments of 1983* (P.L. 98-199) expanded the incentives to local and state governments to provide equal educational opportunities in preschool, early intervention, and transition programs. The *Education of the Handicapped Act Amendments of 1986* (P.L. 99-457) lowered the eligibility for special education services to age three and established the Handicapped Infant and Toddler Programs (birth to age three). These programs provide early intervention services to infants and toddlers who have been diagnosed with physical or mental conditions for which there is a high probability of developmental delay (Center for Special Education Technology: 1991). Under this part of the law, the needs of both the child and the family are considered in the development of an Individualized Family Service Plan (IFSP). The IFSP creates a partnership between the family and early intervention services providers. The IFSP requires an assessment and statement of a family's ability to enhance the child's development; an assessment of the child's functional level; establishment of goals, timelines, and evaluation procedures; identification of an appropriate case manager or service coordinator; and a plan for transition from early intervention to services funded by public school when the child reaches three years.

After the child reaches age three, the special education teacher, health care providers, and the parents work together to develop an IEP, which specifies educational goals, courses of instruction, special equipment, and other services to be provided. The IEP is based on the results of an individualized evaluation and assessment of the child. Schools are required to notify parents in writing any time a decision is made related to the identification of the child's disability, educational needs, development of the IEP, or placement in a special or regular program. Parents have the right to appeal if they disagree with the school's decision and may arrange for an independent evaluation of their child. Both this law and Section 504 of the Rehabilitation Act (see below) provide mechanisms for resolution of disputes. These include formal mediation, due process hearings, and complaint procedures.

In 1990, the name of the Education of the Handicapped Act was changed to the *Individuals with Disabilities Education Act*, referred to as IDEA (P.L. 101-476). IDEA expanded education programs to include services to children with serious emotional problems, attention deficits, autism, and traumatic brain injury. In 1997, IDEA was reauthorized, with amendments, as P.L. 105-17. The amendments require that school personnel provide regular reports on the children's progress, by means such as report cards and by including parents in decisions about their child's placement; educational goals that relate to the general curriculum must be included in the IEP. Guidelines for evaluating students whose behavior has resulted in a disciplinary action require that special education services not be suspended and spell out the steps to assess the situation. Parents who disagree with educators about their child's education are entitled to enter into mediation.

Adolescents with disabilities have special needs as they consider career goals and higher education. Vocational education offers students a combination of classroom instruction and practical job experience to develop the occupational skills needed in the labor market. Vocational education is available in high schools, community colleges, and technical institutes. The *Carl D. Perkins Vocational and Applied Technology Education Act* (P.L. 101-392) provides increased resources to achieve the academic and occupational skills necessary for employment in high technology. Individuals with disabilities are included in this mandate.

Section 504 of the Rehabilitation Act of 1973 prohibits any institution that receives federal funds from discriminating against people with disabilities. Since virtually all postsecondary institutions receive federal funds, they are required to comply with the regulations developed for the enforcement of Section 504 (see Chapter 2, "Laws That Affect People with Disabilities"). Students who qualify for admission into postsecondary education programs must be provided with the services that they need to complete their education (Bowe: 1987). Most universities, colleges, and community colleges have established special offices to serve students with disabilities. Sources of financial assistance for postsecondary students with disabilities are listed below under "Financial Aid for Postsecondary Education."

Some children with disabilities are eligible for monthly Social Security benefits if their family meets a financial means test. In the Sullivan v. Zebley case, the Supreme Court held that the Social Security Administration's eligibility criteria for children during the 1980's did not reflect the intent of Congress and were more stringent for children than for adults; as a result, disability evaluations for children under the age of 18 have been changed. If a child does not qualify for benefits on the basis of medical standards alone, an individual functional assessment must be conducted to determine if the child is capable of functioning at an age appropriate level. Children who were denied benefits from January 1, 1980 to February 11, 1991 may now be eligible and may also receive retroactive benefits. Contact the Social Security Administration [(800) 772-1213 or (800) 325-0778 (TTY)] to determine whether your child is eligible for medical or cash benefits.

In 1997, Congress passed the *Children's Health Insurance Program (CHIP)* (P.L. 105-33), as part of the Balanced Budget Act of 1997 to make available funds for states to provide insurance for uninsured children of low income, working parents. States have the option of expanding their Medicaid plan or developing a new children's health insurance plan. States must submit a plan for approval to the Secretary of Health and Human Services; the law sets standards for what the coverage must include. Eligibility requirements for the program are an income level 200% of the poverty level or 50 percentage points above the Medicaid eligibility limit; and children must not be eligible for Medicaid or other health insurance coverage. States must continue Medicaid eligibility for children who would have lost Supplemental Security Income benefits (see Chapter 2, "Laws That Affect People with Disabilities") because of the change in the definition of childhood disability under the Personal Responsibility and Work Opportunity Act of 1996.

The *Family Opportunity Act of 2001* would allow states to offer a Medicaid buy-in for children with disabilities up to age 18 who would be eligible for SSI disability benefits but for their family income. This plan would cover children whose families earn up to 300% of the federal poverty level ($52,950 for a family of four). As this book went to press, the 106th Congress had not completed action on the bill before adjournment.

Copies of the laws cited above may be obtained from Senators and Representatives. Organizations that advocate on behalf of children and youths with disabilities may also provide them upon request.

References

Bowe, Frank G.
1987 "Section 504: 10 Years Later" American Rehabilitation (April/May/June):2-3;23-24
Center for Special Education Technology
1991 "Update: 1990 Demographic Data" The Marketplace: Report on Technology in Special Education 4:1
Davis, Hilton
1991 "Counselling Families of Children with Disabilities" pp. 223-37 in Hilton Davis and Lesley Fallowfield (eds.) Counselling and Communication in Health Care London: John Wiley & Sons
Davis, Sherry E. et al.
1991 "Developmental Tasks and Transitions of Adolescents with Chronic Illnesses and Disabilities" pp. 70-79 in Robert P. Marinelli and Arthur E. Dell Orto (eds.) The Psychological and Social Impact of Disability New York, NY: Springer Publishing
Fowler, M.G., M.P. Johnson, and S.S. Atkinson
1985 "School Achievement and Absence in Children with Chronic Health Conditions" Journal of Pediatrics 106:4(April):683-687
Gill, Carol J.
1991 "Treating Families Coping with Disability: Doing No Harm" in Rehabilitation Medicine-Adding Life to Years (Special Issue) The Western Journal of Medicine (May) 154:624-625
Gliedman, John and William Roth
1980 The Unexpected Minority: Handicapped Children in America New York, NY: Harcourt Brace Jovanovich
Greenberg, Janice
1994 "Working with Parents" Rehabilitation Digest 25:3(December):7-8
Kaye, H. Stephen
1997 "Education of Children with Disabilities" Disability Statistics Abstract Number 19, July
McInerny, Thomas
1984 "The Role of the General Pediatrician in Coordinating the Care of Children with Chronic Illness" Pediatric Clinics of North America 31:1(February):199-209

National Council on Disability

1990 "The Education of Students with Disabilities: Where Do We Stand?" Journal of Disability Policy Studies 1:1(Spring):103-132

Patterson, Joan M.

1991 "Family Resilience to the Challenge of A Child's Disability" Pediatric Annals 20:9:491-499

Sabbeth, Barbara

1984 "Understanding the Impact of Chronic Childhood Illness on Families" Pediatric Clinics of North America 31:1(February):47-57

Shapiro, Johanna

1983 "Family Reactions and Coping Strategies in Response to the Physically Ill or Handicapped Child: A Review" Social Science and Medicine 17:14:913-931

Teplin, Stuart W.

1988 "Development of the Blind Infant and Child with Retinopathy of Prematurity: The Physician's Role in Intervention," pp. 301-323 in John T. Flynn and Dale L. Phelps (eds.) Retinopathy of Prematurity: Problem and Challenge New York, NY: Alan R. Liss, Inc.

Walker, Deborah Klein

1984 "Care of Chronically Ill Children in School" Pediatric Clinics of North America 31:1(February):221-233

Weiserbs, Barbara and Jay Gottlieb

1992 "Perceived Risk as a Factor Influencing Attitudes Toward Physically Disabled Children" Journal of Developmental and Physical Disabilities 4:4:341-352

Weitzman, Michael

1984 "School and Peer Relations" Pediatric Clinics of North America 31:1(February):59-69

Wenger, Barbara L., H. Stephen Kaye, and Mitchell LaPlante

1996 "Disabilities among Children" Disability Statistics Abstract Number 15, March

Ziegler, Martha

1992 "Parent Advocacy and Children with Disabilities: A History" OSERS News in Print V:1(Summer):4-6

Administration on Developmental Disabilities (ADD)
Administration for Children and Families
U.S. Department of Health and Human Services
Mail Stop: HHH 300-F
370 L'Enfant Promenade, SW
Washington, DC 20447
(202) 690-6590   www.acf.dhhs.gov/programs/add

Works with state governments, local communities, and the private sector to promote self-sufficiency and protect the rights of individuals with developmental disabilities.

American Council on Rural Special Education (ACRES)
Kansas State University
2323 Anderson Avenue, Suite 226
Manhattan, KS 66502
(785) 532-2737   FAX (785) 532-7732
e-mail: acres@ksu.edu   www.ksu.edu/acres

National membership organization for educators who serve students with disabilities in rural areas. Provides scholarships for practicing teachers who work with students with disabilities in rural areas. Membership, regular, $50.00; students, $25.00; includes "Rural Special Education Quarterly" and "RuraLink."

Association on Higher Education and Disability (AHEAD)
University of Massachusetts
100 Morrissey Boulevard
Boston, MA 02125
(617) 287-3880   (617) 287-3882 (TTY)   FAX (617) 287-3881
www.ahead.org

Promotes the full participation of individuals with disabilities in postsecondary education. Special interest groups focus on specific disabilities, technology, Canadian programs, and other topics. Membership, $150.00, includes "Alert" newsletter six times a year and "Journal of Postsecondary Education and Disability;" other membership categories include affiliate, institutional, and student.

Barrier Free Education
Center for Assistive Technology and Environmental Access
Georgia Institute of Technology
490 10th Street, NW
Atlanta, GA 30332
(404) 894-4960 (V/TTY)   FAX (404) 894-9320
e-mail: webmaster@BFE.atlanta.arch.gatech.edu
www.catea.org/barrier_free

This web site is designed to help students in the fields of math and science learn about strategies and adapted equipment that can help them perform experiments and measurements. The site also includes stories about students with disabilities who have been successful using adapted equipment. Provides links to resources. Operates a listserv to exchange information.

Beach Center on Disability
c/o Life Span Institute
University of Kansas
3136 Haworth Hall
1200 Sunnyside Avenue
Lawrence, KS 66045
(785) 864-7600 (V/TTY)   FAX (785) 864-7605
e-mail: beach@dole.lsi.ukans.edu   www.beachcenter.org

A federally funded center that conducts research and training in the factors that contribute to the successful functioning of families with members who have disabilities. A catalogue of publications describes monographs and tapes related to family coping, professional roles, and service delivery. Free

Clearinghouse on Disability Information
Office of Special Education and Rehabilitative Services (OSERS)
U.S. Department of Education
400 Maryland Avenue, SW
Washington, DC 20202
(800) 872-5327   (800) 437-0833 (TTY)   (202) 205-8241
FAX (202)) 401-0689   e-mail: customerservice@inet.ed.gov
www.ed.gov/offices/OSERS

Federal information clearinghouse on disabilities. Answers questions about federal laws, services, and programs for individuals of all ages with disabilities.

Council for Exceptional Children (CEC)
1110 North Glebe Road, Suite 300
Arlington, VA 22201
(888) 232-7733   (703) 620-3660   (703) 264-9446
FAX (703) 264-9494   www.cec.sped.org

A professional membership organization that works to improve the quality of education for children who are gifted or have disabilities. Holds annual conference. Membership dues vary by geographic location. Publishes "Teaching Exceptional Children," a bimonthly journal for special educators; $58.00; and newsletter, "Exceptional Children," published quarterly, $58.00. (CEC's publications office: (800) 232-7323).

EDLAW Center
PO Box 81-7327
Hollywood, FL 33081
(954) 966-4489   FAX (954) 966-8561
e-mail: edlawcenter@edlaw.net   www.edlaw.net

This center provides the text of federal laws pertaining to special education and interpretations of the laws, a state-by-state list of attorneys who specialize in special education, conferences, links to other special education web sites, and discussion groups.

Educational Equity Concepts (EEC)
100 5th Avenue, 2nd Floor
New York, NY 10011
(212) 243-1110 (V/TTY)   FAX (212) 627-0407
e-mail: information@edequity.org   www.edequity.org

Promotes equal educational opportunity and excellence in education for students who have been the subject of bias based on race, gender, disability, or income. Provides information, resources, and referrals. Publishes directories, training kits, and curricula related to disability awareness and inclusion.

ERIC Clearinghouse on Disabilities and Gifted Education (ERIC/EC)
Council for Exceptional Children (CEC)
1110 North Glebe Road, Suite 300
Arlington, VA 22201
(800) 328-0272   e-mail: ericec@ced.sped.org   www.ericec.org

A database of journal articles and books, including those related to the special needs of students with disabilities. AskERIC will answer questions submitted to the electronic mail address: askeric@askeric.org

Insure Kids Now
Children's Health Insurance Program (CHIP)
(877) 543-7669   www.insurekidsnow.gov

This web site provides information on this federal program that encourages states to provide health insurance for uninsured children.

Kids on the Block
9385-C Gerwig Lane
Columbia, MD 21046
(800) 368-5437   (410) 290-9095   FAX (410) 290-9358
e-mail: kob@kotb.com   www.kotb.com

A program that uses puppets to help students understand disabilities and chronic conditions. Various programs available, including blindness, diabetes, and sibling of a child who is disabled.

Lekotek Toy Resource Helpline
National Lekotek Center
(800) 366-7529   (800) 573-4446 (TTY)   www.lekotek.org

Callers to this helpline will receive assistance in choosing toys and activities for children with disabilities. (See "Toy Guide for Differently Abled Kids," in "PUBLICATIONS AND TAPES" section below.)

National Association for the Education of Young Children (NAEYC)
1509 16th Street, NW
Washington, DC 20036
(800) 424-2460   (202) 232-8777   FAX (202) 328-1846
e-mail: naeyc@naeyc.org   www.naeyc.org

Membership organization that advocates for early childhood education programs through professional development, accreditation program, and information services. Membership, $45.00; includes bimonthly journal, "Young Children." Publications include "A Place for Me: Including Children with Special Needs in Early Care and Education Settings," $6.00.

National Information Center for Children and Youth with Disabilities (NICHCY)
PO Box 1492
Washington, DC 20013-1492
(800) 695-0285 (V/TTY)   In the Washington, DC area, (202) 884-8200 (V/TTY)
FAX (202) 884-8441   e-mail: nichcy@aed.org   www.nichcy.org

Provides information and referral, technical assistance, and publications to parents, educators, caregivers, and advocates. Publications are available on the web site.

National Library Service for the Blind and Physically Handicapped (NLS)
1291 Taylor Street, NW
Washington, DC 20542
(800) 424-8567 or (800) 424-8572 (Reference Section)
(800) 424-9100 (to receive application)
(202) 707-5100   FAX (202) 707-0712   e-mail: nls@loc.gov
www.loc.gov/nls

Provides free talking book equipment on loan and recorded and braille books for preschoolers, children, and adults with physical disabilities, visual impairment, or blindness through a regional network of cooperating libraries. "Parents' Guide to the Development of Preschool Children with Disabilities: Resources and Services" lists national organizations; sources for games and toys; materials available in special formats; and a bibliography of articles and books. Free

National Parent Network on Disabilities (NPND)
1130 17th Street, NW, Suite 400
Washington, DC 20036
(202) 463-2299 (V/TTY)   FAX (202) 463-9403   e-mail: npnd@npnd.org
www.npnd.org

A coalition of organizations that serve children with special needs and their families. Provides advocacy regarding federal policy for children with special needs; publishes legislative alerts; and serves as an information and resource network for organizations and parents. Membership, parents or individuals with disabilities, $25.00; professionals, $40.00; parents' groups, $50.00; includes quarterly newsletter, "Networking."

PACER Center (Parent Advocacy Coalition for Educational Rights)
8161 Normandale Boulevard
Minneapolis, MN 55437
(888) 248-0822   (952) 838-9000
In MN, (800) 537-2237   (952) 838-0190 (TTY)
FAX (952) 838-0199   e-mail: pacer@pacer.org   www.pacer.org

A coalition of disability organizations that offers information about laws, procedures, and parents' rights and responsibilities. Publishes "PACESETTER," three times a year, free, and "Early Childhood Connection," for parents of young children with disabilities, two or three times a year, free. Free catalogue of publications.

Parent Education and Assistance for Kids (PEAK)
611 North Weber, Suite 200
Colorado Springs, CO 80903
(800) 284-0251   (719) 531-9400   FAX (719) 531-9452
e-mail: info@peakparent.org   www.peakparent.org

A center that promotes the integration of children with disabilities in the regular classroom. Provides referrals for parents and technical assistance to school systems.

Sibling Support Project
Children's Hospital and Medical Center
PO Box 5371
Seattle, WA 98105
(206) 527-5712   FAX (206) 527-5705
e-mail: dmeyer@chmc.org   www.seattlechildrensorg/sibsupp

Promotes the creation of peer support and education programs for siblings of children with disabilities and chronic conditions. Conducts workshops, produces publications, provides technical assistance, and maintains a database of services for siblings. The Sibshop Model offers recommendations for peer support and education workshops for siblings. Publishes free newsletter, "Sibling Support Project Newsletter." Also available on the web site.

TASH: The Association for Persons with Severe Handicaps
29 West Susquehanna Avenue, Suite 210
Baltimore, MD 21204
(410) 828-8274   (410) 828-1306 (TTY)   FAX (410) 828-6706
e-mail: info@tash.org   www.tash.org

A national advocacy organization that disseminates information to improve the education and increase the independence of individuals with severe disabilities. Holds an annual conference. Publishes a quarterly journal, "Journal of the Association for Persons with Severe Handicaps" and the "TASH Newsletter" (both included with membership). Regular membership, $88.00; associate membership, $45.00.

The Technical Assistance Alliance for Parent Centers
PACER Center (Parent Advocacy Coalition for Educational Rights)
8161 Normandale Boulevard
Minneapolis, MN 55437
(888) 248-0822   (952) 838-9000
In MN, (800) 537-2237   (952) 838-0190 (TTY)   FAX (952) 838-0199
e-mail: alliance@taalliance.org   www.taalliance.org

A federally funded project, the Alliance provides technical assistance to parent training and information centers across the country. Holds regional and national conferences.

Toys for Special Children & Enabling Devices
385 Warburton Avenue
Hastings-on-Hudson, NY 10706
(800) 832-8697   (914) 478-0960
FAX (914) 478-7030   e-mail: customersupport@enablingdevices.com
www.enablingdevices.com

Adapts a range of toys to be used with special switches by children with disabilities. Product catalogue available on the web site.

Wright's Law
c/o The Special Ed Advocate
PO Box 1008
Deltaville, VA 23043
(804) 257-0857   FAX (810) 529-4332
e-mail: webmaster@wrightslaw.com
www.wrightslaw.com

This web site provides information to help parents advocate for children with special needs. It includes information about federal laws. Offers advocacy and law libraries. Publishes "Special Ed Advocate" newsletter; available on the web site only. Peter Wright is an attorney who specializes in special education cases.

Backyards and Butterflies: Ways to Include Children with Disabilities in Outdoor Activities
by Doreen Greenstein, Naomi Miner, and Emilie Kudela
Brookline Books
PO Box 1047
Cambridge, MA 02238-1047
(800) 666-2665   (617) 868-0360   FAX (617) 868-1772
e-mail: milt@brooklinebooks.com   www.brooklinebooks.com

This book provides directions for making outdoor activities accessible to children with disabilities. $14.95

Barnes and Noble

This national bookstore chain has a "Special Needs Collection" for parents and professionals. Includes books on disabilities, such as epilepsy, cerebral palsy, and hearing impairment. Consult a telephone directory to locate the nearest store.

Benefits for Children
Social Security Administration
(800) 772-1213   (800) 325-0778 (TTY)   www.ssa.gov

This publication provides information about obtaining Social Security benefits for children with disabilities. The Social Security Administration distributes many other titles, including those that are available in standard print, alternate formats, and on the web site. Many publications are also available at local Social Security offices. (See Chapter 2, "PUBLICATIONS AND TAPES" for other titles available from the Social Security Administration.)

Children with Disabilities: A Medical Primer
Mark L. Batshaw and Yvonne M. Perret
Paul Brookes Publishing Company
PO Box 10624
Baltimore, MD 21285-9945
(800) 638-3775   FAX (410) 337-8539
e-mail: custserv@pbrookes.com   www.brookespublishing.com

Written by a physician and a social worker, this book describes major types of disability in children, such as hearing impairments, vision impairments, seizure disorders, traumatic brain injury, and AIDS and provides a glossary and resource list. $59.95 plus 10% shipping and handling

Children with Special Needs
by Katharine T. Bartlett and Judith Welch Wegner (eds.)
Transaction Publishers
390 Campus Drive
Somerset, NJ 08073
(888) 999-6778   www.transactionpub.com

This book analyzes the history and implementation of special education following the passage of the Education for All Handicapped Children Act. Includes recommendations for achieving the goals of special education. $44.95

Choosing Home or Residential Care: A Guide for Families of Children with Severe Physical Disabilities
by Marilyn Lash and Paul Kahn
Crotched Mountain Foundation, Book Order
1 Verney Drive
Greenfield, NH 03047
(800) 966-2672   (603) 547-3311   e-mail: info@cmf.org
www.cmf.org

This book discusses the issues that parents face when deciding where their child should be cared for. It covers the emotional impact on the family and the advantages and disadvantages of each setting. Available on the web site only.

The Complete IEP Guide
by Lawrence Siegel
Nolo Press
950 Parker Street
Berkeley, CA 94710
(800) 992-6656   (510) 549-1976   FAX (800) 645-0895
e-mail: order@nolo.com   www.nolo.com

Written for parents of children who are in special education, this book provides detailed information about the Individualized Education Program (IEP) and how to use legal options to resolve disputes with the educational system. $24.95 plus $5.00 shipping and handling

Delicate Threads: Friendships between Children with and without Special Needs in Inclusive Settings
by Debbie Staub
Woodbine House
6510 Bells Mill Road
Bethesda, MD 20817
(800) 843-7323   FAX (301) 897-5838
e-mail: info@woodbinehouse.com www.woodbinehouse.com

Through her observations of seven pairs of children in which one child has a moderate to severe disability, the author describes their friendships and provides practical suggestions to parents and teachers for establishing such relationships. $16.95 plus $4.50 shipping and handling

The Early Intervention Dictionary: A Multidisciplinary Guide to Terminology
by Jeanine G. Coleman
Woodbine House
6510 Bells Mill Road
Bethesda, MD 20817
(800) 843-7323   FAX (301) 897-5838
e-mail: info@woodbinehouse.com   www.woodbinehouse.com

This book defines the medical, therapeutic, and educational terms used in the field of early intervention. $17.95 plus $4.50 shipping and handling

Exam Accommodations Reference Manual
Association on Higher Education and Disability (AHEAD)
University of Massachusetts
100 Morrissey Boulevard
Boston, MA 02125
(617) 287-3880   (617) 287-3882 (TTY)   FAX (617) 287-3881
www.ahead.org

This book discusses the rationale for accommodations in testing and provides examples of accommodations, such as extended time, reader services, and scribe services. Sample forms are also provided. $25.00 plus $5.00 shipping and handling

Exceptional Parent
65 East Route 4
River Edge, NJ 07661
(877) 372-7368   (201) 489-4111   www.eparent.com

This monthly magazine emphasizes problem solving and provides practical information for raising a child with a disability. Includes annual resource guide. $39.95

Families, Friends, Futures
Comforty Media Concepts
2145 Pioneer Road
Evanston, IL 60201
(847) 475-0791   (847) 475-0793
e-mail: comforty@comforty.com   www.comforty.com

Part of the "Inclusion Series," this videotape portrays how inclusion works by observing a 12 year old sixth grader and a three year old in nursery school. The girls' participation in school activities serves as encouragement for their families regarding the girls' futures. 23 minutes. $65.00 plus $10.00 shipping and handling

Family Guide to Assistive Technology
by Katherine Kelker, Roger Holt, and John Sullivan
Brookline Books
PO Box 1047
Cambridge, MA 02238-1047
(800) 666-2665   (617) 868-0360   FAX (617) 868-1772
e-mail: milt@brooklinebooks.com   www.brooklinebooks.com

This book guides parents in obtaining assistive technology for children with disabilities through their special education plans and other resources. $15.95

Friendship-Building Strategies
by Barbara E. Buswell
Parent Education and Assistance for Kids (PEAK)
611 North Weber, Suite 200
Colorado Springs, CO 80903
(800) 284-0251   (719) 531-9400
(719) 531-9452 (V/TTY)   FAX (719) 531-9452
e-mail: info@peakparent.org   www.peakparent.org

A workshop kit that enables parents and professionals to help children with disabilities form friendships. Includes transparencies and bibliography. $89.00 plus $10.75 shipping and handling

A Guide to the Individualized Education Program
Editorial Publications Center
U.S. Department of Education
PO Box 1398
Jessup, MD 20794-1398
(877) 433-7827   (877) 576-7734 (TTY)   FAX (301) 470-1244
www.ed.gov/pubs/edpubs/html

This guide includes information about writing an IEP, IEP team members, and implementation of the IEP. Free. Also available on the web site. To obtain this guide in alternate formats, contact Katie Mincey, Director of the Alternate Format Center, (202) 260-9865; e-mail: Katie_Mincey@ed.gov

The IEP - A Tool for Realizing Possibilities, videotape
Individual Education Plan: Involved Effective Parents, resource guide
Parent Education and Assistance for Kids (PEAK)
611 North Weber, Suite 200
Colorado Springs, CO 80903
(800) 284-0251   (719) 531-9400
(719) 531-9452 (V/TTY)   FAX (719) 531-9452
e-mail: info@peakparent.org   www.peakparent.org

The videotape supports the role of parents in the IEP process and shows children with disabilities included in general education classrooms. 20 minutes. Available in English and Spanish. $15.00 plus $3.75 shipping and handling. The resource guide describes the development of an IEP and the transfer of information from year to year. $10.00 plus $1.50 shipping and handling

Individualized Education Programs
National Information Center for Children and Youth with Disabilities (NICHCY)
PO Box 1492
Washington, DC 20013
(800) 695-0285 (V/TTY)   In the Washington, DC area (202) 884-8200 (V/TTY)
FAX (202) 884-8441   e-mail: nichcy@aed.org   www.nichcy.org

This publication is a verbatim report of the federal regulations regarding IDEA. It describes the purposes and contents of the IEP, the responsibility of the state education agency, the role of parents, and the requirements for holding meetings. Single copy, free. Also available on the web site.

My Brother Matthew
by Mary Thompson
Woodbine House
6510 Bells Mill Road
Bethesda, MD 20817
(800) 843-7323   FAX (301) 897-5838
e-mail: info@woodbinehouse.com   www.woodbinehouse.com

Written for siblings of children with disabilities, this book helps them deal with their emotions and understand their brother's or sister's needs. $14.95 plus $4.50 shipping and handling

National Clearinghouse on Postsecondary Education for Individuals with Disabilities
HEATH Resource Center
2121 K Street, NW, #220
Washington, DC 20037
(800) 544-3284 (V/TTY)   (202) 973-0904   FAX (202) 973-0908
e-mail: help@heath.gwu.edu   www.heath.gwu.edu

A federally funded clearinghouse on the transition from high school to postsecondary education. Publishes newsletter, "Information from HEATH," three times a year; available on the web site only. Publishes "Career Planning and Employment Strategies," "Vocational Rehabilitation Services: A Postsecondary Student Consumer's Guide" and "How to Choose a College: Guide for the Student with a Disability;" free; also available on the web site.

Negotiating the Special Education Maze: A Guide for Parents and Teachers
by Winifred Anderson, Stephen Chitwood, and Deidre Hayden
Woodbine House
6510 Bells Mill Road
Bethesda, MD 20817
(800) 843-7323   FAX (301) 897-5838
e-mail: info@woodbinehouse.com   www.woodbinehouse.com

This book helps parents to understand the IEP process and describes laws such as the Individuals with Disabilities Education Act (IDEA) and the Americans with Disabilities Act (ADA). Includes glossary, reading list, and resource lists. $16.95 plus $4.50 shipping and handling

Opening Doors: Strategies for Including All Students in Regular Education
by C. Beth Schaffner and Barbara E. Buswell
Parent Education and Assistance for Kids (PEAK)
611 North Weber, Suite 200
Colorado Springs, CO 80903
(800) 284-0251   (719) 531-9400
(719) 531-9452 (V/TTY)   FAX (719) 531-9452
e-mail: info@peakparent.org   www.peakparent.org

This book provides practical information on how to include students with disabilities in elementary and secondary classrooms. Discusses curriculum adaptations and behavior supports. $13.00 plus $3.75 shipping and handling

Parenting Children with Special Needs
United Learning
1560 Sherman Avenue, Suite 100
Evanston, IL 60201
(800) 421-2363   (847) 328-6700   FAX (847) 328-6706
e-mail: agc@mcs.net   www.agcmedia.com

This videotape depicts parents' experiences upon learning that their child has a disability, the effects on the family dynamics, the benefits of early intervention, legal requirements, and how to work with health care professionals. 30 minutes. $95.00 plus $3.00 shipping and handling

Parents' Guide: Accessing Parent Groups
by Suzanne Ripley
National Information Center for Children and Youth with Disabilities
PO Box 1492
Washington, DC 20013-1492
(800) 695-0285 (V/TTY)   In the Washington, DC area, (202) 884-8200 (V/TTY)
FAX (202) 884-8441   e-mail: nichcy@aed.org   www.nichcy.org

This publication provides guidelines for locating and/or organizing parent groups; describes community services and how to use them; includes a special section for rural families; and makes recommendations for organizing medical, school, and community services records. Free

Play Helps: Toys and Activities for Children with Special Needs
by Roma Lear
Butterworth-Heinemann
225 Wildwood Avenue
Woburn, MA 01801
(800) 366-2665   FAX (800) 446-6520
e-mail: orders@bh.com   www.bh.com

This book provides practical, affordable ideas for toys and games that will stimulate children with a variety of disabilities. Chapters are organized by the five senses. $39.99 plus $6.00 shipping and handling

Sensitivity and Awareness: A Guide for Developing Understanding among Children
by Norma McPhee with Paddy Favazza and Eleanore Grater Lewis
Jason & Nordic Publishers
PO Box 441
Hollidaysburg, PA 16648
(814) 696-2920   FAX (814) 696-4250
e-mail: turtlebooks@jasonandnordic.com
www.jasonandnordic.com

The activities in this workbook are designed to improve relationships between children with disabilities and children who are not disabled in pre-primary, primary, and middle school classrooms. $14.95 plus $3.50 shipping and handling

Serving Children with Disabilities: A Systematic Look at the Programs
by Laudan Y. Aron, Pamela J. Loprest, and C. Eugene Steuerle
University Press of America
PO Box 191
Blue Ridge Summit, PA 17214-0190
(800) 462-6420   www.univpress.com

This book discusses the major programs available to children with disabilities, including their eligibility criteria and benefits. It also discusses the data needs that are essential to improving the system. Hardcover, $58.50; softcover, $25.50; plus $4.00 shipping and handling.

Sexuality and Me - I'm a Beautiful Person
PACER Center (Parent Advocacy Coalition for Educational Rights)
8161 Normandale Boulevard
Minneapolis, MN 55437
(888) 248-0822   (952) 838-9000
In MN, (800) 537-2237   (952) 838-0190 (TTY)
FAX (952) 838-0199   e-mail: pacer@pacer.org   www.pacer.org

In this videotape, teenagers and young adults discuss issues regarding sexuality and disability. Purchase, $35.00; rental, $10.00.

Sibshops: Workshops for Siblings of Children with Special Needs
by Donald J. Meyer and Patricia F. Vadasy
Paul Brookes Publishing Company
PO Box 10624
Baltimore, MD 21285-9945
(800) 638-3775   FAX (410) 337-8539
e-mail: custserv@pbrookes.com   www.pbrookes.com

This book provides guidance to help the sisters and brothers of children with special needs express their own social and emotional needs. Written for children ages 8 to 13, the book enables professionals and parents to run their own sibshops by suggesting a variety of exercises and group discussion techniques. $32.00 plus $5.00 shipping and handling

Since Owen
by Charles R. Callanan
Johns Hopkins University Press
PO Box 50370
Baltimore, MD 21211-4370
(800) 537-5487   FAX (410) 516-6998   www.press.jhu.edu/press

Written by the father of a child with a disability, this book describes the experience of obtaining an appropriate education and finding resources. $23.95

The Special EDge
Sonoma State University, CalSTAT/CIHS
1801 East Cotati Avenue
Rohnert Park, Ca 94928
(707) 206-0533 ext. 103   FAX (707) 206-9176
e-mail: joyce.rau@cal.state.org   www.cde.ca.gov/spbranch/sed/resource.htm#pubs

This quarterly newsletter provides information on special education issues, such as legislation, family/consumer perspectives, technology, research, and information and resources. Available in standard print, alternate formats, and on the web site.

Steps to Independence: A Skills Training Guide for Parents and Teachers of Children with Special Needs
by Bruce L. Baker and Alan J. Brightman
Paul Brookes Publishing Company
PO Box 10624
Baltimore, MD 21285-0624
(800) 638-3775   FAX (410) 337-8539
e-mail: custserv@pbrookes.com   www.pbrookes.com

A resource guide for teaching independent living. Includes sample activities, self-help sources, and case examples. $28.00 plus $5.00 shipping and handling

Toy Guide for Differently Abled Kids
National Parent Network on Disabilities
1130 17th Street, NW, Suite 400
Washington, DC 20036
(888) 869-7932   www.toysrus.com

A catalogue of toys that are useful for young children with speech, hearing, visual, or mobility impairments. Free

Turtle Books
Jason & Nordic Publishers
PO Box 441
Hollidaysburg, PA 16648
(814) 696-2920   FAX (814) 696-4250
e-mail: turtlebooks@jasonandnordic.com
www.jasonandnordic.com

These books are written for children with disabilities, siblings, and friends who are in pre-school or primary grades. Subjects include disabilities such as communication disorders, deafness, and blindness as well as interacting with children who are not disabled. All books are printed in 18 point large type. Prices vary for hardcover and softcover titles.

Uncommon Fathers: Reflections on Raising a Child with a Disability
by Donald J. Meyer, (ed.)
Woodbine House
6510 Bells Mill Road
Bethesda, MD 20817
(800) 843-7323   FAX (301) 897-5838
e-mail: info@woodbinehouse.com   www.woodbinehouse.com

Written by fathers of children with developmental disabilities, the essays in this book describe the fathers' perspectives of the impact children with disabilities have on their families. $14.95 plus $4.50 shipping and handling

Views From Our Shoes: Growing Up with a Brother or Sister with Special Needs
by Donald J. Meyer (ed.)
Woodbine House
6510 Bells Mill Road
Bethesda, MD 20817
(800) 843-7323   FAX (301) 897-5838
e-mail: info@woodbinehouse.com   www.woodbinehouse.com

This collection of essays was written by the brothers and sisters of individuals with disabilities. Includes glossary of disability terms. $14.95 plus $4.50 shipping and handling

When Parents Can't Fix It: Living with a Child's Disability
by Sharon Thompson and Virginia Cruz
Fanlight Productions
4196 Washington Street, Suite 2
Boston, MA 02131
(800) 937-4113   (617) 469-4999   FAX (617) 469-3379
e-mail: fanlight@fanlight.com   www.fanlight.com

In this videotape, five families describe their experiences raising children with disabilities. Includes discussions of financial and medical issues, effects on the family, and coping strategies. 58 minutes. Purchase, $245.00; rental for one day, $50.00; rental for one week, $100.00; plus $9.00 shipping and handling.

Creating Options: A Resource on Financial Aid for Students with Disabilities
HEATH Resource Center
2121 K Street, NW, #220
Washington, DC 20037
(800) 544-3284 (V/TTY)   (202) 973-0904   FAX (202) 973-0908
e-mail: help@heath.gwu.edu   www.heath.gwu.edu

This guide provides information on federal financial aid programs and state vocational rehabilitation agencies. It also lists private organizations that offer grants and scholarships. Revised annually. Available in standard print, alternate formats, and on the web site. Single copy, free.

Financial Aid for the Disabled and Their Families
by Gail Ann Schlachter and R. David Weber
Reference Service Press
5000 Windplay Drive, Suite 4
El Dorado Hills, CA 95762
(916) 939-9620   FAX (916) 939-9626   www.rspfunding.com

A directory of scholarships, fellowships, loans, and awards for individuals with disabilities. $40.00 plus $5.00 shipping and handling

The Student Guide
Federal Student Aid Information Center
PO Box 84
Washington, DC 20044
(800) 433-3243   www.ed.gov

Updated annually, this booklet describes financial aid available to students with disabilities; includes federal grants, loan, work-study programs, and scholarships; and discusses the rights of students with disabilities. Available in English and Spanish. Also available on audiocassette and on the web site.

Chapter 4

MAKING EVERYDAY LIVING EASIER

Individuals with disabilities and chronic conditions use a wide variety of assistive devices which enable them to continue with their everyday activities. Over 13 million Americans use assistive devices, and over 7 million live in specially adapted homes to accommodate their physical impairments (LaPlante et al.: 1992).

Many ingenious devices have been developed to make independent living safe and comfortable. Often individuals create assistive devices to meet their own needs. In addition to "low tech" devices that make everyday living easier, a wide variety of "high tech" devices is available. While many of these aids enable individuals with disabilities to remain employed, others are useful for transportation and carrying out everyday living in the home and away.

This chapter is divided into two sections: "Environmental Adaptations and Assistive Devices" and "Travel and Recreation."

ENVIRONMENTAL ADAPTATIONS AND ASSISTIVE DEVICES

Environmental adaptations for the home range from a ramp or simple tactile markings on appliances to major renovations, which include the installation of elevators and renovation of kitchens. Lowered kitchen counters and appliances facilitate cooking for individuals who use wheelchairs. Other adaptive design features include accessible routes, light switches, electrical outlets, and thermostats; bathrooms with walls sturdy enough to install grab bars; and kitchens, bathrooms, and entryways with sufficient space to maneuver wheelchairs.

Many architects now specialize in designing buildings and dwelling units that meet the needs of people with disabilities. The state office on disability, the architectural access board, or the local or state professional society of architects should be able to provide a list of qualified architects.

Assistive devices for dressing, such as elastic shoelaces, velcro closures, and buttoning aids, are especially useful for individuals with mobility impairments. Foam hair rollers, water pipe foam insulation, or layers of tape are used to build up the handles of items as varied as toothbrushes, pens, pencils, eating utensils, paint brushes, and crochet hooks.

Remote controls turn on and off lights and televisions and open and close garage doors. Telephones with voice dialers permit the storage of frequently called telephone numbers and automatic dialing. Speaker phones allow individuals with poor motor control or tremors to carry on a telephone conversation comfortably.

Suppliers of personal and home health care aids, recreational products, and mobility aids for more than one type of condition or disability are listed. For suppliers of assistive devices for a specific disability or condition, refer to the chapter that deals with that disability or condition (e.g., vision loss, communication disorders, etc.). Many hospital pharmacies as well as large department and discount stores now sell home health products, such as wheelchairs, bathroom safety devices, canes, and walkers. Some of this equipment may also be available on a rental or loan basis from community health agencies.

References

LaPlante, Mitchell P., Gerry E. Hendershot, and Abigail J. Moss
1992   "Assistive Technology Devices and Home Accessibility Features: Prevalence, Payment, Need, and Trends" <u>Advance Data from Vital and Health Statistics</u> No. 217, Hyattsville, MD: National Center for Health Statistics

ABLEDATA
8630 Fenton Street, Suite 930
Silver Spring, MD 20910
(800) 227-0216   www.abledata.com

This federally funded center responds to telephone, mail, and e-mail inquiries about disabilities, assistive products, and support services. Most publications may be downloaded from the web site.

Architectural and Transportation Barriers Compliance Board (ATBCB)
1331 F Street, NW, Suite 1000
Washington, DC 20004
(800) 872-2253   (800) 993-2822 (TTY)   (202) 272-5434
(202) 272-5449 (TTY)   FAX (202) 272-5447
e-mail: info@access-board.gov   www.access-board.gov

A federal agency charged with developing standards for accessibility. Provides technical assistance, sponsors research, and distributes publications. Publishes a free bimonthly newsletter, "Access Currents." Publications available in standard print, alternate formats, and on the web site.

Center for Universal Design
North Carolina State University
219 Oberlin Road
Raleigh, NC 27695
(800) 647-6777   (919) 515-3082 (V/TTY)   FAX (919) 515-3023
e-mail: cud@ncsu.edu   www.design.ncsu.edu/cud

A federally funded research and training center that works toward improving housing and product design for people with disabilities. Provides technical assistance, training, and publications. Some publications are available on the web site.

GE Answer Center
Louisville, KY 40225
(800) 626-2000   (800) 833-4322 (TTY)
geappliances.com

This consumer information center provides assistance to individuals with disabilities as well as to the general public. Appliance controls marked with braille or raised dots are available for individuals who are blind or visually impaired, free. Two brochures, "Real Life Design" (available in standard print and alternate formats) and "Basic Kitchen Planning for the Physically Handicapped," are free. The center is open 24 hours a day, seven days a week.

National Association of Home Builders (NAHB)
National Research Center, Economics and Policy Analysis Division
400 Prince George's Boulevard
Upper Marlboro, MD 20772
(301) 249-4000   FAX (301) 430-6180   www.nahbrc.org

The research section of the home building industry trade organization produces publications and provides training on housing and special needs.

National Council of State Housing Agencies (NCSHA)
444 North Capitol Street, NW, Suite 438
Washington, DC 20001
(202) 624-7710   FAX (202) 624-5899   www.ncsha.org

Membership organization of state housing agencies. Web site offers a "State Housing Finance Agency Directory" that lists assistance available for home modifications and home ownership programs.

Rural Housing Service National Office
U.S. Department of Agriculture
Room 5037, South Building
14th Street and Independence Avenue, SW
Washington, DC 20250
(202) 720-4323   www.rurdev.usda.gov/rhs

Provides home ownership, renovation, and repair programs for individuals with disabilities who live in rural areas.

U.S. Department of Housing and Urban Development (HUD)
451 7th Street, SW, Room 5240
Washington, DC 20410
(202) 708-1112   (202) 708-1455 (TTY)   www.hud.gov
HUD User Clearinghouse: (800) 245-2691
www.huduser.org (HUD Section 504 One-Stop Web Site)

Operates programs to make housing accessible, including loans for developers of independent living and group homes and loan and mortgage insurance for rehabilitation of single or multifamily units. This agency enforces the Fair Housing Act and will inform callers how to file a complaint with one of the ten regional offices located throughout the country. The HUD User Section 504 web site provides guidance to individuals with disabilities about their rights under Section 504 and information for organizations that receive HUD funds regarding their obligations under Section 504.

Accessible Home Design: Architectural Solutions for the Wheelchair User
PVA Distribution Center
PO Box 753
Waldorf, MD 20604-0753
(888) 860-7244   (301) 932-7834   FAX (301) 843-0159
www.pva.org

This book suggest economical and practical suggestions for making new and renovated homes accessible. $22.95 plus $3.00 shipping and handling

A Consumer's Guide to Home Adaptation
Adaptive Environments Center
374 Congress Street, Suite 301
Boston, MA 02210
(617) 695-1225 (V/TTY)   FAX (617) 482-8099
e-mail: adaptive@adaptenvironments.org
www.adaptenvironments.org

This workbook enables people with disabilities to plan the modifications necessary to adapt their homes. Describes how to widen doorways, lower countertops, etc. $12.00

Designs for Independent Living
The Less Challenging Home
Appliance Information Service (AIS)
Whirlpool Corporation Administrative Center
Benton Harbor, MI 49022
(800) 253-1301   (800) 334-6889 (TTY)   www.whirlpool.com

The first brochure provides information on adaptations for the home environment and major appliances. Free. The second booklet provides suggestions for incorporating accessible design when building or remodeling kitchens and bathrooms. Describes building materials and appliances and includes charts indicating appliance features that are helpful to users with disabilities. Free

Directory of Accessible Building Products
National Association of Home Builders (NAHB)
National Research Center, Economics and Policy Analysis Division
400 Prince George's Boulevard
Upper Marlboro, MD 20772
(301) 249-4000   FAX (301) 430-6180   www.nahbrc.org

This directory describes and illustrates products available for use by individuals with disabilities. $5.00 plus $5.00 shipping and handling

The Do-Able Renewable Home
by John P. S. Salmen
American Association of Retired Persons (AARP)
601 E Street, NW
Washington, DC 20049
(800) 441-2277   (202) 434-2277   www.aarp.org

This booklet describes how individuals with disabilities can modify their homes for independent living. Room-by-room modifications are accompanied by illustrations. Free

Easy Things to Make--To Make Things Easy: Simple Do-It-Yourself Home Modifications for Older People and Others with Physical Disabilities
by Doreen Greenstein
Brookline Books
PO Box 1047
Cambridge, MA 02238-1047
(800) 666-2665   (617) 868-0360   FAX (617) 868-1772
e-mail: milt@brooklinebooks.com   www.brooklinebooks.com

This book describes low-cost home modifications and suggests adaptations for everyday activities. Large print. $15.95

Fair Housing Act Design Manual: A Manual To Assist Designers and Builders in Meeting the Accessibility Requirements of the Fair Housing Act
U.S. Department of Housing and Urban Development
451 7th Street, SW
Washington, DC 20410
HUD USER (800) 245-2691   (202) 708-1112   (202) 708-1455 (TTY)
www.huduser.com

The book provides technical assistance for designers, builders, and developers on meeting accessibility requirements for residences under the Fair Housing Act. Includes resource lists of products and references, plus the text of the Fair Housing Accessibility Guidelines. $5.00

How to Build Ramps for Home Accessibility, Manual
Tips for Building Modular Ramps and Steps, Videotape
Metropolitan Center for Independent Living
1600 University Avenue West, Suite 16
St. Paul, MN 55104-3825
(651) 603-2029   e-mail: jimwi@mcil-mn.org
www.wheelchairramp.org

The manual and videotape provide step-by-step instruction in building modular ramps and steps. Manual, $15.00. May also be downloaded from web site. Videotape, $20.00.

Retrofitting Homes for a Lifetime
National Association of Home Builders (NAHB)
National Research Center, Economics and Policy Analysis Division
400 Prince George's Boulevard
Upper Marlboro, MD 20772
(301) 249-4000   FAX (301) 430-6180   www.nahbrc.org

This publication enables remodelers and homeowners to assess needed modifications; provides an accessibility checklist; suggests financing alternatives; and makes recommendations for working with builders. $15.00 plus $5.00 shipping and handling

SpeciaLiving Magazine
PO Box 1000
Bloomington, IL 61072-1000
(888) 372-3737   (309) 825-8842
e-mail: info@SpeciaLiving.com   www.SpeciaLiving.com

This quarterly magazine features information on accessible housing, recreation, and aids for everyday living. $12.00

Both travel and recreation provide relief from tension, relaxation, and social interactions. Individuals who participate in recreational activities have an increased sense of self-worth and well-being. For individuals who are seriously ill, recreation diverts attention from the illness and provides opportunities for socialization. Some individuals with disabilities need assistance in order to continue with their favorite recreational pastimes. Others may develop an interest in new activities more appropriate to their current condition.

In the aftermath of World War II, rehabilitation programs were developed to treat the men returning home with physical and mental disabilities. Competitive sports were included in the program of the first spinal cord injury center opened in England in 1944 (DePauw and Gavron: 1995). During the 1950s, wheelchair sports expanded from Europe to the United States, and individuals with other disabilities became involved in national and international sports organizations. For men and women who have engaged in sports throughout their lives, the advent of disability seems to signal an end to valued activities. Those who receive care in rehabilitation facilities are more apt to discover the adaptations available in equipment and techniques that make sports opportunities accessible. Sports enthusiasts may choose activities such as skiing, basketball, swimming, running, golf, scuba diving, baseball, horseback riding, archery, and sailing, to name just a few examples.

The Americans with Disabilities Act (ADA) of 1990 mandates accessibility to recreation facilities and athletic programs, from aerobic training classes and local parks to football stadiums and other venues. Advances in technology have led to the development of racing wheelchairs, special hand and foot prostheses, and adapted ski equipment such as sit-skis. All-terrain vehicles (ATVs), adapted with lifts, hand controls, or safety harnesses, enable individuals with mobility impairments to participate in many outdoor recreation activities. Organizations that specialize in adaptive recreation programs are listed below (see "ADAPTIVE SPORTS AND RECREATION ORGANIZATIONS").

The Americans with Disabilities Act requires that fixed route buses and rail transportation be accessible and usable by individuals with disabilities. However, deadlines for implementation of the ADA's regulations vary from six to seven years for private intercity transit to as long as 20 years for Amtrak and commuter rail stations. Many communities offer special transportation services for individuals with disabilities and for elders for a nominal fee. These services enable individuals to shop on their own, participate in recreational activities, visit friends and relatives, and go to the offices of health care providers.

The Federal Aviation Administration requires each airline to submit a company-wide policy for travelers with disabilities. Passengers may call ahead to request early boarding, special seating, or meals which meet dietary restrictions. Airport facilities are designed to offer accessible restrooms, elevators, electric carts or wheelchairs, and first aid stations. The Air Carrier Access Act of 1986 (ACAA) includes regulations that cover the needs of travelers with disabilities, such as access to commuter planes, accessible lavatories, wheelchair storage, and sensitivity training for all airline personnel. Contact the airlines to obtain a written statement of the special services they provide. Individuals who believe that their rights have been denied may file a complaint within 45 days of the incident with the Aviation Consumer

Protection Division, U.S. Department of Transportation, C-75 Room 4107, Washington, DC 20590, (202) 366-2220; e-mail: airconsumer@ost.dot.gov; www.dot.gov/airconsumer

Amtrak offers a 15% discount on most one-way, round trip, and All Aboard America rail fares for individuals with disabilities. Passengers must present proof of disability, such as a certificate of legal blindness or a letter from a physician specifying the nature of the disability. Greyhound allows passengers with disabilities requiring assistance with personal hygiene, eating, medications, or while the bus is in motion to request a free ticket for a companion (certain restrictions apply). There is no charge for service animals for individuals who are visually impaired, blind, deaf, or who have other disabilities.

Travel agencies that plan special trips for people with disabilities are available throughout North America. Many major hotel chains, airlines, and car rental companies provide special assistance to people with disabilities and often have special toll-free numbers for users of teletypewriters (TTYs), also called telecommunication devices for the deaf or TDDs and text telephones or TTs). Some companies offer specially trained travel companions to people with disabilities who need an escort.

Individuals with disabilities and elders are eligible for special entrance passes to federal recreation facilities. The *Golden Access Passport* is a free lifetime pass available to any U.S. citizen or permanent resident, regardless of age, who is blind or permanently disabled. It admits the permit holder and passengers in a single, private, noncommercial vehicle to any parks, monuments, historic sites, recreation areas, and wildlife refuges which usually charge entrance fees. If the permit holder does not enter by car, the Passport admits the permit holder, spouse, and children. The permit holder is also entitled to a 50% discount on charges such as camping, boat launching, and parking fees. Fees charged by private concessionaires are not discounted. Golden Access Passports are available only in person, with proof of disability, such as a certificate of legal blindness. Since the Passport is available at most federal recreation areas, it is not necessary to obtain one ahead of time. A *Golden Age Passport* offers the same benefits to persons age 62 or older, with proof of age.

The Disabled Sportsmen's Access of 1998 (P.L. 105-261) will lead to the accessibility to outdoor recreation programs on military installations for individuals with disability. The outdoor recreation programs include sports such as fishing, trapping, hunting, wildlife observation, boating, and camping.

Rehabilitation hospitals and centers offer driver evaluation services, such as clinical testing and observation to determine an individual's need for adaptive equipment or training. Many U.S. Department of Veterans Affairs Medical Centers (VAMC) offer driver evaluation services, driver training, and information services to veterans with disabilities through the Rehabilitation Medicine Service at their facilities. Major automobile manufacturers offer reimbursement for adaptive equipment installed on new vehicles. Programs for special adaptive equipment offered by automobile manufacturers are listed in the "ORGANIZATIONS" section below.

References

DePauw, Karen P. and Susan J. Gavron
1995 Disability and Sport Champaign, IL: Human Kinetics

Access-Able Travel Service
PO Box 1796
Wheat Ridge, CO 80034
(303) 232-2979   FAX (303) 239-8486
e-mail: bill@access-able.com   www.access-able.com

Provides information on accommodations, access guides, entertainment, tours, and transportation. Free monthly newsletter available by e-mail.

ADED - Association for Driver Rehabilitation Specialists
711 South Vienna Street
Ruston, LA 71270
(800) 290-2344   (318) 257-5055   FAX (318) 255-4175
www.driver-ed.org

Certifies members to conduct driver evaluation and training for individuals with disabilities.

Air Travel Consumer Report
www.dot.gov/airconsumer/disabled.htm

This web site includes information about the rights of passengers with disabilities. The rights of individuals with disabilities regarding new security regulations put in place in late 2001 are described in a fact sheet at www.dot/gov/airconsumer/01-index.htm.

Amtrak
(877) 268-7252   (800) 523-6590 (TTY)   www.amtrak.com

Provides 15% discount on most fares for individuals with disabilities. On-board services and special meals available upon request with advance notice. Request "Access Amtrak: A Guide to Amtrak Services for Travelers with Disabilities." Available in standard print and alternate formats. Free

Architectural and Transportation Barriers Compliance Board (ATBCB)
1331 F Street, NW, Suite 1000
Washington, DC 20004
(800) 872-2253   (800) 993-2822 (TTY)   (202) 272-5434
(202) 272-5449 (TTY)   FAX (202) 272-5447
e-mail: info@access-board.gov   www.access-board.gov

A federal agency charged with developing standards for accessibility. Provides technical assistance, sponsors research, and distributes publications. Publishes a free bimonthly newsletter, "Access Currents." Publications on transportation issues such as over-the-road buses, securement of wheelchair and other mobility aids, and passenger vessels available in standard print, alternate formats, and on the web site.

Auto Channel
(877) 275-4226   www.ican.com

Provides a step-by-step evaluation to enable consumers with disabilities to choose the vehicle that meets their needs.

Automobility Program
DaimlerChrysler Corporation
PO Box 5080
Troy, MI 48007-5080
(800) 255-9877   (800) 922-3826 (TTY)   FAX (810) 597-3501
www.automobility.daimlerchrysler.com

Provides $750 to $1000 reimbursement (on eligible models) on the purchase of alerting devices for people who are deaf or hearing impaired and assistive equipment for vehicles purchased to transport individuals who use wheelchairs.

Ford Mobility Motoring Program
(800) 952-2248   (800) 833-0312 (TTY)   FAX (800) 292-7842
www.ford.com/en/ourServices/specialBuyingPrograms/mobilityMotoringProgram/default.htm

This program funds assistive equipment conversion up to $1000. Provides toll-free information line, free video that describes the program, list of assessment centers that determine equipment needs, and referrals to sources for additional assistance.

General Motors Mobility Assistance Center
100 Renaissance Center, PO Box 100
Detroit, MI 48265-100
(800) 323-9935   (800) 833-9935 (TTY)
www.gm.com/automotive/vehicle_shopping/gm_mobility

This program reimburses customers up to $1000 for vehicle modifications or adaptive driving devices for new or demo vehicles. Includes alerting devices for drivers who are deaf or hearing impaired, such as emergency vehicle siren detectors and enhanced turn signal reminders.

Greyhound Lines, Inc.
PO Box 660362
Dallas, TX 75266-0362
(800) 231-2222 (General Information)
(800) 752-4841 (ADA Assist Line)
(800) 345-3109 (TTY) www.Greyhound.com

Provides assistance to travelers with disabilities upon request. Call ADA Assist line at least 48 hours in advance of travel. Information also available on web site; click on "Travel Planning for Passengers with Disabilities."

Mobility International USA (MIUSA)
PO Box 10767
Eugene, OR 97440
(541) 343-1284 (V/TTY) FAX (541) 343-6812
e-mail: info@miusa.org www.miusa.org

Promotes the participation of individuals with disabilities in international and educational exchange programs, such as workcamps, conferences, and internships. Membership, $35.00, includes semi-annual newsletter, "Over the Rainbow."

MossRehab ResourceNet
www.mossresourcenet.org

This web site offers information on accessible travel for individuals with disabilities. Click on "Accessible Travel."

National Mobility Equipment Dealers Association
11211 North Nebraska Avenue, Suite A-5
Tampa, FL 33612
(800) 833-0427 (813) 977-6603 FAX (813) 977-6402
e-mail: nmeda@aol.com www.nmeda.org

The members of this organization are car dealers, manufacturers, driver evaluators, and insurance companies. Provides local referrals to members who are adaptive equipment dealers and rates members' competencies in equipment installation and conversion.

National Park Service
U.S. Department of the Interior, Office of Public Affairs
1849 C Street, NW, Room 3045
Washington, DC 20240
(202) 208-6843 www.nps.gov

Operates the Golden Access Passport program for people who have disabilities. Free brochure.

Project ACTION Accessible Traveler's Database
www.projectaction.org/paweb/index.htm

This database offers information on accessible transportation services, including accessible car and van rental companies, rural and urban transit operators, major hotel chains, and national toll-free numbers.

Society for Accessible Travel and Hospitality (SATH)
347 Fifth Avenue, Suite 610
New York, NY 10016
(212) 447-7284   FAX (212) 725-8253
e-mail: sathtravel@aol.com   www.sath.org

Advocates for accessibility for individuals with disabilities and serves as a clearinghouse for information on barrier-free travel. Membership, individuals, $45.00; seniors and students, $30.00; includes quarterly newsletter, "Open World for Accessible Travel." Free sample of newsletter is available on request.

Wheelers Accessible Van Rental
(800) 456-1371   www.wheelerz.com

Rents mini-vans accessible to wheelchair users throughout the country.

Access Outdoors
www.accessoutdoors.org

This web site provides information about organizations that offer accessible outdoor recreation experiences, adaptive recreation products, and organizations that provide assistance in creating accessible programs. A service of Wilderness Inquiry.

Achilles Track Club
42 West 38th Street, 4th Floor
New York, NY 10018
(212) 354-0300   FAX (212) 354-3978
e-mail: AchillesClub@aol.com   www.achillestrackclub.org

Promotes running as a recreational activity and competitive sport for individuals with disabilities. Chapters in many states and foreign countries. Membership is free. Publishes newsletter, "The Achilles Heel."

American Canoe Association
7432 Alban Station Boulevard, Suite B-232
Springfield, VA 22150
(703) 451-0141   FAX (703) 451-2245
e-mail: aca@acanet.org   www.acanet.org

Certifies instructors in adaptive paddling course for canoeing, kayaking, and coastal kayaking. Will refer individuals with disabilities to certified instructors in local area. Provides information on equipment adaptations.

Breckenridge Outdoor Education Center
PO Box 697
Breckenridge, CO 80424
(970) 453-6422   FAX (970) 453-4676
e-mail: boec@boec.org   www.boec.org

Offers year-round adaptive outdoor learning experiences for children and adults with disabilities and provides training for therapists and educators.

Challenged Athletes Foundation (CAF)
2148 Jimmy Durante Boulevard, #B
Del Mar, CA 92014
(858) 793-9293
e-mail: execdire@challengedathletes.org
www.challengedathletes.org

The foundation provides grants to individual athletes with disabilities for training, equipment, or travel to competitions.

Disabled Sports, U.S.A.
451 Hungerford Drive, Suite 100
Rockville, MD 20850
(301) 217-0960   (301) 217-0963 (TTY)   FAX (301) 217-0968
e-mail: information@dsusa.org   www.dsusa.org

Nationwide network of chapters sponsors recreational activities, such as skiing, camping, hiking, biking, horseback riding, and mountain climbing. Offers adaptive fitness instructor training to therapists, exercise instructors, and program directors. Membership, $25.00; $40.00, includes subscription to "Challenge Magazine."

Disabled Sports U.S.A. Volleyball
921 North Village Lake Road
DeLand, FL 32724
e-mail: chris@dsusav.org   www.dsusav.org

Promotes the participation of athletes who are amputees or have limb disabilities in volleyball.

Fishing Has No Boundaries
PO Box 175
Hayward, WI 54843
(800) 243-3462   (715) 634-1305
e-mail: info@fhnbinc.org   www.fhnbinc.org

Provides opportunities for individuals with disabilities to fish and teaches them about adaptive devices for fishing. Events sponsored by community organizations.

Handicapped Scuba Association
1104 El Prado
San Clemente, CA 92672
(949) 498-4540   FAX (949) 498-6128
e-mail: hsa@hsascuba.com   www.hsascuba.com

This organization trains and certifies scuba diving instructors to work with individuals with disabilities; teaches able-bodied divers to accompany divers with disabilities; and certifies divers with disabilities in "open water" diving. All contributors become members.

National Ability Center
PO Box 682799
Park City, UT 84068-2779
(435) 649-3991 (V/TTY)   FAX (435) 658-3992
e-mail: nac@xmission.com   www.nationalabilitycenter.org

Offers year-round sports and recreation experiences for children and adults with disabilities.

National Easter Seal Society
230 West Monroe Street, Suite 1800
Chicago, IL 60606
(800) 221-6827   (312) 726-6200   (312) 726-4258 (TTY)
FAX (312) 726-1494   info@easter-seals.org
www.easter-seals.org

Offers 140 camping and recreation facilities for children and adults with disabilities across the U.S. Day, residential, and respite programs are available.

National Sports Center for the Disabled
PO Box 1290
Winter Park, CO 80482
(970) 726-1540   FAX (970) 726-4112
e-mail: info@nscd.org   www.nscd.org

Offers year round recreation programs for children and adults with disabilities and offers training programs for recreation professionals.

National Wheelchair Basketball Association
120 West Madison, Suite 1200
Chicago, IL 60610
(312) 553-0527   FAX (312) 553-0528
e-mail: nwbaed@aol.com www.nwba.org

This organization of more than 175 teams across the U.S. and Canada provides opportunities for organized competition in men's, women's, and youth divisions.

North American Riding for the Handicapped Association (NARHA)
PO Box 33150
Denver, CO 80233
(800) 369-7433   FAX (303) 252-4610
e-mail: narha@narha.com www.narha.org

This professional association promotes therapeutic horseback riding for individuals with disabilities and accredits riding programs. Membership, $40.00, includes membership directory and subscription to two newsletters, "NARHA Strides," published quarterly, and "NARHA News," published eight times a year.

Sailors with Special Needs
United States Sailing Association
15 Maritime Drive, PO Box 1260
Portsmouth, RI 02871
(401) 683-0800   www.ussailing.org/swsn

Promotes competitive and recreational sailing for individuals with disabilities.

United States Golf Association (USGA)
PO Box 708
Far Hills, NJ 07931-0708
(908) 234-2300   www.usga.org

The association's web site lists golf programs for individuals with disabilities. Also provides "A Modification of The Rules of Golf for Golfers with Disabilities," including those who are blind or visually impaired, use canes, crutches, or wheelchairs, have amputations, or have mental retardation.

Universal Wheelchair Football Association
c/o John B. Kraimer
9555 Plainfield Road
Blue Ash, OH 45236
(513) 792-8625   (513) 745-8300 (TTY)   FAX (513) 792-8624
e-mail: john.kraimer@uc.edu   homepages.msn.com/boxseatblvd/madwheelin/uwfa.htm

Promotes the playing of football by individuals with disabilities. Provides rules upon request.

VSA Arts
1300 Connecticut Avenue, NW, Suite 700
Washington, DC 20036
(800) 933-8721   (202) 737-0645 (TTY)   FAX (202) 737-0725
www.vsarts.org

Provides opportunities for individuals with disabilities to participate in fine and performing arts.

Wilderness Inquiry
808 14th Avenue SE
Minneapolis, MN 55414
(800) 728-0719 (V/TTY)   In Minneapolis and St. Paul, (612) 676-9400 (V/TTY)
FAX (612) 676-9401   e-mail: info@wildernessinquiry.org
www.wildernessinquiry.org

Sponsors trips into wilderness areas for individuals with disabilities or chronic conditions. Request schedule of current trips. Available in standard print, alternate formats, and on the web site.

Accessible Gardening for People with Physical Disabilities: A Guide to Methods, Tools, and Plants
by Janeen R. Adil
Woodbine House
6510 Bells Mill Road
Bethesda, MD 20817
(800) 843-7323   FAX (301) 897-5838
e-mail: info@woodbinehouse.com   www.woodbinehouse.com

Written for people with a variety of mobility impairments, this book provides information on making existing gardens more accessible and creating new gardens. Sources for obtaining supplies are included. $16.95 plus $4.50 shipping and handling

Access Travel: Airports
Federal Consumer Information Center
PO Box 100
Pueblo, CO 81002
(888) 878-3256   e-mail: catalog.pueblo@gsa.gov www.pueblo.gsa.gov

This brochure lists facilities and services for people with disabilities in airport terminals worldwide. Free. Also available on the web site.

Challenge
Fanlight Productions
4196 Washington Street, Suite 2
Boston, MA 02131
(800) 937-4113   (617) 469-4999   FAX (617) 469-3379
e-mail: fanlight@fanlight.com www.fanlight.com

This videotape features individuals with disabilities participating in sports such as wheelchair tennis, golf, skiing, and rock climbing. 28 minutes. Purchase, $195.00; rental for one day, $50.00; rental for one week, $100.00; plus $9.00 shipping and handling.

Conditioning with Physical Disabilities
Human Kinetics
1607 North Market Street
PO Box 5076
Champaign, IL 61825-5076
(800) 747-4457   (217) 351-5076   FAX (217) 351-2674
www.humankinetics.com

This illustrated guide describes easy and safe exercises for individuals with physical disabilities. Step-by-step instructions are provided. $23.95

Disability and Sport
by Karen P. DePauw and Susan J. Gavron
Human Kinetics
1607 North Market Street
PO Box 5076
Champaign, IL 61825-5076
(800) 747-4457   (217) 351-5076   FAX (217) 351-2674
www.humankinetics.com

This book reviews the development of the sports movement for individuals with disabilities. Describes sports modifications, lists disability sports organizations, discusses coaching athletes with disabilities, and provides information about publications. Includes biographies of athletes with disabilities. $40.00 plus $5.50 shipping and handling

The Disabled Driver's Mobility Guide
c/o Kay Hamada, Traffic Safety and Engineering
American Automobile Association (AAA)
1000 AAA Drive
Heathrow, FL 32746
(407) 444-7961   FAX (407) 444-7956

This book provides information about adaptive equipment, driver training, and travel information services. $8.95 plus $3.00 shipping and handling

Games for People with Sensory Impairments: Strategies for Including Individuals of All Ages
by Lauren J. Lieberman and Jim F. Cowart
Human Kinetics
1607 North Market Street
PO Box 5076
Champaign, IL 61825-5076
(800) 747-4457   (217) 351-5076   FAX (217) 351-2674
www.humankinetics.com

This book describes program adaptations and instructional strategies for 70 games for individuals with vision or hearing impairment. $19.00 plus $5.50 shipping and handling

Guide to Accredited Camps
American Camping Association (ACA)
5000 State Road 67 North
Martinsville, IN 46151
(800) 428-2267   (317) 342-8456   FAX (317) 342-2065
e-mail: customerservice@aca-camps.org
www.aca-camps.org

This guide of ACA-accredited camps includes special programs for campers with disabilities.
$10.95 plus $4.00 shipping and handling

Guide to Summer Camps and Summer Schools
Porter Sargent Publishers, Inc.
c/o IDS
300 Bedford Street, Building B, Suite 213
Manchester, NH 03101
(800) 342-7470   e-mail: orders@portersargent.com
www.portersargent.com

This guide to summer educational and recreation programs includes special programs for individuals with disabilities. Hardcover, $45.00 plus $6.50 shipping and handling; softcover, $27.00 plus $6.50 shipping and handling.

Guide to Wheelchair Sports and Recreation
PVA Distribution Center
PO Box 753
Waldorf, MD 20604-0753
(888) 860-7244   (301) 932-7834   FAX (301) 843-0159
www.pva.org

This book describes the wide range of wheelchair sports and lists manufacturers of equipment, Paralyzed Veterans of America chapters that offer such sports, and programs for children. Available in English and Spanish. Free plus $3.00 shipping and handling

New Horizons for the Air Traveler with a Disability
U.S. Department of Transportation
www.faa.gov/acr.acess.htm

This brochure provides information about the Air Carrier Access rules and other regulations that affect air travelers. Available on the web site only.

Sports 'N Spokes
2111 East Highland Avenue, Suite 180
Phoenix, AZ 85016
(888) 888-2201   FAX (602) 224-0507   www.pva.org

A bimonthly magazine that features articles about sports activities for people who use wheelchairs. Eight issues, $21.00

Wheelchair Basketball Book and Videotapes
PVA Distribution Center
PO Box 753
Waldorf, MD 20604-0753
(888) 860-7244   (301) 932-7834   FAX (301) 843-0159
www.pva.org

This instruction manual and videotape series covers individual skills and team play. Available in English and Spanish. Complete set, $75.00 plus $6.00 shipping and handling; separately: book, $21.95; video I, individual skills, $29.95; video II, team play, $29.95; plus $3.00 shipping and handling each.

A World of Options: A Guide to International Exchange, Community Service, and Travel for Persons with Disabilities
by C. Bucks (ed.)
Mobility International USA (MIUSA)
PO Box 10767
Eugene, OR 97440
(541) 343-1284 (V/TTY)   FAX (541) 343-6812
e-mail: info@miusa.org   www.miusa.org

This book lists educational exchange programs, international workcamps, and accessible travel opportunities. Personal experiences are used to describe these programs. Members, $30.00; nonmembers, $35.00.

RESOURCES FOR ASSISTIVE DEVICES

The following vendors sell assistive devices that help people remain independent. Those that specialize in a specific type of product have a notation under the listing. Otherwise, their product line is broad, usually including personal, health care, and recreation aids and devices for the home. Unless otherwise noted, the catalogues are free.

Abilitations
One Sportime Way
Atlanta, GA 30340
(800) 850-8602   FAX (800) 845-1535
www.abilitations.com

Access to Recreation
8 Sandra Court
Newbury Park, CA 91320
(800) 634-4351   (805) 498-7535   FAX (805) 498-8186
e-mail: dkrebs@gte.net   www.accesstr.com

Sells assistive devices that help people with disabilities enjoy sports and recreational activities, such as swimming aids, fishing equipment, fitness equipment and home gyms, golf clubs, wheelchair ramps, bowling aids, and adapted games.

Access with Ease
PO Box 1150
Chino Valley, AZ 86323
(800) 531-9479   (520) 636-9469   FAX (520) 636-0292
e-mail: kmjc@northlink.com   www.shop.store.yahoo.com/capability/info.html

Dynamic Living, Inc.
1265 John Fitch Boulevard, #9
South Windsor, CT 06074
(888) 940-0605   FAX (860) 291-8884
e-mail: info@dynamic-living.com www.dynamic-living.com

Enrichments
Sammons Preston
PO Box 5071
Bollingbrook, IL 60440
(800) 323-5547   FAX (800) 547-4333
e-mail: sp@sammonspreston.com   www.sammonspreston.com

Independent Living Aids, Inc. (ILA)
200 Robbins Lane
Jericho, NY 11753
(800) 537-2118   FAX (516) 752-3135
e-mail: can-do@independentliving.com
www.independentliving.com

LS & S Group
PO Box 673
Northbrook, IL 60065
(800) 468-4789   (800) 317-8533 (TTY)   FAX (847) 498-1482
e-mail: lssgrp@aol.com   www.lssgroup.com

Medic Alert
PO Box 1009
Turlock, CA 95381
(800) 432-5378   In CA, (209) 668-3333
FAX (209) 669-2495   e-mail: postmaster@medicalert.org
www.medicalert.org

Medical identification bracelet for people with chronic conditions.

Radio Shack/Tandy Corporation
500 One Tandy Center, 100 Throckmorton Street
Fort Worth, TX 76102
(800) 843-7422   (817) 415-3700   www.radioshack.com

Radio Shack products for individuals with disabilities, such as talking watches and clocks and assistive listening aids, are included in the company's regular catalogues.

Rolli-Moden Designs
12225 World Trade Drive, Suite T
San Diego, CA 92128
(800) 707-2395   (858) 676-1825   FAX (858) 676-0820
e-mail: rm@rolli-moden.com   www.rolli-moden.com

Sells dress and casual clothing and accessories designed for wheelchair users. Free catalogue.

Sears Home HealthCare Catalog
7700 Brush Hill Road
Hinsdale, IL 60521
(800) 326-1750   (800) 733-7249 (TTY)

Sells health care and rehabilitation products.

Chapter 5

COMMUNICATION DISORDERS

Because impaired communication can result in social isolation, hearing disorders and speech disorders may have severe effects on individuals. Although speech impairments are sometimes caused by disease, individuals with profound hearing impairments often have speech impairments as well. It is for this reason that both of these communication disorders have been combined into one chapter.

HEARING DISORDERS

Hearing disorders are among the most prevalent conditions resulting in disability in the United States. Although estimates of the number of people with hearing disorders vary widely as do the definitions of impairment used in the studies, there is no doubt that this population is growing. One study suggests that over 20 million Americans age three or older have some hearing loss. Some of these individuals have only a slight hearing loss, but 11.5 million have bilateral hearing loss, and 4.8 million have a loss so severe that they cannot understand normal conversation (Ries: 1994). The National Center for Health Statistics (1999) indicates that in 1996, the prevalence rate of hearing impairments was 83.4 per thousand population. Hearing disorders are most common among elders. For those under age 18, the rate was 12.6 per thousand, while for those 75 years or older, the rate was 369.8 per thousand.

Labels such as profound, severe, moderate, and mild hearing impairments have not been clearly defined. Relatively few individuals are totally deaf, unable to perceive any sound whatsoever. People who have severe or profound hearing impairments may be able to hear some sounds, although their residual hearing is usually not useful for communication. People who have moderate or mild hearing impairments or who are hard of hearing have residual hearing that is useful for communication. Usually these individuals supplement their remaining functional hearing with the use of assistive devices and visual cues.

CAUSES AND TYPES OF HEARING IMPAIRMENT AND DEAFNESS

Congenital hearing disorders may result from viral infections; from the effects of certain drugs taken by the mother during pregnancy; or from problems that occur during labor or delivery. Congenital conditions such as Down syndrome, cystic fibrosis, and cerebral palsy may also cause hearing loss (Strome: 1989). One type of Usher syndrome causes congenital deafness, progressive vision loss, and sometimes mental retardation.

Otosclerosis involves the formation of spongy bone, often resulting in the fixation of the ossicles, which are the small bones of the middle ear. This condition can impede the vibrations from passing through this area, thereby causing hearing impairment. Otosclerosis is a progressive disease that often begins in the teenage years or early twenties. Surgery to improve this condition is called stapedectomy; the stapes or stirrup of the middle ear is replaced with a synthetic device capable of vibrating.

Otitis media is an inflammation of the middle ear that is very common in children, although it can occur at any age. Medications usually prevent otitis media from causing permanent hearing loss, but in some cases the inflammation may be chronic, causing permanent damage.

Meningitis is an inflammation of the meninges, which are the membranes that cover the brain and the spinal cord. Hearing loss is sometimes a complication of meningitis, although prompt diagnosis and medication can usually prevent it.

Hereditary conditions, *trauma*, and the *exposure to loud noise* over a long period of time may also cause hearing impairment. Other possible causes of hearing loss include *stroke* and the *side effects of drugs*, including diuretics used to lower blood pressure and anti-cancer drugs.

There are three major types of hearing loss: conductive, sensorineural, and central. Hearing loss that includes both conductive and sensorineural impairments is referred to as mixed hearing loss.

Conductive hearing loss is an impairment that prevents sound waves from traveling through the outer or middle ear, on the way to the inner ear. This type of impairment reduces the sound, similar to the reduction of sound that results from using ear plugs. Increased amplification of sound enables the person with this type of hearing loss to understand speech in its normal quality (Price and Snider: 1983). Hearing aids are especially effective with this type of hearing loss.

Sensorineural hearing loss results from damage to the cochlea in the inner ear or to the surrounding hair cells that transmit electrical signals to the nerve fibers and the brain. For this reason, many people with this type of hearing impairment are told that they have "nerve deafness." This type of hearing loss is the kind most frequently found in the older population.

Tinnitus, considered a sensorineural disorder, is the ringing or buzzing sensation that occurs in the ears in the absence of any external sound. There is a variety of causes for tinnitus, including the use of certain medications. Although there is rarely a cure for tinnitus, there are ways to alleviate its effects. A tinnitus masker substitutes a more acceptable sound for the sound produced by tinnitus. Because hearing loss often accompanies tinnitus, hearing aids are sometimes effective in alleviating the effects. Tinnitus instruments combine a tinnitus masker with a high frequency emphasis hearing aid. Since each has a separate volume control, the individual can adjust the devices to partially or completely cover up the tinnitus. Other treatments that are frequently prescribed are drugs, surgery, biofeedback, and relaxation techniques.

Vestibular disorders are the result of disease or damage in the inner ear and affect both orientation and balance. They include Meniere's disease, labyrinthitis, and vertigo. They may be caused by ear infections, blows to the head, whiplash, or stroke-related loss of blood flow to the inner ear or brain. Damage to the inner ear may result in dizziness, nausea, and balance disorders. Hearing loss ranges from mild to total deafness.

Central hearing loss is the result of damage to nerves in the pathway to the brain or in the brain itself. Although sound levels are not affected, speech discrimination is impaired. Central hearing loss is often a secondary result of other medical conditions, including stroke, head injuries, or vascular problems.

The cochlear implant is an inner ear prosthesis used to restore a degree of hearing function in individuals who are profoundly deaf. Electrodes are implanted to bypass the damaged hair cells surrounding the cochlea and stimulate nerve fibers in the ear. After implantation, speech and language professionals devise a rehabilitation plan to help the individual learn to use the implant as effectively as possible. Originally limited to use in adults, the cochlear implant was approved by the Food and Drug Administration (FDA) for use in children in 1990. The general criteria for selecting individuals with profound deafness to receive the implant include the ineffectiveness of hearing aids in improving auditory recognition, no medical contraindications, and realistic expectations of the results.

The original cochlear implants, using a single channel to stimulate the hair cells, enabled recipients to hear environmental sounds, such as the ring of a telephone or doorbell, traffic noise, and household appliances but not to discriminate speech. Auditory cues such as pitch, when used in conjunction with speechreading, improved the individual's ability to understand speech. Improved speechreading was the most common result of the earlier generation of cochlear implants (U.S. Department of Health and Human Services: 1988).

Recent advances in technology have expanded the capabilities of cochlear implants. Now they use multiple channels to transmit sound, with the result that many recipients have not only improved speechreading abilities but are also able to recognize speech based solely on auditory recognition. The success of the implant varies with the type of recipient. The most successful are individuals who have developed speech prior to losing their hearing. It is not understood why some individuals are more successful than others in understanding speech following cochlear implantation.

A panel of experts appointed by the National Institutes of Health has recommended that the use of cochlear implants be expanded (NIH Consensus Development Panel on Cochlear Implants in Adults and Children: 1995). The panel recommended that adults with severe hearing impairments who receive only marginal benefits from hearing aids be considered as candidates for cochlear implants.

In 2000, the FDA approved a new device for adults with moderate to severe sensorineural hearing loss. The Vibrant Soundbridge is a surgically implanted hearing device that converts sound into vibrations that are transmitted to the middle ear. Several other implantable middle ear devices are under development.

HEARING LOSS IN CHILDREN

One of every 1,000 children is born totally deaf (National Institute on Deafness and Other Communication Disorders: 1989). Congenital hearing loss is usually diagnosed after parents or other care providers have noticed that the child fails to respond to sounds and has not developed speech as expected. Children whose hearing loss is congenital or who experience hearing loss prior to development of language (prelingual) must learn to communicate without the ability to mimic the speech they hear from family members and others. Parents and special teachers for children who are deaf or hearing impaired must help these children to communicate through the use of sign language, speechreading or lipreading, finger spelling, and oral communication. There is still much to learn about how children who are congenitally deaf or prelingually deaf acquire language and communication skills.

It is essential that children who have hearing impairments be diagnosed early and that intervention begin at once. Sophisticated techniques, such as the auditory evoked potential which measures the brain's response to sound, allow the diagnosis of hearing impairments in very small infants. According to Bess (1993), less than 3% of all newborns in the United States are screened for hearing impairment and the average age for diagnosing the impairment is 2 to 2 1/2 years. Unilateral hearing impairments or impairments that are less than profound are often not diagnosed immediately (Radcliffe: 1993). Physicians must respond to parents' requests for diagnostic tests and not assume that parents are misguided when they say that their children do not respond to sound. Parents are usually the individuals who have the most knowledge about their child's behavior.

At one time, children who were deaf were forbidden to use sign language or other manual communication, in an effort to integrate them totally into the hearing world; this philosophy is referred to as oral communication or oralism. Today, many advocate "total communication," a philosophy espousing the use of all types of communication methods that enable individuals who are deaf or hearing impaired to communicate with each other as well as with people who have normal hearing.

Most children who are deaf are born to parents with normal hearing. Parents in this situation help their children and themselves by learning alternative means of communication, such as sign language. Sign language has a different structure than oral English. It is a language based on concepts, with the same gesture having several different meanings depending upon its position in relation to the body. Finger spelling, often used in conjunction with sign language, is a system in which each letter of the alphabet is spelled out (Mitchell: 1980). Sign supported speech denotes a communication method using both spoken English and simultaneous signs. Sign supported speech differs from other types of sign languages because it has been specially developed to support the structure and grammar of spoken English. Cued speech is a method that uses hand motions to supplement speechreading. Eight handshapes represent groups of consonant sounds, and four positions about the face represent vowel sounds (Schwartz: 1987). Speechreading, sometimes called lipreading, is a supportive visual process that assists in understanding language. Because many consonants appear as similar mouth shapes, it is impossible to decipher most of spoken English through speechreading alone.

An analysis (Allen: 1993) of the Annual Survey of Hearing Impaired Children and Youth in the United States for the school year 1990-1991 revealed that the majority of students with the least severe hearing loss attended a local public or private school and spent three or more hours daily integrated with students with normal hearing. Only 10% of students who were profoundly deaf were placed in local public or private schools where they spent three or more hours daily with students with normal hearing; nearly two-fifths of these students (39%) were placed in special residential schools for students who are deaf. As students get older, the proportion attending nonintegrated residential schools increases.

Parents and professionals continue to debate over the benefits and disadvantages of including students who are deaf or hearing impaired in regular classrooms. (see Chapter 3, "Children and Youths" for a discussion of federal laws regarding the education of children with disabilities). How students fare in this environment will depend upon numerous factors, including the onset and severity of the hearing impairment, the student's proficiency in communicating, the support services available, and the school staff's ability to provide appropriate assistance for the student. Teachers in regular classrooms should be educated by vocational rehabilitation professionals, audiologists, or educators who specialize in working with students who are deaf or hearing impaired. Teachers should understand that they must face the class when speaking; keep their mouth visible; provide good lighting; let students who are deaf or hearing impaired sit at the front of the room; and use visual aids whenever possible (Mitchell: 1980). In some cases, it is necessary for an interpreter to be present both in the classroom and during other school activities.

Students who are integrated into regular classrooms may encounter problems because they are "different" from their peers. The school years are times when conformity is valued greatly and wearing a hearing aid, speaking differently, or needing an interpreter in the classroom may present difficult situations. Programs to sensitize other students in the classroom to the experience of living with a disability may begin to bring about attitude change and greater acceptance of students who are different. Explaining the nature of the hearing impairment; having students with normal hearing spend time with a simulated hearing loss; and discussing sign language, hearing aids, and the role of interpreters can help to break the ice with classmates. Support services for students who are deaf or hearing impaired include speech and language therapy, audiological services, the services of a classroom aide or interpreter, and environmental adaptations, such as carpeting and acoustical tile.

Students who are interested in pursuing postsecondary education may receive guidance from a vocational or guidance counselor at school or from a rehabilitation counselor at the state vocational rehabilitation department. There are many publications available that describe the support services available for students with disabilities at technical institutes, junior colleges, and four year colleges and universities (see "PUBLICATIONS AND TAPES" section below). Several postsecondary institutions receive federal funding for programs specifically for students who are deaf or hearing impaired (see "ORGANIZATIONS" section below).

A report issued by the Commission on Education for the Deaf (1988) concluded that the education of deaf students did not meet acceptable standards. The Commission studied a wide variety of issues, including the availability of elementary, secondary, and postsecondary education and appropriate support services; the qualifications of teachers, audiologists, speech therapists, and interpreters; and the quality of outreach services and research provided by federally funded institutions, such as Gallaudet University and the National Technical Institute for the Deaf. Other studies indicate that educational achievements of students who are deaf fall behind those of their peers with normal hearing (Johnson et al.: 1989).

HEARING LOSS IN ELDERS

Hearing loss is most common among people 65 years or older. Most elders experience sensorineural hearing loss, which is not amenable to medical treatment. However, there are many adaptive devices that can help elders cope successfully with hearing loss. The adjustments and psychological effects are much different for people who lose hearing later in life than for those who have congenital or prelingual hearing impairment. For elders, hearing loss is often one of several impairments that they must learn to cope with. A major issue for many elders is acceptance of the fact that they do indeed have a hearing loss. For those elders who live alone, hearing loss may become a threat to safety, as they may be unable to hear a fire alarm or other important alerting devices, such as doorbells. (For a more detailed discussion about hearing loss in elders and services available to help them, see Resources for Elders with Disabilities, described in "PUBLICATIONS AND TAPES" section below.)

PSYCHOLOGICAL ASPECTS OF HEARING LOSS

The effects of deafness and hearing impairment are different for people whose disability occurred congenitally or prelingually than for those whose hearing loss was acquired after they developed speech. Higgins (1980) has described the subculture created by individuals who are prelingually deaf or hearing impaired. These individuals are able to identify with others who have experienced isolation, rejection, and frustration in communications. People who become deaf later in life are audiologically deaf, but not socially deaf, according to Higgins. These individuals are as likely to stigmatize people who are deaf as are members of the hearing community.

When a child who is deaf or hearing impaired is born to parents with normal hearing (which is true in the overwhelming number of cases), the amount of change required within the family can be overwhelming. According to Luterman (1987), not only do some parents deny the deafness or hearing impairment for a while, but they may also view the child as fragile. As is often the case when a disabling or chronic condition is present in children, the parents may tend to focus all of their attention on that child to the neglect of their other children. They often must work with a variety of professionals, including physicians, audiologists, and special educators. This process can be very time consuming, resulting in the need to restructure the normal activities of work and home life.

For those individuals whose hearing loss occurred later in life, adjustment in virtually all areas of everyday living is necessary. Tasks that were once taken for granted, such as answering the doorbell or talking on the telephone, now seem to be insurmountable obstacles. As a result, depression is a very common consequence of hearing loss. Studies suggest that people with hearing loss are more likely to be depressed and have low life satisfaction than peers with normal hearing (Glass: 1986). Two factors that frequently undergo change as a result of hearing loss are job satisfaction and relationships with significant others (Weinberger: 1980). Fear of progressive hearing loss and dependency is also a common and natural psychological reaction.

Social withdrawal is another psychological reaction that sometimes accompanies hearing loss. Because some people find it difficult to accept their hearing loss and to seek out appropriate treatment, they try to function as they always did but are unable to do so. Their behavior is often interpreted as mentally inappropriate by family members and friends who are not aware that hearing loss has occurred. In such instances, family members and friends may also withdraw from social encounters. The withdrawal of family and friends reinforces the individual's self-devaluation. In extreme cases, individuals whose hearing loss has not been diagnosed are inappropriately hospitalized for mental disorders.

The ability to hear sound but not to understand words and meanings leads some individuals to believe that speakers are mumbling or speaking too softly. This reaction is often accompanied by a denial that hearing loss has occurred. When individuals deny that they have experienced hearing loss, they will be unwilling to seek assistance from professionals who can provide assistive devices or training to improve their communication. Such a situation often causes frustration for family members and friends of the person with hearing loss and may result in increased tensions within the individual's family setting.

PROFESSIONAL SERVICE PROVIDERS

Otologists are physicians who specialize in diseases of the ear. Physicians who specialize in treatment of the ear, nose, and throat are called *otorhinolaryngologists*. These physicians diagnose and manage diseases that cause hearing problems. For many conditions, medical or surgical treatment results in restoration of hearing. Unfortunately, for most people who experience sensorineural hearing loss, there is no cure. In order to determine if a condition may be improved with medical or surgical intervention, all individuals with hearing loss should be examined by an otologist or otorhinolaryngologist. In cases where there is no effective medical or surgical treatment to restore lost hearing, the physician should refer the patient to an audiologist or a hearing aid dispenser for evaluation for assistive devices.

Audiologists have special training to administer tests to determine the level of functional hearing; to prescribe hearing aids and other devices; to train patients to use the prescribed devices; to refer patients to other professionals and resources; and to train patients in auditory and visual communication (American Speech-Language-Hearing Association: 1988). In the case of children, audiologists must work not just with other health care professionals and parents, but also with the school staff to ensure that children have the best assistive devices for the physical setting and that teachers are knowledgeable about the children's needs. Audiologists have either a masters or doctoral degree in audiology and are certified by the American Speech-Language-Hearing Association; in addition, most states license audiologists to practice within the state (Weinstein: 1989). Many audiologists practice in otologists' offices. Others practice in their own private offices, in a hospital or clinic setting, or in a rehabilitation agency.

Hearing aid dispensers sell hearing aids to individuals and are not trained in the diagnosis or treatment of conditions that affect hearing. Some hearing aid dispensers do perform basic audiometric tests. Many individuals are referred to dispensers by audiologists. The U.S. Food and Drug Administration requires a medical evaluation prior to the fitting of hearing aids. Although individuals may sign a waiver that permits hearing aid dispensers to fit a hearing aid without a medical evaluation, it is wise to be examined by a physician to determine whether the condition that is causing the hearing loss may be amenable to medical intervention and whether the underlying condition is causing other medical problems.

Speech therapists may also play a role in the rehabilitation of individuals with hearing loss. Individuals who are congenitally or prelingually deaf or hearing impaired need special training to learn how to speak. Individuals with hearing loss can no longer hear their own voices, so they must learn how to modulate their voices properly. Speech therapists receive certificates of clinical competence (CCC) from the American Speech-Language-Hearing Association.

Teachers of the deaf receive special training in university programs located throughout the country. They receive certification from the Council on Education of the Deaf. They may work in special schools for students who are deaf or in public schools. Regular classroom teachers who have students who are deaf or hearing impaired in their classes should receive training in techniques that maximize the educational environment for these students.

Interpreters facilitate communication between individuals who are deaf or hearing impaired and individuals with normal hearing who are not fluent in sign language. The interpreter may be viewed as a translator and does not contribute any of his or her own comments to the conversation. The language the interpreter uses should be chosen by the person who is deaf or hearing impaired. It may be American Sign Language; another type of sign language that is correlated with spoken English; or oral interpreting, which uses natural lip movements without speech.

Rehabilitation counselors help individuals with hearing disorders prepare for independent living and for job placement. Rehabilitation includes prescription of appropriate assistive devices, training in the use of these devices, training in techniques such as speechreading or sign language to enhance communication, and counseling for both the individual with hearing loss and family members. Rehabilitation counselors may help to locate the appropriate assistive listening devices necessary to perform the requirements of a specific position and help the employer to modify the environment for individuals who are deaf or hearing impaired.

Since hereditary conditions are responsible for some types of hearing impairment, *genetic counselors* may play an important role. Genetic counselors are specially trained and often work in a multidisciplinary team of physicians, social workers, and nurses. They obtain information about the family's medical history and the pregnancy history of the mother. Audiograms and physical examinations for family members may help the geneticist determine the cause of the hearing impairment. Geneticists are sometimes able to explain the hereditary process by which the genes causing deafness or hearing impairment were passed on to succeeding generations. Knowing whether a hearing impairment is hereditary and the probability of passing it on to offspring can be a valuable asset in family planning.

WHERE TO FIND SERVICES

Many states have special offices to provide services to individuals who are deaf or hearing impaired. These agencies often provide assistive devices, interpreters, vocational counseling, special educational programs, and counseling and advocacy. The specific services and the populations served vary by state. Individuals should contact the state government information operator, the state office serving individuals with disabilities, or the state department of vocational rehabilitation services to determine if an office for people who are deaf or hearing impaired exists in their state. In addition, state offices of vocational rehabilitation provide services for individuals who are deaf or hearing impaired and are interested in retaining their current positions or receiving training for new careers. Some state agencies, private agencies, university programs, and adult education courses teach sign language to family members of individuals who are deaf or hearing impaired.

Local agencies providing services to people who are deaf or hearing impaired include hospitals with otology or otolaryngology departments; private agencies that specialize in services and rehabilitation for individuals who are deaf or hearing impaired; independent living centers; audiologists and otologists in private practice or at speech and hearing clinics; hearing aid dispensers (listed in the Yellow Pages); universities that have graduate programs for audiologists or speech therapists; and Veterans Affairs Medical Centers. Some general rehabilitation facilities provide special rehabilitation for people who are deaf or hearing impaired.

Most children who are totally deaf or profoundly hearing impaired spend at least some time in special residential schools for students who are deaf (Schein and Delk: 1974), which are often state supported institutions. Other educational options for children who are deaf or hearing impaired include special day schools; special classes within a regular school; and inclusion in a regular classroom, often with the assistance of a speech therapist, interpreter, classroom aide, or resource room teacher. Local education agencies are required to provide services for children and youths with disabilities (see Chapter 3, "Children and Youths"). Parents may benefit by joining support groups composed of parents of children who are deaf or hearing impaired or other formal organizations that provide counseling and referral for parents.

Public libraries are a good source of directories of local agencies. In addition, some libraries and museums have special programs for people with hearing disorders. An increasing number of performances and social events have special amplification devices available for people with hearing loss. (see "ASSISTIVE DEVICES" section below)

ENVIRONMENTAL ADAPTATIONS

Most children who are deaf or hearing impaired will receive prescriptions for hearing aids and other assistive devices from audiologists and school personnel. As they move through the school system or change schools, re-evaluation of hearing aids, other assistive devices, and the environment should be carried out on a regular basis. Those individuals who have congenital disorders are likely to remain stable, but requirements of given tasks may change, creating the need for changes in the adaptive equipment.

It is not uncommon for people with acquired hearing loss to resist the use of adaptive equipment. Meeting with other people who have successfully adapted to the use of hearing aids or other devices may encourage those who are resistant to seek out these devices themselves. Purchasing hearing aids and other devices that include a trial period may also encourage resistant individuals.

People with acquired hearing loss should consider the wide variety of options available to improve their communication skills. For example, they should consider speechreading, a technique that maximizes visual cues from lip movements and other body gestures as well as learning to think about the context of the speech. Individuals should always face the speaker during a conversation in order to see these visual cues.

Environmental adaptations should also be made at health care providers' offices, hospitals, rehabilitation centers, senior citizen centers, and any facility that is designed for group use, such as theaters, churches, and the like. New buildings and those being renovated should have good acoustics. For example, curtains and carpets absorb background noise (Dion: 1989). Amplification systems and assistive listening devices should be installed.

Family, friends, and service providers should all learn how to communicate effectively with people with hearing loss. The following tips will save much frustration when holding a conversation with someone who is deaf or hearing impaired:

- Be certain that the person knows that you are speaking to him or her.
- Always face the person throughout the conversation so that he or she may get visual cues. Be certain that your mouth is visible throughout the conversation, even if the person with hearing loss is not an experienced lipreader.
- Be certain that background noises have been eliminated. For example, radios, and televisions should not be playing and water should not be running.
- Speak clearly at a level just slightly above normal, but do not shout.
- If the person does not understand what you are saying, rephrase the sentence.
- Ask the person if he or she has understood you.
- When speaking to a person through an interpreter, look directly at the person and speak in the same way as you would in any other conversation. Do not say to the interpreter, "Ask him or her..."

ASSISTIVE DEVICES

The types of devices most appropriate to a given individual depend upon not only the type and severity of the hearing impairment but also the individual's usual activities. The variety of assistive devices available to help people with hearing loss communicate effectively is constantly expanding. Major organizations such as Self Help for Hard of Hearing People, the American Speech-Language-Hearing Association, and the Laurent Clerc National Deaf Education Network and Clearinghouse at Gallaudet University (see "ORGANIZATIONS" section below) publish information about a wide range of devices. For those individuals who are not able to afford the devices they need, financial assistance is often available through a state agency or through local service organizations. Assistive devices are available on display at local rehabilitation agencies.

The most common device, the *hearing aid*, is used by 3.6 million Americans or 43% of those who cannot understand normal speech (Ries: 1994). Hearing aids have undergone considerable improvement in recent years, and there are many types and models to choose from. The reluctance on the part of many people to use hearing aids may be attributed in part to denial of hearing loss, the high cost of some hearing aids, the failure of many medical insurance policies to cover the cost, and improper training in the use of hearing aids.

Because hearing aids amplify sound, they amplify background noises as well as conversation. The amplification of background noise is a common reason that some people do not find hearing aids useful. Some hearing aids are designed to screen out certain frequencies and background noises; however, no model is capable of enhancing speech and eliminating background noise perfectly. Advances in hearing aid technology have resulted in a new generation of digitally programmed hearing aids. Audiologists are able to program digital hearing aids so that amplification is specific to the individual's hearing loss at various frequencies. Experts recommend that people with hearing loss purchase hearing aids with a 30 day trial period, so they may be returned or adjusted if not satisfactory. Because the level of hearing impairment may change, individuals should be re-evaluated on a regular basis and whenever a decrease in hearing ability is noticed.

Assistive listening devices (ALDs) are alternative devices for situations where hearing aids are not sufficient. ALDs transmit sound waves directly into the ears of people with hearing loss. They utilize microphones close to the source of the sound, amplifiers, and headsets. Three types of ALDs are infrared, FM, and hard-wired systems. The first two types of systems are useful in group situations and are currently available in large group settings, such as theaters and churches, while the hard-wired system is often useful in the home and may be installed inexpensively (Weinstein: 1989).

Teletypewriters (TTYs), also called telecommunication devices for the deaf (TDDs) or text telephone (TTs), transmit printed messages across telephone lines. They utilize computers with screens and keyboards as well as a modem, which serves as the communication device. TTYs may only be used when there is a TTY at the other end of the telephone line. Telephone relay service (TRS) enables parties to communicate by phone when one party does not have a TTY; there is no additional charge for this service. A communications assistant relays the conversation from text to voice and from voice to text. The Americans with Disabilities Act requires that all common carriers provide nationwide 24-hour TRS service. Telephone companies can provide information about installing a TTY. A special operator is available for directory assistance and placing credit card, collect, person-to-person and third party calls. The local telephone directory includes the toll-free number for this service in a section on services for customers with disabilities.

Telephone amplifiers make communication with the outside world available to many individuals with hearing loss. Available in a variety of models, some are easy to use and produce high quality sound, while others are difficult to use and produce inferior sound. Hand-held telephone amplifiers and volume controls attach to phones at home and are useful when traveling. Some states provide telephone amplifiers to qualified users at no charge; the state office that serves individuals who are deaf or hearing impaired should know if the state provides these devices. These devices have become so commonplace that many stores and mail order catalogues that sell phone equipment stock amplifiers as well as TTYs. Federal law in the United States requires that telephones with cords and cordless telephones be compatible with hearing aids.

Visual alerting systems are available to use as smoke or fire detectors and as indicators that the telephone or doorbell is ringing. Automobile manufacturers offer special alerting devices, such as emergency vehicle siren detectors and enhanced turn signal reminders for drivers who are deaf or hard of hearing (see Chapter 4, "TRAVEL AND TRANSPORTATION ORGANIZATIONS" section). *Vibrators* are available to substitute for an audible signal from an alarm clock. A digital telephone answering machine is available with adjustable tone control and adjustable speed that enables individuals to maximize the clarity of replayed messages.

Hearing dogs are used in ways that are similar to guide dogs for people with vision impairments. Dogs are trained to lead their owners to the source of sound and enable people with hearing loss, especially those who live alone, to maintain their independence and security.

Closed captioned television programs, which were relatively rare just a few years ago, are becoming more common, with all major network programs in prime time now closed captioned. Closed captioning provides a print output of the program's speech on the television screen. The Television Decoder Circuitry Act (P.L. 101-431) mandates that all television sets with screens 13 inches or larger be manufactured with built-in decoders for closed captions. For older television models not equipped with closed captioning, closed captioned programs are accessible through decoders, which are available through a variety of outlets and cost about two-hundred dollars or less. Section 713 of the Telecommunications Act of 1996 (P.L. 104-104) requires that video services be accessible to individuals with hearing impairments via closed captioning.

Interpreted captioning is a system that enables people with hearing loss who are not fluent in sign language or speechreading to understand the conversation at group meetings (Grant and Walsh: 1990). There are several methods of interpreted captioning, including visual recording, where a volunteer uses large sheets of paper to record the meeting in words, symbols, and graphics, and computer assisted real time captioning (CART), where an operator types the dialogue from a meeting into a computer. The computer display may be presented in enlarged form by projection onto a screen or wall; alternatively, large print software may be sufficient to enable members of the group to read the proceedings.

References

Allen, Thomas E.
1993 "Subgroup Differences in Educational Placement for Deaf and Hard of Hearing Students" American Annals of the Deaf 137:5:381-388

American Speech-Language-Hearing Association
1988 Position Statement "The Role of Speech-Language Pathologists and Audiologists in Working with Older Persons" ASHA 30(March):80-84

Bess, Fred H.
1993 "Early Identification of Hearing Loss: A Review of the Whys, Hows, and Whens" The Hearing Journal 46:6(June):22-25

Commission on Education of the Deaf
1988 Toward Equality A Report to the President and the Congress of the United States Washington D.C.: U.S. Government Printing Office

Dion, Betty
1989 "Designing a Barrier-Free Environment" Rehabilitation Digest (Spring):12-14

Glass, Laurel E.
1986 "Rehabilitation for Deaf and Hearing-Impaired Elderly" pp. 218-236 in Stanley J. Brody and George E. Ruff (eds.) Aging and Rehabilitation New York, NY: Springer

Grant, Nancy C. and Birrell Walsh
1990 "Interpreted Captioning: Facilitating Interactive Discussion Among Hearing Impaired Adults" International Journal of Technology and Aging 3(Fall/Winter)2:133-144

Higgins, Paul C.
1980 Outsiders in a Hearing World Beverly Hills, CA: Sage Publications

Johnson, Robert E., Scott K. Liddell, and Carol J. Erting
1989 Unlocking the Curriculum: Principles for Achieving Access in Deaf Education Washington D.C.: Gallaudet Research Institute

Luterman, David

1987 Deafness in the Family Boston: Little Brown, College Hill Publications

Mitchell, Joyce Slayton

1980 See Me More Clearly New York, NY: Harcourt, Brace, Jovanovich

National Center for Health Statistics

1999 Vital and Health Statistics, Current Estimates from the National Health Interview Survey Series 10, No. 200 DHHS Pub. No. (PHS) 99-1528, Hyattsville, MD: Public Health Service

National Institute on Deafness and Other Communication Disorders

1989 National Strategic Research Plan Bethesda, MD: National Institutes of Health

NIH Consensus Development Panel on Cochlear Implants in Adults and Children

1995 "Cochlear Implants in Adults and Children" JAMA 274:24(December 27):1955-1961

Price, Lloyd L. and Robert M. Snider

1983 "The Geriatric Patient: Ear, Nose and Throat Problems" in William Reichel (ed.) Clinical Aspects of Aging Baltimore, MD: Williams and Wilkins

Radcliffe, Donald

1993 "In Identifying Hearing Loss in Infants, Time is of the Essence" The Hearing Journal 46:4(April):13-21

Ries, Peter W.

1994 "Prevalence and Characteristics of Persons with Hearing Trouble: United States, 1990-1991" Vital and Health Statistics, Series 10, No. 188 National Center for Health Statistics Hyattsville, MD: Public Health Service

Schein, Jerome D. and Marcus T. Delk, Jr.

1974 The Deaf Population of the United States Silver Spring, MD: National Association of the Deaf

Schwartz, Sue

1987 Choices in Deafness: A Parents Guide Rockville, MD: Woodbine House

Strome, Marshall

1989 "Hearing Loss and Hearing Aids" Harvard Medical School Health Letter 14(April):6:5-8

U.S. Department of Health and Human Services

1988 "Cochlear Implants" National Institutes of Health Consensus Development Conference Statement 7(May 4):2

Weinberger, Morris

1980 "Social and Psychological Consequences of Legitimating a Hearing Impairment" Social Science and Medicine 14A:213-222

Weinstein, Barbara

1989 "Geriatric Hearing Loss: Myths, Realities, Resources for Physicians" Geriatrics 44(April):42-59

Alexander Graham Bell Association for the Deaf
3417 Volta Place, NW
Washington, DC 20007
(800) 432-7543   (202) 337-5220   (202) 337-5221 (TTY)
FAX (202) 337-8314   e-mail: info@agbell.org   www.agbell.org

A membership organization that provides services and support for people who are deaf or hearing impaired. Sponsors conferences and workshops. Special section for parents of children who are deaf or hearing impaired and special publications addressing children's needs. Membership, parents, $40.00; regular membership, $50.00; includes "Volta Review," a professional journal and "Volta Voices," a magazine. Members receive a 15% discount on most publications.

American Society for Deaf Children (ASDC)
PO Box 3355
Gettysburg, PA 17325
(800) 942-2732 (V/TTY)   (717) 334-7922 (V/TTY)   FAX (717) 334-8808
e-mail: asda@deafchildren.org   www.deafchildren.org

A membership organization for parents of children who are deaf, ASDC provides resource materials, makes referrals, and holds a biennial meeting. Individual/family membership, $40.00, includes quarterly newsletter, "Endeavor." Sample issue available on the web site.

American Speech-Language-Hearing Association (ASHA)
10801 Rockville Pike
Rockville, MD 20852
(800) 638-8255 (V/TTY)   FAX (301) 897-7355
e-mail: actioncenter@asha.org   www.asha.org

A professional organization of speech-language pathologists and audiologists. Toll-free HELPLINE offers answers to questions about conditions and services as well as referrals. Provides information on communication problems and a free list of certified audiologists and speech therapists for each state. Also available on the web site. Web site also lists self-help groups for individuals with hearing disorders.

American Tinnitus Association (ATA)
PO Box 5
Portland, OR 97207-0005
(800) 634-8978   (503) 248-9985   FAX (503) 248-0024
e-mail: tinnitus@ata.org   www.ata.org

Membership organization that carries out and supports research and education on tinnitus and other ear diseases. Provides audiocassettes of environmental sounds that may provide relief from tinnitus. Membership, $25.00, includes subscription to quarterly magazine, "Tinnitus Today" and informational brochures.

Association of Late-Deafened Adults (ALDA)
1131 Lake Street, #204
Oak Park, IL 60301
(877) 348-7537 (V/FAX)   (708) 358-0135 (TTY)   e-mail: info@alda.org
www.alda.org

Sponsors a network of self-help groups for adults throughout the U.S. and Canada who became deaf as adults. Provides information and consultations for professionals and the public. Membership, $20.00; $15.00, age 62 or older; includes newsletter, "ALDA News."

Canine Companions for Independence
PO Box 446
2965 Dutton Avenue
Santa Rosa, CA 95402
(800) 572-2275, connects to nearest regional center
(866) 224-3647, connects to national headquarters
www.caninecompanions.org

Trains and places hearing dogs with individuals who are hearing impaired or deaf. Services are free.

Center for Hereditary Hearing Loss
Center for the Study and Treatment of Usher Syndrome
Boys Town National Research Hospital
555 North 30th Street
Omaha, NE 68131
(800) 835-1468 (V/TTY)   FAX (402) 498-6331
www.boystownhospital.org/parents/info/index.asp

This center studies the hereditary aspects of hearing impairment. Disseminates information to professionals and families.

Cochlear Implant Association, Inc. (CIAI)
5335 Wisconsin Avenue, NW, Suite 440
Washington, DC 20015
(202) 895-2781 (V/TTY)   FAX: (202) 895-2782
e-mail: info@cici.org   www.cici.org

A membership organization that provides support and information to individuals prior to and following cochlear implantation. Assists with the formation of local CICI chapters. Membership, individuals, $25.00; families, $25.00; professionals, $60.00; includes quarterly newsletter, "CONTACT."

Council for Exceptional Children (CEC)
1110 North Glebe Road, Suite 300
Arlington, VA 22201
(888) 232-7733   (703) 620-3660   (703) 264-9446
FAX (703) 264-9494   www.cec.sped.org

A professional membership organization that works toward improving the quality of education for children who have disabilities or are gifted. Membership fees vary by geographic location. Special division for communicative disabilities and deafness; membership, $20.00. Publishes "Communications Disorders Quarterly," $39.00.

Dogs for the Deaf
10175 Wheeler Road
Central Point, OR 97502
(541) 826-9220 (V/TTY)   FAX (541) 826-6696
e-mail: info@dogsforthedeaf.org   www.dogsforthedeaf.org

Trains dogs that provide assistance to individuals who are hearing impaired or deaf. These dogs respond to a variety of sounds, such as doorbells, smoke alarms, alarm clocks, etc. One week of training is provided at the recipient's home. All services are free.

Federal Communications Commission (FCC)
445 12th Street, SW
Washington, DC 20554
(888) 225-5322   (888) 835-5322 (TTY)   (202) 418-0190
(202) 418-2555 (TTY)   e-mail: fccinfo@fcc.gov   www.fcc.gov

Responsible for developing regulations for telecommunication issues related to federal laws, including the ADA and the Telecommunications Act of 1996.

Gallaudet Research Institute (GRI)
Gallaudet University
800 Florida Avenue, NE
Washington, DC 20002
(202) 651-5400 (V/TTY)   e-mail: grioffice@gallaudet.edu
gri.gallaudet.edu

Conducts research on all aspects of deafness and hearing impairment. Publishes newsletter, "Research at Gallaudet," which reviews research findings. Free. Also available on the web site. Some publications are available on the web site.

Gallaudet University
800 Florida Avenue, NE
Washington, DC 20002
(202) 651-5000 (V/TTY)   www.gallaudet.edu

The recipient of federal funding, Gallaudet is a university for students who are deaf. It also operates special model educational programs for students in elementary and secondary school. Classes are taught in sign language, and a wide range of support services is available. Conducts outreach programs through distribution of educational materials developed at Gallaudet, workshops, seminars, and consultations with school departments throughout the country.

Hear Now
6700 Washington Avenue South
Eden Prairie, MN 55344
(800) 648-4327 (V/TTY)   FAX (952) 828-6946
www.sotheworldmayhear.org

Provides hearing aids to people with limited financial resources. Nonrefundable application processing fee of $39.00 per hearing aid. Recycles donated, used hearing aids.

Helen Keller National Center for Deaf-Blind Youths and Adults (HKNC)
111 Middle Neck Road
Sands Point, NY 11050
(516) 944-8900   (516) 944-8637 (TTY)   FAX (516) 944-7302
www.helenkeller.org/national

Offers evaluation, vocational rehabilitation training, counseling, job preparation, placement, and related services through ten regional offices.

Laurent Clerc National Deaf Education Network and Clearinghouse
Gallaudet University
800 Florida Avenue, NE, Washington, DC 20002
(202) 651-5051   (202) 651-5052 (TTY)   FAX (202) 651-5054
e-mail: clearinghouse.infotogo@gallaudet.edu
clerccenter.gallaudet.edu

The Center provides information on a wide variety of topics related to deafness and hearing loss in children. The web site includes a directory of organizations related to deafness and hearing loss and a list of Clerc Center publications. Publications are available only on the web site.

Lexington School and Center for the Deaf, Inc.
30th Avenue and 75th Street
Jackson Heights, NY 11370
(718) 899-8800 (V/TTY)   (718) 350-3201 (V/TTY)   FAX (718) 899-3433
e-mail: info@hearingresearch.org   www.hearingresearch.org

A federally funded program that develops and evaluates hearing aids and other assistive listening devices. Publications for consumers, service providers, and researchers. Free publications list. Also available on the web site.

MEDLINEplus: Hearing Disorders and Deafness
www.nlm.nih.gov/medlineplus/hearingdisorders.html

This web site provides links to sites for general information about hearing disorders and deafness, symptoms and diagnosis, treatment, prevention/screening, specific conditions/aspects, children, seniors, organizations, and research. Some information is available in Spanish. Provides links to MEDLINE research articles and related MEDLINEplus pages.

National Association of the Deaf (NAD)
814 Thayer Avenue
Silver Spring, MD 20910
(301) 587-1788   (301) 587-1789 (TTY)
FAX (301) 587-1791   e-mail: nadinfo@nad.org   www.nad.org

A membership organization with state chapters throughout the U.S. Advocates for its members and serves as an information clearinghouse. Special programs for youths and special sections for senior citizens, federal employees, and sign language instructors. Holds national and regional conventions. Membership, individuals, $30.00; seniors (over 60), $15.00.

National Institute on Deafness and Other Communication Disorders (NIDCD)
Building 31, Room 3C35
31 Center Drive, MSC 2320
Bethesda, MD 20892
(301) 496-7243   (301) 402-0252 (TTY)
FAX (301) 402-0018   www.nidcd.nih.gov

Federal agency that funds basic research studies on problems of hearing, balance, voice, language, and speech.

National Institute on Deafness and Other Communication Disorders Information Clearinghouse
1 Communication Avenue
Bethesda, MD 20892
(800) 241-1044   (800) 241-1055 (TTY)   FAX (301) 907-8830
e-mail: nidcdinfo@nidcd.nih.gov   www.nidcd.nih.gov

Maintains a database of references and responds to requests for information from the public and professionals. Publishes newsletter, "Inside NIDCD Information Clearinghouse," free. Free publications list.

National Technical Institute for the Deaf (NTID)
Rochester Institute of Technology
Lyndon Baines Johnson Building
52 Lomb Memorial Drive
Rochester, NY 14623
(716) 475-6400 (V/TTY)   FAX (716) 475-6500
e-mail: ntidmc@rit.edu   www.rit.edu

A federally funded technical college created for deaf students within a larger institution for students with normal hearing. Students may enroll in courses in the other colleges within the Rochester Institute of Technology.

Registry of Interpreters of the Deaf (RID)
333 Commerce Street
Alexandria, VA 22314
(703) 838-0030   (703) 838-0459 (TTY)   FAX (703) 838-0454
e-mail: info@rid.org   www.rid.org

The national certifying organization for interpreters. Establishes guidelines for professional interpreters. Produces guide of training programs for interpreters throughout the country. Maintains a list of interpreters and postsecondary institutions that offer interpreter training programs.

Rehabilitation Research and Training Center for Persons Who Are Deaf or Hard of Hearing
University of Arkansas
4601 West Markham Street
Little Rock, AR 72205
(501) 686-9691 (V/TTY)   FAX (501) 686-9698
e-mail: rehabres@cavern.uark.edu
www.uark.edu/deafrtc

A federally funded research center that focuses on enhancing the transition from school to work for people who are deaf or hearing impaired. Also addresses communication and adjustment skills. Sponsors workshops, conferences, and graduate training programs.

Rehabilitation Research & Training Center for Persons Who Are Hard of Hearing or Late Deafened
California School of Professional Psychology
6160 Cornerstone Court East
San Diego, CA 92121
(858) 623-2777   (800) 432-7619 (TTY)   FAX (858) 642-0266
e-mail: rrtc@cspp.edu   www.hearinghealth.org

A federally funded research center that focuses on maintaining the employment status and addressing the personal adjustment needs of persons who are hard of hearing or late deafened. Projects include research on pre- and post-surgical adjustment of cochlear implant recipients and mental health issues of persons who are deaf-blind.

Self Help for Hard of Hearing People (SHHH)
7910 Woodmont Avenue, Suite 1200
Bethesda, MD 20814
(301) 657-2248   (301) 657-2249 (TTY)   FAX (301) 913-9413
e-mail: national@shhh.org   www.shhh.org

National membership organization with local and regional chapters. Provides information, support, and individual referrals. Membership, individuals, $25.00; professionals, $50.00; includes subscription to bimonthly magazine, "Hearing Loss: The Journal of Self Help for Hard of Hearing People."

TDI
8630 Fenton Street, Suite 604
Silver Spring, MD 20910
(301) 589-3786   (301) 589-3006 (TTY)   FAX (301) 589-3797
e-mail: info@tdi-online.org   www.tdi-online.org

Membership organization that lobbies for improved telecommunication for individuals who are deaf or hearing impaired. Publishes "National Directory and Resource Guide" annually. Membership, $25.00, includes directory listing and quarterly newsletter, "GA-SK."

University of California San Francisco Center on Deafness
3333 California Street, Suite 10
San Francisco, CA 94143
(415) 476-4980   (415) 476-7600 (TTY)   FAX (415) 476-7113
e-mail: UCCD@itsa.ucsf.edu

A federally funded research and training center that focuses on the mental health needs of people who are deaf. Sponsors conferences and graduate training. Articles available documenting findings of research projects.

U.S. Department of Veterans Affairs (VA)
Prosthetics Division, local VA Medical Centers
(800) 827-1000 (connects with regional office)   www.va.gov

Provides free hearing aids to eligible veterans and Tele-Caption decoder for veterans with hearing loss that is service related. In some cases, the VA will pay for cochlear implants.

Vestibular Disorders Association
PO Box 4467
Portland, OR 97208-4467
(800) 837-8428   (503) 229-7705   FAX (503) 229-8064
e-mail: veda@vestibular.org   www.vestibular.org

Provides support and information to individuals who experience dizziness, inner-ear balance disorders, vertigo, and related hearing problems. Produces publications and videotapes. Membership, individuals or families, $25.00; professionals, $40.00; includes quarterly newsletter, "On the Level," and new member information packet.

Publications focusing specifically on assistive devices are listed in "RESOURCES FOR ASSISTIVE DEVICES" section below.

<u>American Annals of the Deaf Annual Reference Issue</u>
Publications and Marketing
Gallaudet University
Fowler Hall 409
800 Florida Avenue, NE
Washington, DC 20002
(202) 651-5530 (V/TTY)   FAX (202) 651-5869
e-mail: mary.carew@gallaudet.edu sehs.gallaudet.edu/annals

The annual reference issue is published each spring and lists special schools and programs throughout the U.S. and Canada for individuals who are deaf or deaf-blind. $27.00

<u>Captioned Media Program</u>
1447 East Main Street
Spartanburg, SC 29307
(800) 237-6213   (800) 237-6819 (TTY)   FAX (800) 538-5636
e-mail: info@cfv.org   www.cfv.org

Offers lending library of videotapes with open captions (no need for decoders). Free

<u>The Challenge of Educating Together Deaf and Hearing Youth: Making Mainstreaming Work</u>
by Paul C. Higgins
Charles C. Thomas Publisher
2600 South First Street
Springfield, IL 62704
(800) 258-8980   (217) 789-8980   FAX (217) 789-9130
e-mail: books@ccthomas.com   www.ccthomas.com

This book discusses the controversy over mainstreaming students who are deaf; the advantages of mainstreaming; student placement; and social relations between students who are deaf and those with normal hearing. Hardcover, $43.95; softcover, $30.95; plus $5.95 shipping and handling.

<u>Choices in Deafness: A Parents Guide to Communication Options</u>
by Sue Schwartz
Woodbine House
6510 Bells Mill Road
Bethesda, MD 20817
(800) 843-7323   FAX (301) 897-5838
e-mail: info@woodbinehouse.com   www.woodbinehouse.com

This book discusses the various services children who are deaf or hearing impaired need; the choices in communication; and case studies of parents and children who have successfully adapted to deafness or hearing impairment. $16.95 plus $4.50 shipping and handling

<u>Cochlear Implants</u>
National Institute on Deafness and Other Communication Disorders Information Clearinghouse
1 Communication Avenue
Washington, DC 20892
(800) 241-1044   (800) 241-1055 (TTY)   FAX (301) 907-8830
e-mail: nidcdinfo@nidcd.nih.gov   www.nidcd.nih.gov

This publication includes information describing how the cochlear implant works, recent articles on the subject, resources, and an annotated bibliography. Free. Also available on the web site.

<u>College and Career Programs for Deaf Students</u>
Gallaudet Research Institute
Gallaudet University
800 Florida Avenue, NE
Washington, DC 20002
(800) 451-8834 (V/TTY)   (800) 995-0513   (202) 651-5575 (V/TTY)
gri.gallaudet.edu

This book describes admissions, costs, degrees available, and support services for students who are deaf at postsecondary programs throughout the U.S. and Canada. $12.95 plus $7.00 postage. Portions of the book are available on the web site.

<u>Communication Options for Children Who Are Deaf or Hard-of-Hearing</u>
National Institute on Deafness and Other Communication Disorders Information Clearinghouse
1 Communication Avenue
Washington, DC 20892
(800) 241-1044   (800) 241-1055 (TTY)   FAX (301) 907-8830
e-mail: nidcdinfo@nidcd.nih.gov   www.nidcd.nih.gov

This fact sheet describes the diagnosis of hearing loss in newborns and young children and discusses communication alternatives. Free. Also available on the web site.

Coping with Hearing Loss
by Susan V. Rezen and Carl Hausman
Self Help for Hard of Hearing People (SHHH)
7910 Woodmont Avenue, Suite 1200
Bethesda, MD 20814
(301) 657-2248   (301) 657-2249 (TTY)   FAX (301) 913-9413
e-mail: national@shhh.org   www.shhh.org

This book discusses causes of hearing loss, problems experienced by people with hearing loss, solutions for these problems, information about hearing aids, and tips on speechreading. $19.95 plus $4.45 shipping and handling

Coping with Hearing Loss and Hearing Aids
by Debra A. Shimon
Thomson Learning
7625 Empire Drive
Florence, KY 41042
(800) 347-7707   FAX (859) 647-5023
www.thomsonlearning.com

This book discusses the effects of hearing loss, how hearing aids work, and how to buy a hearing aid. $22.95

Deaf or Hard-of-Hearing: Tips for Working with Your Doctor
American Academy of Family Physicians
11400 Tomahawk Creek Parkway
Leawood, KS 66211-2672
(913) 906-6000   e-mail: fp@aafp.org   www.aafp.org
familydoctor.org

This fact sheet provides communication tips for individuals who are deaf and use sign language and those who are hard of hearing or deaf and rely on spoken language. Free. Also available on the web site.

Directory: Information Resources for Human Communication Disorders
National Institute on Deafness and Other Communication Disorders Information Clearinghouse
1 Communication Avenue
Washington, DC 20892
(800) 241-1044   (800) 241-1055 (TTY)   FAX (301) 907-8830
e-mail: nidcdinfo@nidcd.nih.gov   www.nidcd.nih.gov

This directory provides a listing and description of organizations throughout the country that deal with communication disorders. Free. Also available on the web site.

Facilitating the Transition of Deaf Adolescents to Adulthood: Focus on Families
Rehabilitation Research and Training Center for Persons Who Are Deaf or Hard of Hearing
University of Arkansas
4601 West Markham Street
Little Rock, AR 72205
(501) 686-9691 (V/TTY)   FAX (501) 686-9698
e-mail: rehabres@cavern.uark.edu
www.uark.edu/deafrtc

This book discusses how parents and professionals can work together to help adolescents and what rehabilitation counselors can do for this age group. $15.00

Hearing Aids
National Institute on Deafness and Other Communication Disorders Information Clearinghouse
1 Communication Avenue
Washington, DC 20892
(800) 241-1044   (800) 241-1055 (TTY)   FAX (301) 907-8830
e-mail: nidcdinfo@nidcd.nih.gov   www.nidcd.nih.gov

This fact sheet discusses types of hearing loss and four basic styles of hearing aids. Provides tips for purchasing hearing aids and how to care for them. Free. Also available on the web site.

Hearing Loss and Older Adults
National Institute on Deafness and Other Communication Disorders Information Clearinghouse
1 Communication Avenue
Washington, DC 20892
(800) 241-1044   (800) 241-1055 (TTY)   FAX (301) 907-8830
e-mail: nidcdinfo@nidcd.nih.gov   www.nidcd.nih.gov

This fact sheet describes hearing loss and devices that may be helpful. Includes a checklist that individuals can use to evaluate their hearing and a resource list. Free. Also available on the web site.

Hear: Solutions, Skills, and Sources for Hard of Hearing People
by Anne Pope
Self Help for Hard of Hearing People (SHHH)
7910 Woodmont Avenue, Suite 1200
Bethesda, MD 20814
(301) 657-2248   (301) 657-2249 (TTY)   FAX (301) 913-9413
e-mail: national@shhh.org   www.shhh.org

This book describes how the ear works and what can go wrong and offers practical communication strategies. $19.95 plus $4.45 shipping and handling

How the Student with Hearing Loss Can Succeed in College
by Carol Flexer, Denise Wray, Ron Leavitt, and Robert Flexer
Alexander Graham Bell Association for the Deaf
3417 Volta Place, NW
Washington, DC 20007
(800) 432-7543   (202) 337-5220   (202) 337-5221 (TTY)
FAX (202) 337-8314   e-mail: info@agbell.org   www.agbell.org

This book provides information for students who plan to attend universities. Includes information about support services, financial aid, and technological services. $28.95 plus $9.00 shipping

Infants & Toddlers with Hearing Loss: Family-Centered Assessment and Intervention
by Jackson Roush and Noel D. Matkin (eds.)
York Press, Inc.
PO Box 504
Timonium, MD 21094
(800) 962-2763   FAX (410) 560-6758   e-mail: york@abs.net

This book discusses methods for identifying and managing hearing loss using a multidisciplinary team. Development of the Individualized Family Service Plan is addressed. $38.50 plus $3.50 shipping and handling

I See What You're Saying: Lipreading Program
by Mary Kleeman
Alexander Graham Bell Association for the Deaf
3417 Volta Place, NW
Washington, DC 20007
(800) 432-7543   (202) 337-5220   (202) 337-5221 (TTY)
FAX (202) 337-8314   e-mail: info@agbell.org   www.agbell.org

This videotape and manual provide instruction in lipreading for adults with hearing loss. Includes many examples in noisy and quiet environments. 54 minutes. $49.95 plus $9.00 shipping and handling

Legal Rights: The Guide for Deaf and Hard of Hearing People
Gallaudet University Press
Chicago Distribution Center
11030 South Langley Avenue
(800) 621-2736   (888) 630-9347 (TTY)   FAX (800) 621-8476
gupress.gallaudet.edu

This book discusses the legal rights of people with hearing impairments in situations such as employment, education, and health care. Federal and state statutes included. $29.95 plus $4.00 shipping and handling

Living Well with Hearing Loss
by Debbie Huning
John Wiley and Sons
1 John Wiley Drive
Somerset, NJ 08875
(800) 225-5945   (908) 469-4400   FAX (908) 302-2300
www.wiley.com

Written by an audiologist, this book provides practical information about communications, hearing aids, and other issues pertinent to individuals with hearing loss and their families. $12.95

Living with Hearing Loss: The Sourcebook for Deafness and Hearing Disorders
by Carol Turkington and Allen E. Sussman
Facts on File
132 West 31st Street, 17th Floor
New York, NY 10001
(800) 322-8755, extension 4228 FAX (800) 678-3633   www.factsonfile.com

This book provides information about types of hearing loss in children and adults, treatment, choosing hearing aids, other assistive devices, and organizations that serve individuals who are deaf or hearing-impaired. $16.95 plus $4.00 shipping and handling

Missing Words: The Family Handbook on Adult Hearing Loss
by Kay Thomsett and Eve Nickerson
Gallaudet University Press
Chicago Distribution Center
11030 South Langley Avenue
(800) 621-2736   (888) 630-9347 (TTY)   FAX (800) 621-8476
gupress.gallaudet.edu

Written by a woman who is deaf and her daughter, this book describes how families can adjust to a member's hearing loss. Ms Nickerson, the recipient of a cochlear implant, describes the barriers she encountered in everyday life after becoming deaf and her psychological responses as well as her experience adjusting to the cochlear implant. Includes communication methods and information on hearing aids and cochlear implants. $29.95 plus $4.00 shipping and handling

The Noise in Your Ears: Facts About Tinnitus
National Institute on Deafness and Other Communication Disorders Information Clearinghouse
1 Communication Avenue
Washington, DC 20892
(800) 241-1044   (800) 241-1055 (TTY)   FAX (301) 907-8830
e-mail: nidcdinfo@nidcd.nih.gov   www.nidcd.nih.gov

This fact sheet describes the causes of tinnitus and possible treatments and lists resources for further information. Also available in large print. Free. Also available on the web site.

Questions Teachers Ask: A Guide for the Mainstream Classroom Teacher with a Hearing-Impaired Student
by Julie W. Otto and Victoria J. Kozack
Central Institute for the Deaf
4560 Clayton Avenue
St. Louis, MO 63110
(314) 977-0133   (314) 977-0000 (V/TTY)   FAX (314) 977-0023
e-mail: dgushleff@cid.wustl.edu   www.cid.wustl.edu

Using a question and answer format, this book provides tips for teachers who have hearing-impaired students in their classrooms. Includes information about assistive devices. $15.00 plus $3.00 shipping and handling

Resources for Elders with Disabilities
Resources for Rehabilitation
22 Bonad Road
Winchester, MA 01890
(781) 368-9094   FAX (781) 368-9096
e-mail: orders@rfr.org   www.rfr.org

A large print resource directory that describes services and products that help elders with disabilities to function independently. Includes chapters on hearing loss, stroke, vision loss, Parkinson's disease, arthritis, diabetes, and osteoporosis. $49.95 plus $5.00 shipping and handling. (See order form on last page of this book.)

See What I'm Saying
by Thomas Kaufman
Fanlight Productions
4196 Washington Street, Suite 2
Boston, MA 02131
(800) 937-4113   (617) 469-4999   FAX (617) 469-3379
e-mail: fanlight@fanlight.com   www.fanlight.com

This videotape shows how the acquisition of communication skills affects an elementary school student who is deaf and her family and peers. 31 minutes. Open captioned. Purchase, $195.00; rental for one day, $50.00; rental for one week, $100.00; plus $9.00 shipping and handling.

Self-Advocacy for Students Who Are Deaf or Hard of Hearing
by Kristina M. English
Pro-Ed
8700 Shoal Creek Boulevard
Austin, TX 78757
(800) 897-3202   FAX (800) 397-7633   www.proedinc.com

This book presents strategies that enable post-secondary students to advocate for themselves in education and employment. $31.00 plus 10% shipping and handling

Telecommunications Relay Services: An Informational Handbook
Federal Communications Commission (FCC)
445 12th Street, SW
Washington, DC 20554
(888) 225-5322   (888) 835-5322 (TTY)   (202) 418-0190
(202) 418-2555 (TTY)   e-mail: fccinfo@fcc.gov   www.fcc.gov

A booklet that describes how telecommunications relay services work. Lists telephone numbers to reach communication assistants and to obtain information about this service in each state. Free. Also available on the web site; click on "Disabilities Issues."

Tinnitus: Questions and Answers
by Jack A. Vernon and Barbara Tabachnick Sanders
Allyn & Bacon
160 Gould Street
Needham Heights, MA 02494
(800) 278-3525   www.ablongman.com

Using a question and answer format, this book discusses topics such as the causes of tinnitus, medications, masking devices, tinnitus instruments, support groups, and resources. $28.00 plus $5.99 shipping and handling

Toward Effective Public School Programs for Deaf Students: Context, Process, and Outcomes
by Thomas N. Kluwin, Donald E. Moore, and Martha Gonter Gaustad (eds.)
Teachers College Press
PO Box 20
Williston, VT 05495-0020
(800) 575-6566   FAX (802) 864-7626
e-mail: tcporders@aidcvt.com   www.tc.columbia.edu

Based on a longitudinal study of 15 school systems, this book discusses mainstreaming students who are deaf into public schools. Various models are described, and practical recommendations are included. $22.95

Usher Syndrome
National Institute on Deafness and Other Communication Disorders Information Clearinghouse
1 Communication Avenue
Washington, DC 20892
(800) 241-1044   (800) 241-1055 (TTY)   FAX (301) 907-8830
e-mail: nidcdinfo@nidcd.nih.gov   www.nidcd.nih.gov

This fact sheet describes the three types of this major cause of deaf-blindness. Includes resource list. Free. Also available on the web site.

You and Your Deaf Child: A Self-Help Guide for Parents of Deaf and Hard of Hearing Children
by John W. Adams
Gallaudet University Press
Chicago Distribution Center
11030 South Langley Avenue
(800) 621-2736   (888) 630-9347 (TTY)   FAX (800) 621-8476
gupress.gallaudet.edu

This book provides information and support for parents, describes language development, and offers suggestions for behavior management. $29.95 plus $4.00 shipping and handling

When Your Child is Deaf
by David Luterman with Mark Ross
York Press, Inc.
PO Box 504
Timonium, MD 21094
(800) 962-2763   FAX (410) 560-6758   e-mail: york@abs.net
www.yorkpress.com

This book provides guidelines to help parents cope with the diagnosis of a child's hearing loss. It describes audiological procedures, amplification, education, and emotional responses. $20.25 plus $4.00 shipping and handling

Listed below are publications and organizations that provide information about assistive devices and catalogues that specialize in devices for people with hearing loss. For generic catalogues that sell some assistive devices for people with hearing loss, see Chapter 4, "RESOURCES FOR ASSISTIVE DEVICES" section. For a listing of programs that offer special alerting devices in automobiles, see Chapter 4, "TRAVEL AND TRANSPORTATION ORGANIZATIONS" section.

<u>Alerting and Communication Devices for Deaf and Hard of Hearing People</u>
Laurent Clerc National Deaf Education Network and Clearinghouse
800 Florida Avenue, NE
Washington, DC 20002
(202) 651-5051 (V/TTY)   FAX (202) 651-5054
e-mail: clearinghouse.infotogo@gallaudet.edu
clerccenter.gallaudet.edu

A basic guide to the major categories of assistive devices. Available on web site only.

<u>Ameriphone</u>
12082 Western Avenue
Garden Grove, CA 92841
(800) 874-3005   (800) 772-2889 (TTY)   (714) 897-0808
FAX (714) 897-4703   e-mail: customerservice@ameriphone.com
www.ameriphone.com

Produces adaptive telephone equipment and television caption decoders.

<u>Assistive Listening Systems</u>
Architectural and Transportation Barriers Compliance Board (ATBCB)
1331 F Street, NW, Suite 1000
Washington, DC 20004
(800) 872-2253   (800) 993-2822 (TTY)   (202) 272-5434
(202) 272-5449 (TTY)   FAX (202) 272-5447
e-mail: info@access-board.gov   www.access-board.gov

Describes assistive listening systems. Available in versions for consumers, providers, and installers. Free. Also available on the web site.

Communication Access for Persons with Hearing Loss: Compliance with the Americans with Disabilities Act (ADA)
by Mark Ross (ed.)
York Press, Inc.
PO Box 504
Timonium, MD 21094
(800) 962-2763   FAX (410) 560-6758   e-mail: york@abs.net
www.yorkpress.com

This book explains the communications access provisions of the Americans with Disabilities Act and describes communication aids, such as FM, infrared, and induction loop systems, amplification devices, interpreters, alerting and signaling devices, and devices to help people with both hearing and vision loss. $37.50 plus $4.00 shipping and handling

Food and Drug Administration (FDA)
Office of Consumer Affairs
5600 Fishers Lane
Rockville, MD 20857
(888) 463-6332   (301) 827-4420   FAX (301) 443-9767
e-mail: execsec@oc.fda.gov   www.fda.gov

Distributes publications about hearing aids, which are regulated by the FDA. Free list of current titles.

General Hearing Instruments, Inc.
PO Box 23748
New Orleans, LA 70183-0748
(800) 824-3021   (504) 733-3767   FAX (504) 733-3799
www.generalhearing.com

Sells tinnitus products, such as tinnitus maskers, tinnitus instruments, and low-level noise generators.

Harris Communications
15155 Technology Drive
Eden Prairie, MN 55344
(800) 825-6758   (800) 825-9187   FAX (952) 906-1099
www.harriscomm.com

Sells products for individuals who are deaf and hard of hearing, such as TTYs, warning devices, clocks and wake-up alarms, assistive listening devices, telephones, and books, videotapes, and CDs. Free catalogue.

LS & S Group Inc. Catalogue
PO Box 673
Northbrook, IL 60065
(800) 468-4789   (847) 498-9777
e-mail: lssgrp@aol.com   www.lssgroup.com

This catalogue includes a variety of devices including clocks, telephones, amplifiers, TTYs, alerting systems, and assistive listening systems. Free

Oval Window Audio
33 Wildflower Court
Nederland, CO 80466
(303) 447-3607 (V/TTY/FAX)   e-mail: info@ovalwindowaudio.com
www.ovalwindowaudio.com

Produces induction assistive listening devices and visual and vibrotactile technology.

Phonic Ear
3880 Cypress Drive
Petaluma, CA 94954
(800) 227-0735   FAX (707) 781-9145   www.phonicear.com

Produces the Easy Listener, a personal FM amplification system.

Sound Advice About Hearing Aids
Federal Trade Commission (FTC)
Bureau of Consumer Protection
600 Pennsylvania Avenue, NW
Washington, DC 20580
(877) 382-4357   (202) 382-4357   (202) 326-2502 (TTY)
FAX (202) 326-2572   www.ftc.gov

This publication makes suggestions for consumers who are considering purchasing a hearing aid; discusses federal and state standards that apply to the sale of hearing aids; and where to file a complaint, if necessary. Free

Symphonix Devices, Inc.
2331 Zanker Road
San Jose, CA 95131
(800) 833-7733   FAX (408) 273-1795   www.symphonix.com

Sells the Vibrant Soundbridge, a surgically implanted hearing device that converts sound into vibrations that are transmitted to the middle ear.

Using a TTY
Architectural and Transportation Barriers Compliance Board (ATBCB)
1331 F Street, NW, Suite 1000
Washington, DC 20004
(800) 872-2253   (800) 993-2822 (TTY)   (202) 272-5434
(202) 272-5449 (TTY)   FAX (202) 272-5447
e-mail: info@access-board.gov   www.access-board.gov

A brochure with basic information about TTYs (also called TDDs or TTs). Free

Williams Sound Corporation
10399 West 70th Street
Eden Prairie, MN 55344
(800) 328-6190   FAX (952) 943-2174   www.williamsound.com

Sells assistive listening devices for personal use and assistive listening systems for group listening. Free catalogue.

SPEECH DISORDERS

More than 2.5 million Americans over the age of 15 have difficulty speaking so that their speech is understood. This disability affects 1% of the population age 15 to 64 years and 3.5% of the population 65 years or over (U.S. Bureau of the Census: 1986). The inability to communicate effectively creates a barrier to all types of social interactions, including education and employment.

CAUSES AND TYPES OF SPEECH IMPAIRMENTS

There are four types of speech impairments. *Disorders of articulation* include omission, distortion, substitution, or addition of sounds. These disorders may be either functional with no known organic cause, or they may have organic origins, such as cerebral palsy, brain damage, or cleft palate (Kriegman: 1978). *Disorders of the voice* involve defects of pitch and volume. These disorders are sometimes caused by abnormal growths on the vocal cords or by hearing impairments.

Disorders of time and rhythm of sound production result in speech that is difficult to listen to and is sometimes unintelligible. Stuttering is the most common type of disorder of time and rhythm. Stuttering is an involuntary hesitation in producing sounds or an involuntary repetition of the same sound. About 2.5 million Americans, or 1% of the population, stutter (Fraser: 1990). The cause of stuttering is unknown; although it has often been attributed to psychological problems, some researchers believe that the muscles used in speech and vocal cord regulation are responsible (U.S. Department of Health and Human Services: 1991).

Aphasia or *dysphasia* is the inability to recognize and use symbols and expressions. There are many different types of aphasia. In expressive aphasia, speech is slow and labored, and words connecting nouns and verbs are often missing; the individual is aware of his or her difficulties. In receptive aphasia, the person has difficulty understanding speech and in monitoring his or her own conversation; he or she is often unaware of these difficulties. Global aphasia consists of both expressive and receptive aphasia (Zezima: 1994). Some individuals with aphasia are able to speak fluently, but their understanding of speech is impaired. Others comprehend written and oral language but are nonfluent (Albert and Helm-Estabrooks: 1988). In most cases, aphasia is caused by strokes, but brain tumors and head injuries may also cause aphasia.

As noted above, many speech impairments are the result of *deafness* or *severe hearing impairment*. Teaching speech to children who are congenitally or prelingually deaf is a slow, laborious process. Visual cues help children to understand conversations. The delay in acquisition of language may affect the child's ability to keep pace with standard educational objectives. The individual never develops the same speaking skills that individuals with normal hearing do (Bowe: 1978). Children who are deaf have different articulation, frequency, and voice quality patterns than children with normal hearing (Bernstein et al.: 1990).

Cancer of the larynx is another cause of speech impairment. In advanced stages of the disease, the larynx, which contains the vocal cords, is removed surgically. Individuals whose larynx has been removed (often referred to as laryngectomees) must learn new ways of speaking, or they may use an artificial larynx. Artificial larynxes enable an early return to work while speech training is taking place; they also enable individuals whose surgery has been extensive or who do not have the motivation to learn a new way of speaking to continue oral communication.

Esophageal speech is a method that uses belches to form sounds. Although esophageal speech does not result in smooth sounds, it is the first step in learning pharyngeal speech. In pharyngeal speech, the individual blocks the air that enters the nose and mouth with quick tongue actions, causing it to vibrate against the pharynx (the empty space in the throat above the larynx). Pharyngeal speech requires a great deal of patience and practice before the speech approaches the sounds of normal speech.

A *cleft palate* is a split or fissure in the roof of the mouth. Cleft palate interferes with the formation of consonants, which are formed by pressure of the tongue on the roof of the mouth. Cleft palate is usually corrected by surgery. However, even individuals who have undergone successful surgery may still have speech impairments.

Cerebral palsy, a condition in which nerve tissues in the brain are defective or injured, results in partial paralysis and lack of muscle control. There are many varieties of cerebral palsy; those that cause respiratory problems frequently result in speech impairments. Because cerebral palsy is a central nervous system disorder, the effects on speech are generally those involving the motor mechanisms of speech (Weiss and Lillywhite: 1981).

PSYCHOLOGICAL ASPECTS OF SPEECH IMPAIRMENTS

The psychological responses to speech impairments vary with the type of impairment. Parents of children who are deaf or hearing impaired or who have cerebral palsy may find it overwhelming to learn about these conditions and the services available to help their children. At the same time, they must learn to cope with necessary changes in the family's way of living. Individuals who have cancer must learn to speak in a different way while they are facing the possible recurrence of the disease. Laryngectomees and individuals who stutter fear that they will be unable to communicate in everyday situations and worry about embarrassment. In addition, people who cannot speak fear that they will not be able to obtain help in case of an emergency. People with aphasia often have multiple disorders, since aphasia is usually caused by strokes or traumatic brain injuries. Depression is common and natural under these circumstances. Many people assume that individuals who cannot communicate verbally also lack normal intelligence. This inaccurate stereotype leads to further loss of self-esteem for the person who is nonverbal.

PROFESSIONAL SERVICE PROVIDERS

Speech-language pathologists aid in the recovery or maintenance of speech or language function. Speech-language pathologists conduct screenings to detect possible speech impairments. After an assessment of the condition, they design and implement programs to treat language difficulties. Often the test results obtained by speech-language pathologists will help the medical staff in caring for the individual with aphasia. Speech-language pathologists may have sub-specialties, so it is important to find one who has experience in the specific condition. Speech-language pathologists are certified by the American Speech-Language-Hearing Association (ASHA) and receive a certificate of clinical competence (CCC).

Other service providers who work with speech-language pathologists include *audiologists,* who help to determine whether hearing impairment is a contributory factor; *special educators,* who may help the speech-language pathologists determine the appropriate educational program for children; and *otolaryngologists,* who diagnose and treat the physical conditions affecting the ears and throat. *Social workers* may help individuals with speech impairments to locate appropriate service providers. Both social workers and *psychologists* provide counseling to help individuals overcome fears, embarrassment, and denial; accept changes; and learn how to cope effectively. *Rehabilitation counselors* help individuals find services and assistive devices that enable them to remain independent and find appropriate job placements.

WHERE TO FIND SERVICES

Both speech-language pathologists and audiologists work in schools, speech and hearing clinics, and private practices. Many colleges and universities that train speech-language pathologists and audiologists also operate clinics where they provide services to the public. The American Speech-Language-Hearing Association (ASHA) provides a free list of certified speech-language pathologists and audiologists in each state. Public school systems generally hire both speech-language pathologists and audiologists as regular staff members to provide services to students. State supported vocational rehabilitation agencies, otolaryngology departments, and rehabilitation units at hospitals also offer these services.

ASSISTIVE DEVICES

Devices that enable people with speech impairments to communicate are referred to as augmentative communication devices. Communication boards depict symbols that represent words or ideas; people who are unable to speak may point to the symbols to communicate. Speech synthesizers (which are also used by people who are visually impaired or blind) are artificial voices that utilize modern technology; they may be built into a communication board, or they may be part of a computer system. When part of a computer system, they may be used with a variety of options, such as printers, keyboards, and headpointers for people with limited mobility.

Portable communication aids operate on batteries and enable the user to locate words or phrases that are pronounced by a speech synthesizer. For people who have mobility impairments as well as speech impairments, switches are available to facilitate the use of these devices. Different types of switches are designed for operation by different parts of the body. For example, puff switches are activated by blowing into a mouthpiece; others may be operated by the hands or the feet; and still others may be mounted on wheelchairs.

Personal computers with speech synthesizers may be used in conjunction with software programs to train individuals with speech impairments to improve their verbal skills. These programs help with articulation, stuttering, pitch, and rate, and provide evaluative feedback of the individual's speech. Special programs have been developed for impairments caused by various conditions, such as aphasia and brain injury, and for children. Special instructional programs for children who have not developed speech use pictures along with communication boards that say the word associated with the picture. Some speech synthesizers connected to computers enable individuals with speech impairments to communicate over the telephone. Teletypewriters (TTYs), also called telecommunication devices for the deaf (TDDs) or text telephones (TTs), may also be used for phone communication by anyone who is unable to speak.

Portable speech amplifiers are available for people who have had laryngectomies. Devices to help people who have had laryngectomies learn to use their esophageal voice and artificial larynxes are also available.

References

Albert, Martin and Nancy Helm-Estabrooks
1988   "Diagnosis and Treatment of Aphasia, Part II" JAMA 259:8(February 26):1205-1210
Bernstein, Lynne E., Moise H. Goldstein, and James J. Mahshie
1990   "Speech Training Aids for Hearing-Impaired Individuals: Overview and Aims" Journal of Rehabilitation Research 25(4):53-62
Bowe, Frank
1978 Handicapping America New York, NY: Harper and Row
Fraser, Malcolm
1990 Self-Therapy for the Stutterer Memphis, TN: Speech Foundation of America
Kriegman, Lois
1978 "Speech and Language Disorders" pp. 541-559 in Robert M. Goldenson (ed.) Disability and Rehabilitation Handbook New York, NY: McGraw Hill
U.S. Bureau of the Census
1986 Disability, Functional Limitation, and Health Insurance Coverage: 1984/85 Current Population Reports, Series P-70, No. 8 Washington, DC: U.S. Government Printing Office
U.S. Department of Health and Human Services
1991 "Update on Stuttering" Stuttering: Hope through Research Washington, DC: National Institute on Deafness and Other Communication Disorders
Weiss, Curtis E. and Herold S. Lillywhite
1981 Communicative Disorders: Prevention and Early Intervention St. Louis, MO: C.V. Mosby
Zezima, Michele and Michael
1994 "Louder than Words: Treating Aphasia and Agnosia" Advance/Rehabilitation 3:8 (September):27-28

ORGANIZATIONS

American Cleft Palate-Craniofacial Association (ACPA)
104 South Estes Drive, Suite 204
Chapel Hill, NC 27514
(800) 242-5338   (919) 933-9044   FAX (919) 933-9604
e-mail: cleftline@aol.com   www.cleftline.org

A membership organization for professionals who treat patients with cleft palate and craniofacial deformities. Operates the Cleft Palate Foundation, which educates the public and disseminates publications to parents of children with cleft palates and to adults with cleft palates. Membership, $150.00, includes bimonthly "The Cleft Palate-Craniofacial Journal." Offers free publications. Also available on the web site.

American Speech-Language-Hearing Association (ASHA)
10801 Rockville Pike
Rockville, MD 20852
(800) 638-8255   FAX (301) 897-7355
e-mail: actioncenter@asha.org   www.asha.org

A professional organization of speech-language pathologists and audiologists. Toll-free HELPLINE offers answers to questions about conditions and services as well as referrals. Provides information on communication problems and a free list of certified audiologists and speech therapists for each state. Also available on the web site. Web site also lists self-help groups for individuals with speech and language disorders.

Council for Exceptional Children (CEC)
1110 North Glebe Road, Suite 300
Arlington, VA 22201
(888) 232-7733   (703) 620-3660   (703) 264-9446
FAX (703) 264-9494   www.cec.sped.org

A professional membership organization that works toward improving the quality of education for children who have disabilities or are gifted. Membership fees vary by geographic location. Special division for communicative disabilities and deafness; membership, $20.00. Publishes "Communications Disorders Quarterly," $39.00.

International Association of Laryngectomees (IAL)
8900 Thornton Road
Box 99311
Stockton, CA 95209
(866) 425-3678   FAX (209) 472-0516
e-mail: IAL@larynxlink.com   www.larynxlink.com

Sponsors self-help groups throughout the U.S. and disseminates information through its publications and videotapes. Newsletter, "IAL News," published three times a year, free.

MEDLINEplus: Speech and Communication Disorders
www.nlm.nih.gov/medlineplus/speechcommunicationsdisorders.html

This web site provides links to sites for general information about speech and communication disorders, symptoms and diagnosis, specific conditions/aspects, children, organizations, clinical trials, and research. Some information is available in Spanish. Provides links to MEDLINE research articles and related MEDLINEplus pages.

National Aphasia Association
29 John Street, Suite 1103
New York, NY 10038
(800) 922-4622   (212) 267-2812   e-mail: naa@aphasia.org
www.aphasia.org

Promotes public awareness, publishes public education brochures, and develops community programs for people with aphasia. Maintains list of health care professionals who will make referrals to local resources. Publishes a variety of inexpensive fact sheets and "Aphasia Community Group Manual," for organizers of local aphasia support groups, $30.00. Membership, $25.00, includes quarterly newsletter.

National Center for Stuttering
200 East 33rd Street
New York, NY 10016
(800) 221-2483   (212) 532-1460   FAX (212) 683-1372
e-mail: martin.schwartz@nyu.edu   www.stuttering.com

Trains stutterers to use new technique of breathing to relax vocal cords. Provides training for speech professionals. Hotline answers questions about stuttering.

National Craniofacial Association (FACES)
PO Box 11082
Chattanooga, TN 37401
(800) 332-2373   (423) 266-1632   FAX (423) 267-3124
e-mail: faces@faces-cranio.org   www.faces-cranio.org

Provides financial assistance to children and adults for travel for reconstructive facial surgery; sponsors support groups; and provides information and referral. Publishes quarterly newsletter, "Faces;" requests $10.00 donation to defray expenses.

National Easter Seal Society
230 West Monroe Street, Suite 1800
Chicago, IL 60606
(800) 221-6827   (312) 726-6200   (312) 726-4258 (TTY)
FAX (312) 726-1494   info@easter-seals.org
www.easter-seals.org

Promotes research, education, and rehabilitation for people with physical disabilities and
speech and language problems. Sponsors Easter Seal Stroke Clubs for people who have had
strokes, their families, and friends.

National Institute of Neurological Disorders and Stroke (NINDS)
Building 31, Room 8A06
31 Center Drive, MSC 2540
Bethesda, MD 20892
(800) 352-9424   (301) 496-5751   FAX (301) 402-2186
e-mail: braininfo@ninds.nih.gov   www.ninds.nih.gov

A federal agency that supports basic and clinical research on brain and nervous system
disorders.

National Institute on Deafness and Other Communication Disorders (NIDCD)
Building 31, Room 3C35
31 Center Drive, MSC 2320
Bethesda, MD 20892
(301) 496-7243   (301) 402-0252 (TTY)
www.nidcd.nih.gov

A federal agency that funds basic research studies on problems of hearing, balance, voice,
language, and speech.

National Institute on Deafness and Other Communication Disorders Information Clearinghouse
1 Communication Avenue
Bethesda, MD 20892
(800) 241-1044   (800) 241-1055 (TTY)   FAX (301) 907-8830
e-mail: nidcdinfo@nidcd.nih.gov   www.nidcd.nih.gov

Maintains a database of references, answers requests for information from the public and
professionals, and publishes biannual newsletter, "Inside NIDCD Information Clearinghouse."
Free

National Stroke Association (NSA)
9707 East Easter Lane
Englewood, CO 80112
(800) 787-6537   (303) 649-9299   FAX (303) 649-1328
e-mail: info@stroke.org   www.stroke.org

Assists individuals with stroke and educates their families, physicians, and the general public about stroke. Membership, $25.00. Publishes bimonthly newsletter, "Stroke Smart," $12.00. Publications are available on the web site.

National Stuttering Association
5100 East La Palma Avenue, Suite 208
Anaheim Hills, CA 92807
(800) 364-1677   FAX (714) 693-7554
e-mail: NSAstutter@aol.com   www.nsastutter.org

A membership organization of individuals who stutter, their families, and service providers. Sponsors self-help groups, holds conferences, and publishes self-help guides, videotapes, and audiocassettes. Membership, regular, $35.00; students, $20.00; includes monthly newsletter, "Letting GO."

Stroke Connection
American Heart Association
7272 Greenville Avenue
Dallas, TX 75231
(888) 478-7653   www.strokeassociation.org

Coordinates a network of more than 1200 stroke clubs and groups. The Stroke Group Registry provides referrals to these groups; (800) 553-6321. Sponsors "Common Threads PenFriends," which matches stroke survivors, caregivers, and family members. Bimonthly newsletter, "Stroke Connection Magazine," $12.00. A courtesy subscription is available to any stroke survivor unable to pay. Also available on the web site.

Stuttering Foundation of America
3100 Walnut Grove Road, Suite 603
Memphis, TN 38111
(800) 992-9392   (901) 452-7343   FAX (901) 452-3931
e-mail: stutter@vantek.net   www.stutteringhelp.org

Dedicated to the prevention of stuttering in children and improved treatment for adults. Hotline answers questions about stuttering. Provides information packet and referrals for parents of children who stutter. Maintains a national list of referrals. Conducts conferences for professionals. Produces numerous inexpensive publications and videotapes about stuttering.

United Cerebral Palsy Association (UCP)
1660 L Street, NW, Suite 700
Washington, DC 20036
(800) 872-5827   (202) 842-1266
e-mail: natl@ucp.org   www.ucp.org

Member groups throughout the country provide treatment, information, education, and counseling. Web site links user to resources in his or her state, including education, housing, sports and leisure, employment, parenting and families, and transportation.

U.S. Society for Augmentative and Alternative Communication (USSAAC)
PO Box 21418
Sarasota, FL 34276
(941) 312-0992   e-mail: USSAAC@home.com   www.ussac.org

A membership organization that advocates for augmentative and alternative communication for individuals who do not speak. Conducts public awareness activities; provides information and referrals and professional education. Membership, consumers/families, $27.00; professionals, $53.00; includes quarterly newsletter, "Speak Up."

Aphasia
National Institute on Deafness and Other Communication Disorders Information Clearinghouse
1 Communication Avenue
Washington, DC 20892
(800) 241-1044   (800) 241-1055 (TTY)   FAX (301) 907-8830
e-mail: nidcdinfo@nidcd.nih.gov   www.nidcd.nih.gov

This fact sheet describes the causes of aphasia, diagnosis, and treatment. Includes resource list. Free. Also available on the web site.

Aphasia Community Group Manual
National Aphasia Association
Response Center
351 Butternut Court
Millersville, MD 21108
(800) 922-4622   FAX (4100) 729-5724   www.aphasia.org

This manual provides information on how to start a group, including needs assessment, recruiting members, ideas for programs, and resources. $30.00 plus $3.00 shipping and handling

Augmentative and Alternative Communication
by David R. Beukelman and Pat Mirenda
Paul Brookes Publishing Company
PO Box 10624
Baltimore, MD 21285-0624
(800) 638-3775   FAX (410) 337-8539
e-mail: custserv@pbrookes.com   www.pbrookes.com

This book discusses the communication needs of children and adults with disabilities and methods of implementing augmentative and alternative communication. $59.95 plus 10% shipping and handling

Coping with Aphasia
by Jon C. Lyon
Thomson Learning
7625 Empire Drive
Florence, KY 41042
(800) 347-7707   FAX (859) 647-5023
www.thomsonlearning.com

This book deals with the causes and medical treatments of aphasia as well as the emotional aspects. $53.00

Directory: Information Resources for Human Communication Disorders
National Institute on Deafness and Other Communication Disorders Information Clearinghouse
1 Communication Avenue
Washington, DC 20892
(800) 241-1044   (800) 241-1055 (TTY)   FAX (301) 907-8830
e-mail: nidcdinfo@nidcd.nih.gov   www.nidcd.nih.gov

This directory provides a listing and description of organizations throughout the country that deal with communication disorders. Free. Also available on the web site.

Foundations of Spoken Language for Hearing-Impaired Children
by Daniel Ling
Alexander Graham Bell Association for the Deaf
3417 Volta Place, NW
Washington, DC 20007
(800) 432-7543   (202) 337-5220   (202) 337-5221 (TTY)
FAX (202) 337-8314   e-mail: info@agbell.org   www.agbell.org

This textbook describes advances in the techniques of teaching spoken language to children who are hearing impaired. $44.95 plus $9.00 shipping and handling

A Handbook on Stuttering
by Oliver Bloodstein
Thomson Learning
7625 Empire Drive
Florence, KY 41042
(800) 347-7707   FAX (859) 647-5023
www.thomsonlearning.com

This book presents a review of the research on the causes, incidence, and treatment of stuttering. $67.95

If Your Child Stutters: A Guide for Parents
Stuttering Foundation of America
3100 Walnut Grove Road, Suite 603
Memphis, TN 38111
(800) 992-9392   (901) 452-7343   FAX (901) 452-3931
e-mail: stutter@vantek.net   www.stutteringhelp.org

A guide that enables parents to provide appropriate help for children who stutter. Available in English, Spanish, and French. $1.00

Lookin' for Me
National Aphasia Association
29 John Street, Suite 1103
New York, NY 10038
(800) 922-4622   (212) 267-2812   e-mail: naa@aphasia.org
www.aphasia.org

This videotape features interviews with three individuals with aphasia. It emphasizes how to communicate with people who have aphasia. 22 minutes. $10.00

Managing Stroke: A Guide to Living Well After Stroke
by Paul R. Rao, Mark N. Ozer, and John E. Toerge (eds.)
National Rehabilitation Hospital
102 Irving Street, NW
Washington, DC 20010
(202) 877-1776   (202) 829-5180   www.nrhrehab.org

This book provides information on the medical, financial, and psychological aspects of living with stroke. Includes guidance for choosing a rehabilitation program. $13.95 plus $4.00 shipping and handling

Parents and Teachers: Partners in Language Development
by Audrey Simmons-Martin and Karen Glover Rossi
Alexander Graham Bell Association for the Deaf
3417 Volta Place, NW
Washington, DC 20007
(800) 432-7543   (202) 337-5220   (202) 337-5221 (TTY)
FAX (202) 337-8314   e-mail: info@agbell.org   www.agbell.org

This book describes strategies for teaching language to school age children in both the school and at home. $27.95 plus $9.00 shipping and handling

Parents, Families, and the Stuttering Child
by Lena Rustin (ed.)
Thomson Learning, Florence, KY

This book focuses on the preschool children and school age children who stutter and how the family can help. Out of print

Self-Therapy for the Stutterer
by Malcolm Fraser
Stuttering Foundation of America
3100 Walnut Grove Road, Suite 603
Memphis, TN 38111
(800) 992-9392   (901) 452-7343   FAX (901) 452-3931
e-mail: stutter@vantek.net   www.stutteringhelp.org

A self-help guide that enables adults who stutter to overcome the problems on their own. Available in English and Spanish. $3.00

Stroke Survivors
by William H. Bergquist, Rod McLean and Barbara A. Kobylinski
Jossey-Bass Publishers, San Francisco, CA

This book uses the personal histories of stroke survivors to describe the stroke experience, the recovery and rehabilitation process, and the viewpoints of caregivers. Out of print

Stuttering and Your Child: A Videotape for Parents
Stuttering Foundation of America
3100 Walnut Grove Road, Suite 603
Memphis, TN 38111
(800) 992-9392   (901) 452-7343   FAX (901) 452-3931
e-mail: stutter@vantek.net   www.stutteringhelp.org

This videotape provides parents, teachers, and health care providers with information about what to expect when a child stutters and how to help children speak more clearly with less stuttering. 30 minutes. $10.00

Talk with Me
by Ellyn Altman
Alexander Graham Bell Association for the Deaf
3417 Volta Place, NW
Washington, DC 20007
(800) 432-7543   (202) 337-5220   (202) 337-5221 (TTY)
FAX (202) 337-8314   e-mail: info@agbell.org   www.agbell.org

This book discusses the early decisions that affect speech, language, auditory, and emotional development of children with hearing impairments. $22.95 plus $7.50 shipping and handling

Telecommunications Relay Services: An Informational Handbook
Federal Communications Commission (FCC)
445 12th Street, SW
Washington, DC 20554

(888) 225-5322   (888) 835-5322 (TTY)   (202) 418-0190
(202) 418-2555 (TTY)   e-mail: fccinfo@fcc.gov   www.fcc.gov

A booklet that describes how telecommunications relay services work. Lists telephone numbers to reach communication assistants and to obtain information about this service in each state. Free. Also available on the web site; click on "Disabilities Issues."

RESOURCES FOR ASSISTIVE DEVICES

All catalogues are free unless otherwise noted.

Ablenet
1081 Tenth Avenue, SE
Minneapolis, MN 55414
(800) 322-0956   FAX (612) 379-9143
www.ablenetinc.com

Mail order catalogue of communication aids; switches and control units for off-the-shelf appliances; and battery powered toys. Produces videotapes and conducts technology workshops.

Attainment Company, Inc.
PO Box 930160
Verona, WI 53593-0160
(800) 327-4269   FAX (608) 845-7880
e-mail: info@attainmentcompany.com
www.attainmentcompany.com

Mail order catalogue of augmentative communication devices.

Communication Aids for Children and Adults
Crestwood Company
6625 North Sidney Place
Milwaukee WI 53209
(414) 352-5678   FAX (414) 352-5679
e-mail: crestcomm@aol.com   www.communicationaids.com

Mail order catalogue with a wide variety of teaching aids for children and adults with speech impairments, toys, switches, and other products for people who have both speech and mobility impairments.

Communication Skill Builders
19500 Bull Verde
San Antonio, TX 78270
(800) 866-4446   FAX (800) 232-1223
www.psychcorp.com

Mail order catalogue with a wide variety of products for children and adults with speech impairments and evaluative tools for professionals.

Don Johnston, Inc.
26799 West Commerce Drive
Volo, IL 60073
(800) 999-4660   (847) 740-0749   FAX (847) 740-7326
e-mail: info@donjohnston.com   www.donjohnston.com

Mail order catalogue of communication boards, speech synthesizers used in conjunction with software programs that teach speech, adapted computer equipment, and publications.

Dynavox Systems
2100 Wharton Street, Suite 400
Pittsburgh, PA 15203
(888) 697-7332   (412) 381-4883   FAX (412) 381-5241
e-mail: sales@dynavoxsys.com   www.dynavoxsys.com

Produces augmentative communication hardware and software, communication boards, and accessories.

Imaginart Communication Products
307 Arizona Street
Bisbee, AZ 85603
(800) 828-1376   FAX (800) 737-1376
e-mail: imaginart@compuserve.comwww.imaginartonline.com

Mail order catalogue of augmentative communication devices for children and adults; special products for people with traumatic brain injury, aphasia, and cleft palate; videotapes; and books.

Prentke Romich Company
1022 Heyl Road
Wooster, OH 44691
(800) 262-1933   FAX (330) 263-4829
e-mail: sales@prentrom.com   www.prentrom.com

Produces augmentative communication systems and alternative computer access devices. Provides training in the use of their products.

Words+
1220 West Avenue J
Lancaster, CA 93534
(800) 869-8521   (661) 723-6523   FAX (661) 723-2114
e-mail: info@words-plus.com   www.words-plus.com

Produces augmentative communication hardware and software, communication boards, and accessories.

Chapter 6

DIABETES

Diabetes mellitus is a term that applies to a variety of disorders related to the production or utilization of insulin, a substance that is necessary to metabolize the glucose (a sugar) that the body needs for energy. As a result of diabetes, the body is unable to maintain normal glucose levels. *Hypoglycemia* is a condition where the level of glucose is too low. It occurs when the individual does not eat soon enough or eats too little, uses too much insulin, or engages in overactivity. Hypoglycemia may lead to an insulin reaction; symptoms may include feeling shaky or sweaty, headache, hunger, irritability, and dizziness. Insulin shock sometimes occurs if an insulin reaction is not treated quickly; in these cases individuals may lose consciousness. *Hyperglycemia* is a condition where the level of glucose in the blood is too high. Symptoms include extreme thirst, a dry mouth, excessive urination, blurred vision, and lethargy. Sometimes when an individual who has had an insulin reaction takes food high in sugar to replace glucose in the body, too much glucose is released, resulting in high blood glucose levels (hyperglycemia). The combination of too much sugar without enough insulin to use it properly may gradually lead to diabetic coma if warning signs are not monitored; diabetic coma usually occurs only in individuals with insulin-dependent diabetes.

As the prevalence of diabetes has increased, it has become a major health problem in the United States and an important contributor to the cost of health care. From 1980 to 1996, the number of individuals with diagnosed diabetes increased 26% (Centers for Disease Control and Prevention: 1999). Over 10 million Americans age 20 or older, or 5.1% of the population, have been diagnosed with diabetes; an additional 5.4 million have the disease but have not been diagnosed (Harris et al.: 1998). Diabetes is an age-related disease, occurring in 18.4% of those age 65 or over (Centers for Disease Control and Prevention: 1997). African-Americans and Hispanics have higher rates of diabetes than whites. Unfortunately, the data sources for determining rates of diabetes among other minority groups are inadequate and do not provide accurate estimates. It is known that among Native Americans, rates vary by tribe and that the Pima Indians of Arizona have the highest recorded prevalence - more than 50% of adults age 35 or over have diabetes (Centers for Disease Control and Prevention: 1997).

Diabetes was the second most frequent primary diagnosis for individuals who visited internal medicine specialists in 1989 (Schappert: 1992). Direct medical expenses for diabetes care totaled 44.1 billion dollars in 1997. Factoring in the cost of lost work productivity and premature mortality increased the cost of the disease by an additional 54 billion dollars. On a per capita basis, individuals with diabetes spent on average $10,071 in 1997 for medical care compared to $2,669 for individuals without diabetes (American Diabetes Association: 1998).

Diabetes and its complications are responsible for many hospital stays and have a large economic impact on society. Ng et al. (2001) found that individuals with diabetes lost about one-third of their annual earnings, due in large part to the complications caused by the disease.

Currently, there is no cure for diabetes; however, there are means to control the disease and to decrease the risk of the numerous associated complications. Early diagnosis and intervention are crucial steps in maintaining proper control of diabetes.

Transplantations of the pancreas (the gland responsible for secreting insulin), although no longer considered experimental, are performed only in a select group of patients. Currently, transplantations are performed on patients who have end-stage renal disease, have had or plan to have a kidney transplant as well, have serious clinical difficulty with insulin injections, and do not present an excessive risk for this type of surgery (American Diabetes Association: 2001). When successful, pancreas transplantation results in the elimination of insulin injections. Rejection of transplanted tissue and the need for large amounts of immunosuppressive drugs are important factors that have prevented this type of transplantation from becoming standard procedure. Because people with diabetes are especially prone to infection, transplantation involves more risks for this population than for other individuals. Research to improve the management of diabetes through innovative administration of insulin and drugs that improve the body's use of insulin are ongoing. Transplantation of islet cells that are responsible for insulin production in the pancreas is also under investigation.

TYPES OF DIABETES

The two major types of diabetes mellitus are referred to as type 1 and type 2. In *type 1*, the pancreas does not produce insulin. Individuals with type 1 diabetes must take regular injections of insulin. For this reason, type 1 is also referred to as insulin-dependent diabetes mellitus (IDDM). This variant of the disease was formerly called juvenile-onset diabetes, because it is usually diagnosed at a young age. Symptoms of type 1 diabetes include extreme thirst, weight loss despite increased appetite, weakness and fatigue, and blurred vision.

Approximately five to ten percent of Americans who have diabetes have type 1 (Centers for Disease Control and Prevention: 1998). In addition to daily insulin injections, individuals with type 1 diabetes must carefully watch their diet and coordinate meals with insulin doses to maintain a balanced glucose level. Insulin may be injected by syringe or by "jet injectors" that do not use actual needles. Some individuals, especially those who are on erratic schedules that prevent them from eating on a regular schedule, use insulin pumps that automatically provide insulin throughout the day. The use of insulin pumps often results in improved control of blood glucose levels over other methods. Prior to eating, pump users determine the amount of insulin they need and program the pump to release that amount.

In *type 2* diabetes, the body produces some insulin but does not produce enough or does not utilize it properly. Because type 2 diabetes usually does not require insulin injections, it is also referred to as noninsulin-dependent diabetes mellitus (NIDDM). This type of the disease is often called adult-onset or maturity-onset diabetes, because it is most frequently diagnosed after age forty. It is estimated that over 90% of the cases of diabetes in the United States are type 2 (Centers for Disease Control and Prevention: 1998). It has been estimated that type 2 diabetes may be present for up to 12 years before it is diagnosed (Harris et al.: 1992).

Although the causes of type 2 diabetes are not known, obesity (80 to 90% of all individuals with type 2 diabetes are obese) and a family history of diabetes are predisposing factors. Symptoms of type 2 diabetes include fatigue, frequent urination, excessive thirst, and vaginal infections in women. Individuals who have these symptoms should make an appointment for a physical examination. However, diabetes is sometimes present when no symptoms are evident (Williams: 1983). Tests for glucose in urine or a blood glucose test conducted during a routine physical examination are often the first indications of diabetes.

In many cases, type 2 diabetes can be controlled through both diet and exercise. For obese individuals who have diabetes, a change in diet and reduction of caloric intake may make a dramatic difference in blood glucose levels. Research suggests that individuals with type 2 diabetes may lower their blood glucose and insulin levels throughout the day by increasing the frequency and decreasing the size of their meals. This strategy slows the rate of carbohydrate absorption. A possible disadvantage is that obese individuals who use this dietary plan may have a tendency to gain weight (Jenkins: 1995).

A subtype of diabetes caused by a defect in the mitochondrial DNA has recently been discovered. Called maternally inherited diabetes and deafness (MIDD) because the mitochondrial DNA is inherited only from the mother, this type of diabetes is associated with deafness and may be either type 1 or type 2 diabetes (Kobayashi et al.: 1997). Approximately 1.5% of the people that have diabetes have MIDD (Paquis-Flucklinger et al.: 1998), although it is highly likely that they are unaware of the type of diabetes they have. In most cases, individuals with this type of diabetes are not obese. If they have type 2 diabetes, they usually do not need insulin in the early stages of the disease, although they may need it as the disease progresses. Protein in the urine, a sign of kidney disease, is sometimes diagnosed in individuals with MIDD; this clinical symptom is caused by the mutation, not the diabetes (Jansen et al.: 1997). A study of individuals with MIDD found that subjects treated with a dietary supplement, coenzyme Q10, had better outcomes in terms of beta cell production (the cells produced by the pancreas that are responsible for insulin production) and hearing than members of a control group (Suzuki et al.: 1998).

Diet and exercise for people with any type of diabetes should be planned with a physician's advice to ensure that all medical conditions are taken into account. The goals of dietary restrictions are to control the intake of glucose (carbohydrates) and to reduce total body weight for those with type 2 diabetes. Policy recommendations from the American Diabetes Association (1994) indicate that the use of simple sugars, such as sucrose (table sugar) is not off limits and that they do not cause greater or more rapid rises in blood glucose than other carbohydrates. Scientific evidence suggests that sucrose has a similar effect on blood glucose as bread, rice, and potatoes. It is important to keep in mind the total amount of carbohydrates consumed; simple sugars must be used in place of other carbohydrates in the diet. Federal law that mandates nutritional labeling of foods makes the calculation much easier, as the amount of carbohydrates per serving must be indicated on the food label. In order to control the amount of carbohydrates, many foods, including desserts and candies, are sweetened with artificial sweeteners. The American Diabetes Association has produced many publications about diet for people with diabetes, including "Exchange Lists" (developed jointly with the American Dietetic Association), which list foods with similar caloric and nutrient contents (see "PUBLICATIONS AND TAPES" section below).

Exercise helps the body to burn off the glucose and thus is an important part of the plan to control diabetes. In some individuals with type 2 diabetes, the muscle cells that are receptors for glucose do not work efficiently; exercise enables muscle cells to use the glucose efficiently without requiring more insulin (Cantu: 1982). Exercise also reduces fat, which is known to reduce the body's sensitivity to insulin. After consulting with a physician, even individuals who have been sedentary can begin a gradual exercise program by starting to take brief daily walks. A regular exercise regimen has been shown to be useful in reducing the required levels of daily insulin injections.

When diet and exercise are insufficient to control type 2 diabetes, oral medications are prescribed. Sulfonylureas are a type of medication that causes the pancreas to produce increased amounts of insulin. Side effects of this type of medication include hypoglycemia and hyperinsulinemia, a condition in which too much insulin is in the bloodstream. Hyperinsulinemia is a risk factor for vascular disease and heart attack. In addition, sulfonylureas often fail to work after a number of years, as the pancreas can no longer produce sufficient insulin. When this occurs, individuals must begin injecting insulin.

Several drugs that use different mechanisms to control diabetes were approved in the 1990s by the Food and Drug Administration. One drug that has been available throughout much of the world since the late 1950s, metformin (Glucophage), was approved for use in the United States in 1995. Although it is not clear exactly how metformin works, it decreases the amount of glucose produced by the liver and increases the muscles' uptake of glucose, thereby lowering blood glucose levels. Metformin has no serious side effects, unless the individual has kidney disease at the outset. Another drug approved by the Food and Drug Administration is acarbose, a carbohydrase inhibitor. Carbohydrases are the enzymes that break down carbohydrates and turn them into glucose. The side effects of acarbose are bloating, gas, and diarrhea, which may subside after six months of taking the drug (American Diabetes Association: 1995). Troglitazone (Rezulin), approved by the FDA in the 1990s, has been implicated in a small number of liver problems and fatalities and has been removed from the market.

Although testing urine for sugar was previously used to monitor blood glucose levels, this method is not as accurate as testing the blood directly. People with both types of diabetes use home blood glucose monitoring equipment to measure glucose levels; this involves putting a drop of blood from the fingertip on a specially treated strip designed to react to the glucose and placing the strip in the monitor. The color of the strip indicates the level of glucose that is present. A digital display or speech output indicates the blood glucose level, and some monitors even record the date and time of the reading. Illness, even a simple cold, can affect how the body uses insulin; glucose monitoring is even more important at these times. Log booklets enable individuals to keep a record of their blood glucose levels and to analyze their diets and schedules to determine what causes them to have varying levels of blood glucose. Home blood glucose monitors are inexpensive and are quite compact, making them suitable for travel and to take to work or school.

Both types of diabetes have the same potential long term health effects. It is essential that everyone with diabetes be aware of the proper management of their disease and all of the potential complications. Complications of diabetes include greater risks of heart disease, stroke, infections, and kidney disease; circulatory problems that can be especially problematic for legs and feet (resulting in amputation in extreme cases); neuropathy or nerve disease which may cause tingling, numbness, double vision, pain, or dizziness; and vision problems. Good control of blood glucose levels can help to prevent these long term complications.

Among the leading vision problems caused by diabetes is diabetic retinopathy. Visual impairment occurs when the small blood vessels in the retina are damaged and fail to nourish the retina adequately. One consequence of this process is bleeding inside the eye. If detected early, diabetic retinopathy can sometimes be treated successfully by laser therapy. In other cases, complex surgical procedures are performed in the attempt to restore useful vision. To manage their diabetes, many people with visual impairments use a wide range of adapted equipment, such as glucometers, scales, and thermometers with speech output; syringe magnifiers; special insulin gauges; and special syringes that automatically measure insulin doses.

The Diabetes Control and Complications Trial (DCCT) (1993) reported the results of a study which monitored 1,441 individuals with type 1 diabetes who were assigned to receive either conventional therapy (one or two injections of insulin daily) or intensive therapy (three or more injections of insulin daily). Results indicate that the intensive therapy group had a significantly lower incidence of retinopathy, nephropathy, and neuropathy. The chief adverse effect of intensive therapy was increased episodes of severe hypoglycemia. In a follow-up study, the DCCT investigators (2000) reported that the effects of intensive therapy continued to decrease the rates of retinopathy and nephropathy four years later.

A British study carried out over a period of 20 years (UK Prospective Diabetes Study Group: 1998a) found that intensive control had similar benefits for individuals with type 2 diabetes. Individuals whose diabetes was controlled by sulfonylureas or insulin also had increased episodes of hypoglycemia. Obese individuals treated with metformin had even lower risks for diabetes complications and fewer episodes of hypoglycemia than individuals treated with sulfonylureas or insulin (UK Prospective Diabetes Study Group: 1998b).

Currently, the National Institute of Diabetes and Digestive and Kidney Diseases is conducting national studies to see if both types of diabetes can be prevented. Close relatives of individuals who have type 1 diabetes and who have a greater than 50% risk of developing the disease are randomly assigned to an experimental group that receives two daily doses of insulin injections plus a four day hospital stay each year to receive intravenous insulin. Those who have a 25 to 50% risk of developing the disease are randomly assigned to an experimental group that receives oral medication, such as insulin and other beta cell materials. Each trial includes a control group that does not receive treatment (Diabetes Dateline: 1994). Individuals with impaired glucose tolerance are subjects in a study to learn how to prevent type 2 diabetes. Members of minority groups with high rates of type 2 diabetes, obese individuals, and women who have had gestational diabetes are assigned to test groups who undergo behavioral modification of diet and exercise or receive oral anti-diabetes medications (Diabetes Dateline: 1996).

DIABETES IN CHILDREN

Approximately 123,000 children and teenagers have diabetes (Centers for Disease Control and Prevention: 1998). Childhood diabetes (type 1 or IDDM) is often first diagnosed by a family physician, usually after an acute episode marked by extreme thirst, unexplained weight loss, and/or frequent urination. Children with diabetes are often referred to a pediatric diabetes specialist or to a specialty clinic for training in the management of their condition.

In recent years, there has been a noticeable increase in type 2 diabetes in children and adolescents. Although little is known about this variant of the disease, most of the children are overweight or obese, have a family history of type 2 diabetes, and are over the age of ten. The early age at which the disease occurs suggests that these children are at greater risk for complications of diabetes, which are directly related to duration of the disease. Children who are not ill when they are first diagnosed may be treated with diet and exercise, although most progress to using drugs to treat their hyperglycemia (American Diabetes Association: 1999).

Children with diabetes should be taught to accept the major responsibility for control of their disease. School personnel should be informed about the student's diabetes and should know the warning signs of an insulin reaction and what measures to take if an insulin reaction occurs. Generally, there is no need to avoid participation in sports; however, extra carbohydrates may be needed after strenuous activity.

Diabetes may be especially difficult to manage during the teenage years, when peer pressure is strong and body image takes on new emphasis. Health care providers have noted and research (Weissberg-Benchell et al.: 1995) has confirmed that teenagers often avoid proper diabetes self-management, including skipping insulin shots, eating inappropriate food, and falsifying blood glucose readings. Parents frequently underestimate these behaviors. When diabetes is out of control in adolescence, puberty may be delayed and growth slowed (Davis et al.: 1991). Hamp's review (1984) found that diabetes in youths was likely to be in good control if the diabetes regimen was part of the family routine; the family was highly cohesive; parents treated the child with diabetes and siblings equally; the family supported the child in diabetes self-management; and familial and financial situations were stable.

It has often been suggested that children and youths with type 1 diabetes are at higher risk for depression than the general population. A study (Kovacs et al.: 1997) confirmed that this is indeed the case. Following 92 children from the onset of their diabetes for as long as ten years, Kovacs and her colleagues concluded that youngsters with diabetes are most likely to experience depression in the first year following their diagnosis. By ten years after diagnosis, 42.4% had experienced at least one episode of psychiatric disorder, including depression, anxiety, or behavior disorder. Depression was the most common disorder, with 27.5% of the subjects experiencing a major depressive episode. These findings suggest that both parents and health care providers should be alert to changes in youngsters' behavior following diagnosis of diabetes and seek appropriate counseling.

Children and teenagers with diabetes often attend a "diabetes camp" where they can meet others with diabetes. In such a setting, youths can learn how to cope effectively and discuss their feelings about diabetes. Attendance at a camp also provides the family with a respite period.

It is not uncommon for parents to feel guilty about their child's condition, especially when the child must undergo painful tests and treatments. Feelings of guilt on the part of the parents may result in poor judgment regarding their decisions about the child; in addition, the child may sense the guilt and in turn feel guilty for causing this problem for his or her parent (Finston: 1993). Other children in the family may feel neglected when parents are concentrating on the care of a sibling with diabetes.

Parents should not allow their emotions to interfere with rational management for their child's diabetes care. Not only should they have an agreement with each other about helping their child manage his or her diabetes, they should not allow the child to manipulate them in order to avoid blood glucose testing or monitoring. When one parent is manipulated by the child, it affects not only the child's health, but also the relationship between the parents, causing friction in their marriage (Rosin: 1997). Professional counselors or family support groups may help parents cope with these feelings and also offer valuable practical information and emotional support.

DIABETES IN ELDERS

Over six million Americans (18.4%) age 65 years or older have diabetes (Centers for Disease Control and Prevention: 1998). Over half of the elders who have diabetes have experienced long term reduction in their activity (Centers for Disease Control and Prevention: 1997). The prevalence rate of diabetes in African-American adults age 65 to 74 is consistently higher than in white Americans of the same age. As might be expected, the rate of severe complications is also higher; amputations, visual impairment, and kidney disease are more prevalent in African-Americans than in whites (National Institute of Diabetes and Digestive and Kidney Disease: 1990).

The costs of the supplies used to monitor diabetes control have been a barrier for some individuals, especially those on limited or fixed incomes. Beginning July 1, 1998, Medicare will pay for the cost of supplies for all beneficiaries who have diabetes, whether or not they take insulin. Supplies include blood glucose monitors, lancets, test strips, insulin, etc.

Elders, especially those who live alone, must understand the importance of their diet in diabetes control. If they receive meals-on-wheels or attend a senior meal site, they should make known their special dietary needs. Senior health programs which include screenings for hypertension, diabetes, and vision problems; foot care programs; and exercise classes may help reduce the incidence of diabetes complications. (For a more detailed description of diabetes in elders, see Resources for Elders with Disabilities, described in "PUBLICATIONS AND TAPES" section below.)

PSYCHOLOGICAL ASPECTS OF DIABETES

Although shock, fear, and depression are normal reactions to diabetes at first, these emotions may subside once the individual understands how to control the disease. Many people feel a loss of control over their bodies. Because diabetes affects so many parts of the body, it also affects many aspects of daily life. In addition to prescribed changes in diet and exercise, individuals with diabetes must always be aware of the symptoms that indicate hyperglycemia or hypoglycemia. Individuals who must take daily injections of insulin may have to overcome a fear of needles; talking with others who have experienced this fear and overcome it may prove extremely valuable.

Changes in daily routines are never accepted readily. For individuals with diabetes, changes in lifestyle and the need to monitor glucose may cause great stress. Social events and travel must be carefully planned to ensure that meals will comply with special diets.

The diagnosis of diabetes may result in the fear that most food is off limits and that it will be impossible to enjoy eating. The knowledge that people with diabetes should eat what is considered a healthy diet for the general public as long as they keep track of their carbohydrate intake may prove comforting to individuals who have recently been diagnosed with diabetes. In addition, a number of food manufacturers cater to the dietary needs of individuals with diabetes by producing foods that are low in carbohydrates; their products are often available in the dietetic food section of supermarkets. Perseverance in tracking down the right foods will allow for an interesting and varied diet; however, the shock and depression that follow the diagnosis of diabetes may limit the individual's emotional endurance. Support from a family member or close friend can help the person with diabetes to carry out this endeavor.

Public libraries are a good source for the myriad cookbooks that have been written especially for people with diabetes. Discovering the variety of interesting recipes, including those for dessert and candies, should prove to be a psychological boost for the person who fears being restricted to bland meals.

The fears and lifestyle changes mentioned above put individuals with diabetes at risk for depression. A study by Anderson et al. (2001) reviewed a large number of studies to determine if individuals with diabetes experienced depression at higher rates than individuals without the disease. Indeed, individuals with diabetes were twice as likely to experience clinical depression (requiring treatment) as those without the disease; women and those whose diabetes was not in control were most likely to experience depression.

Children with type 1 diabetes usually adjust quickly to insulin injections, and even young children learn to administer their own insulin. Adolescents with diabetes may worry about being different from their peers at a time of life when conformity is highly valued. It is common for all adolescents to worry about school, social life, and the future; for adolescents with diabetes, this additional factor makes the stress greater.

Parents of children with type 1 diabetes must cope with the knowledge that their child has a chronic disease; they may have the same feelings as an adult who has just been diagnosed as having diabetes. Although the exact cause of diabetes is still unknown, parents often feel guilty that their child may have inherited traits that put him or her at risk for diabetes. Families must adjust to the strict schedule of meals, injections, and monitoring necessary to manage their child's diabetes. Parents must try not to be over-protective and should allow their children to participate in normal recreational activities.

Diligent efforts to control glucose by following the recommended dosages of insulin or diets do not always result in the desired response. Individuals whose glucose is out of control should learn not to feel guilty; they may need to have their dosage and diet modified by a health care professional.

A common response to adult-onset or type 2 diabetes is that "It's just a touch of diabetes." This response can be extremely dangerous when the individual fails to properly monitor and control the disease. Individuals with diabetes and their family members must discuss the disease and its potential effects so that they understand the importance of the prescribed dietary regimen, exercise, and blood glucose monitoring. It should not be assumed that children or elders with diabetes are not capable of caring for themselves properly solely because of their age. Family members should be instructed to allow these individuals to have the maximum responsibility possible for caring for themselves.

PROFESSIONAL SERVICE PROVIDERS

Because diabetes is a systemic disease, it has a wide range of effects. As a result, many types of health care professionals are involved in caring for people with diabetes.

Family physicians and *internists* are the physicians in charge of coordinating the various aspects of care for individuals with diabetes. *Diabetologists* (endocrinologists) are physicians who specialize in the treatment of individuals with diabetes. *Nephrologists* are physicians who treat people with kidney disease, which is a common complication of diabetes. *Ophthalmologists* are physicians who specialize in diseases of the eye. If diabetic retinopathy is detected, individuals are often referred to subspecialists called retina and vitreous specialists.

Certified diabetes educators (CDE) are health care professionals certified by the American Association of Diabetes Educators to teach individuals with diabetes how to effectively manage their disease. Certified diabetes educators may be physicians or nurses. Many are dieticians or nutritionists who help people with diabetes plan a diet to control their blood glucose levels.

Psychologists, *social workers*, and other counselors help people with diabetes and their family members adjust to the regimen prescribed to control the diabetes.

WHERE TO FIND SERVICES

In some areas, special treatment centers for diabetes and dialysis centers for people with kidney disease are available. The special physicians listed above practice in hospitals or have private practices. Affiliates of the American Diabetes Association (ADA) exist in every state. These affiliates may provide publications, educational programs, sponsor camps for children with diabetes, and make referrals to local resources. The national office (described in the "ORGANIZATIONS" section below) can provide the address and phone number of local affiliates. The ADA also has information about support groups that individuals can join. Understanding that others with diabetes continue to live fulfilling lives can be an extremely important benefit of attending support groups. People with diabetes who have vision problems may obtain services from public or private rehabilitation agencies serving individuals who are visually impaired or blind (see Chapter 11, "Visual Impairment and Blindness").

ASSISTIVE DEVICES

Individuals with insulin-dependent diabetes use a variety of devices to administer their insulin, such as syringes; insulin pens which combine the insulin dose and injector; needle-free jet injectors; and insulin pumps, which automatically deliver insulin slowly throughout the day and night through a plastic tube attached to a needle. Equipment to measure blood glucose is necessary for both type 1 and type 2 diabetes. Some private health insurance policies will pay some of the costs for glucose monitors and test strips. It is wise to check with the insurance carrier before purchasing such equipment. (See section above "Diabetes in Elders" regarding Medicare's policy.)

Supplies and equipment to help individuals with diabetes to monitor and manage their disease are usually available at pharmacies or medical supply stores. Mail order catalogues also sell these supplies.

HOW TO RECOGNIZE AN INSULIN REACTION AND GIVE FIRST AID

Individuals experiencing an insulin reaction may feel shaky or dizzy, sweat profusely, complain of a headache, or act irritable. Suggestions for giving first aid to individuals who have had an insulin reaction are:

> • Give the individual some food, such as orange juice, milk, or even sugar itself, to replace the low blood sugar level. Many individuals with diabetes carry sugar packets, glucose tablets, or candy with them for use in emergencies.
> • If the individual is unconscious, rub honey or another sugary substance into the mouth, between the teeth and cheek.

Frequent insulin reactions should be reported to the physician. It is recommended that individuals with diabetes wear a medical identification bracelet so that emergency care personnel will know that they have diabetes.

References

American Diabetes Association
2001 "Pancreas Transplantation for Patients with Diabetes Mellitus" Diabetes Care 24(January):Supplement 1:S93
2000 "Consensus Statement: Type 2 Diabetes in Children and Adolescents" Diabetes Care 23:3(March):381-389
1998 "Economic Consequences of Diabetes Mellitus in the U.S. in 1997" Diabetes Care 21:2(February):296-309
1995 "Surge Protector" Diabetes Forecast 48:5(May):23-24
1994 "Nutrition Recommendations and Principles for People with Diabetes Mellitus" Diabetes Care 17:5(May):519-522
Anderson, Ryan J. et al.
2001 "The Prevalence of Comorbid Depression in Adults with Diabetes: A Meta-analysis" Diabetes Care 24:6(June):1069-1078
Cantu, Robert C.
1982 Diabetes and Exercise New York, NY: E.P. Dutton
Centers for Disease Control and Prevention
1999 Diabetes Surveillance 1999 Atlanta, GA: Public Health Service
1998 National Diabetes Fact Sheet: National Estimates and General Information on Diabetes in the United States Atlanta, GA: Centers for Disease Control and Prevention
1997 National Diabetes Fact Sheet: National Estimates and General Information on Diabetes in the United States Atlanta, GA: Centers for Disease Control and Prevention

Davis, Sherry E. et al.

1991 "Developmental Tasks and Transitions of Adolescents with Chronic Illnesses and Disabilities" pp. 70-79 in Robert P. Marinelli and Arthur E. Dell Orto (eds.) The Psychological and Social Impact of Disability New York, NY: Springer Publishing

Diabetes Control and Complications Trial Research Group

2000 "Retinopathy and Nephropathy in Patients with Type 1 Diabetes Four Years after a Trial of Intensive Therapy" New England Journal of Medicine 342:6(February 10):381-389

1993 "The Effect of Intensive Treatment of Diabetes on the Development and Progression of Long-Term Complications in Insulin-Dependent Diabetes Mellitus" New England Journal of Medicine 329:14(September 30):977-986

Diabetes Dateline

1996 "Volunteers Sought for NIDDK Studies" Diabetes Dateline Fall p. 4

1994 "NIDDK Launches Study to Prevent Insulin-Dependent Diabetes" Diabetes Dateline May pp. 1-2

Finston, Peggy

1993 "Quitting the Self-Blame Game" Diabetes Forecast 46:12(December):46-49

Hamp, Melissa

1984 "The Diabetic Teenager" pp. 217-238 in Robert W. Blum (ed.) Chronic Illness and Disabilities in Childhood and Adolescence Orlando, FL: Grune and Stratton

Harris, Maureen I. et al.

1998 "Prevalence of Diabetes, Impaired Fasting Glucose, and Impaired Glucose Tolerance in U.S. Adults" Diabetes Care 21:4(April):518-524

Harris, Maureen I. et al.

1992 "Onset of NIDDM Occurs at Least 4-7 Years before Clinical Diagnosis" Diabetes Care 15:7(July):815-819

Jansen, J.J. et al.

1997 "Mutation in Mitochondrial tRNA (Leu(UUR)) Gene Associated with Progressive Kidney Disease" Journal of the American Society of Nephrology 8:7(July):1118-1124

Jenkins, David J.A.

1995 "Nutritional Principles and Diabetes" Diabetes Care 18:11(November):1491-1498

Kobayashi, Tetsuro et al.

1997 "In Situ Characterization of Islets in Diabetes with a Mitochondrial DNA Mutation at Nucleotide Position 3243" Diabetes 46:1(October):1567-15710

Kovacs, Maria et al.

1997 "Psychiatric Disorders in Youths with IDDM: Rates and Risk Factors" Diabetes Care 20:1(January):36-44

National Institute of Diabetes and Digestive and Kidney Diseases

1990 Diabetes-Related Programs for Black Americans: A Resource Guide NIH Publication No. 90-1585 Bethesda, MD: National Diabetes Information Clearinghouse

Ng, Ying Chu, Philip Jacobs, and J.A. Johnson

2001 "Productivity Losses Associated with Diabetes in the U.S," Diabetes Care 24:2(February):257-261

Paquis-Flucklinger, V. et al.

1998 "Importance of Searching for mtDNA Defects in Patients with Diabetes and Hearing Deficit" Diabetologia 41:740-741

Rosin, Lindsay

1997 "Family Matters" Diabetes Forecast 50:2(February):65-66, 68

Schappert, Susan M.

1992 "Office Visits for Diabetes Mellitus: United States, 1989" Advance Data from Vital and Health Statistics, No. 211, DHHS Pub. No. (PHS) 92-1250. Hyattsville, MD: Public Health Service, March 24, 1992

Suzuki, S. et al.

1998 "The Effects of Coenzyme Q10 Treatment on Maternally Inherited Diabetes and Deafness and Mitochondrial DNA 3243 (A to G) Mutation" Diabetologia 41:5(May):584-588

UK Prospective Diabetes Study Group

1998a "Intensive Blood-Glucose Control with Sulphonylureas or Insulin Compared with Conventional Treatment and Risk of Complications in Patients with Type 2 Diabetes" The Lancet 352(September 12):837-853

1998b "Effect of Intensive Blood-Glucose Control with Metformin on Complications in Overweight Patients with Type 2 Diabetes" The Lancet 352(September 12):854-865

Weissberg-Benchell, Jill et al.

1995 "Adolescent Diabetes Management and Mismanagement" Diabetes Care 18:1(January):77-82

Williams, T. Franklin

1983 "Diabetes Mellitus in Older People" pp. 411-415 in William Reichel (ed.) Clinical Aspects of Aging Baltimore, MD: Williams and Wilkins

American Association of Diabetes Educators (AADE)
100 West Monroe, Suite 400
Chicago, IL 60603
(800) 338-3633   (312) 424-2426   FAX (312) 424-2427
e-mail: mhorner@aadenet.org   www.aadenet.org

Membership organization for health care professionals who work with people with diabetes. Holds annual meeting. Membership, $110.00, includes a bimonthly journal, "The Diabetes Educator," $45.00. Journal only, $55.00.

American Association of Kidney Patients (AAKP)
3505 East Frontage Road, Suite 315
Tampa, FL 33607
(800) 749-2257   (813) 636-8100   FAX (813) 636-8122
e-mail: info@aakp.org   www.aakp.org

Advocates on behalf of patients with kidney disease; sponsors local patient and family support groups; holds conferences and seminars. Membership, patients/families, $25.00; professionals, $35.00; includes quarterly newsletter, "aakpRENALIFE." Also available on the web site.

American Diabetes Association (ADA)
1701 North Beauregard Street
Alexandria, VA 22311
(800) 342-2383   In the Washington, DC, (703) 549-1500
FAX (703) 836-7439   e-mail: customerservice@diabetes.org
www.diabetes.org

National membership organization with local affiliates. Publications for both professionals and consumers, including cookbooks and guides for the management of diabetes (see "PUBLIC-ATIONS AND TAPES" section below). Membership, $28.00, which includes membership in a local affiliate, discounts on publications, a subscription to "Diabetes Forecast" (Also available on cassette from the National Library Service. See Chapter 11, "Visual Impairment and Blindness"). The January issue includes a resource guide to diabetes products. Many local affiliates offer their own publications, sponsor support groups, and conduct professional training programs. The web site includes featured articles from "Diabetes Forecast" and the medical journal "Diabetes Care" as well as basic information on diabetes. Publications ordered through the web site receive a discount. A toll-free hotline [(800) 342-2383)] offers information on diabetes and a packet of information.

American Dietetic Association (ADA)
216 West Jackson Boulevard
Chicago, IL 60606
(800) 877-1600   (312) 899-0040   FAX (312) 899-1758
e-mail: hotline@eatright.org   www.eatright.org

Consumers may receive a referral to a registered dietitian or receive information about nutrition on the telephone or on the web site. Available in English and Spanish.

American Kidney Fund
6110 Executive Boulevard, Suite 1010
Rockville, MD 20852
(800) 638-8299   (301) 881-3052   FAX (301) 881-0898
e-mail: helpline@akfinc.org   www.kidneyfund.org

Provides public and professional education and financial aid to individuals who have chronic kidney problems.

Amputee Coalition of America (ACA)
National Limb Loss Information Center
900 East Hill Avenue, Suite 285
Knoxville, TN 37915
(888) 267-5669   (865) 524-8772   FAX (865) 525-7917
e-mail: info@amputee-coalition.org www.amputee-coalition.org

Provides education and support services to individuals with amputations through a network of peer support groups, educational programs for health professionals, and a database of resources. Membership, individuals, $25.00; professionals, $50.00; includes bimonthly magazine, "In-Motion." Guides for organizing peer support groups and peer visitation programs also available.

CDC Division of Diabetes Translation
PO Box 8728
Silver Spring, MD 20910
(877) 232-3422   FAX (301) 562-1050
e-mail: diabetes@cdc.gov   www.cdc.gov/diabetes

The Centers for Disease Control Division of Diabetes Translation conducts research related to the prevalence of diabetes; assesses clinical practices in order to develop optimal treatment; and works with state health departments to develop diabetes control programs.

Diabetes Action Network, National Federation of the Blind
1412 I-70 Drive SW, Suite C
Columbia, MO 65203
(573) 875-8911   FAX (573) 875-8902
www.nfb.org/diabetes.htm

A national support and information network. Publishes a quarterly magazine, "Voice of the Diabetic," which includes personal experiences, medical information, recipes, and resources. Available in standard print, four-track audiocassette, and on the web site. Nonmembers may also obtain free subscriptions but are encouraged to pay $20.00. Also available, "Diabetes Resources: Equipment, Services and Information," a list of adaptive equipment; available in standard print and alternate formats, $5.00. Order from: National Federation of the Blind, 1800 Johnson Street, Baltimore, MD 21230. Also available on the web site.

Diabetes Exercise and Sports Association (DESA)
formerly International Diabetic Athletes Association
PO Box 1935
Litchfield Park, AZ 85340
(800) 898-4322   (623) 535-4593   FAX (623) 535-4741
e-mail: desa@diabetes-exercise.org www.diabetes-exercise.org

An organization that provides education for individuals with diabetes who participate in sports and fitness activities, family members, and service providers through conferences, workshops, and publications. Membership, individuals, $30.00; corporate, $150.00; includes quarterly newsletter, "The Challenge."

Diabetes-Sight.org
www.diabetes-sight.org

Sponsored by Prevent Blindness America, this web site provides information for individuals and professionals about prevention of vision loss due to diabetes. Includes interactive tools such as a quiz, vision loss simulation, and tour of the eye's anatomy as well as research summaries and preferred practice guidelines.

Juvenile Diabetes Research Foundation International (JDRF)
120 Wall Street, 19th Floor
New York, NY 10005
(800) 533-2873   (212) 785-9500   FAX (212) 785-9595
e-mail: info@jdrf.org   www.jdrf.org

Supports research and provides information to individuals with diabetes and their families. Chapters in many states and affiliates in other countries. Membership, $25.00, includes quarterly magazine, "Countdown," "Countdown for Kids," and discounts on books.

MEDLINEplus: Diabetes
www.nlm.nih.gov/medlineplus/diabetes.html

This web site provides links to sites for general information about diabetes, symptoms and diagnosis, treatment, alternative therapy, clinical trials, disease management, organizations, and research. Includes an interactive tutorial. Some information available in Spanish.

National Diabetes Education Program (NDEP)
National Institute of Diabetes and Digestive and Kidney Diseases (NIDDKD)
31 Center Drive, MSC 2560
Washington, DC 20892
(800) 438-5383   (301) 496-3583   www.ndep.nih.gov

A joint project of the National Institutes of Health and the Centers for Disease Control and Prevention, this program aims to prevent the increase in diabetes in this country through partnerships with other organizations that will provide public information about the disease. The web site has information about diabetes, and the program has produced public information materials, including cookbooks.

National Diabetes Information Clearinghouse (NDIC)
1 Information Way
Bethesda, MD 20892
(800) 860-8747   (301) 654-3327   FAX (301) 907-8906
e-mail: ndic@info.niddk.nih.gov   www.niddk.nih.gov/health/diabetes/ndic.htm

Responds to information requests from the public and professionals. Maintains a database of publications and brochures. Publishes newsletter, "Diabetes Dateline," free. Free list of publications (see "PUBLICATIONS AND TAPES" section below). Also available on the web site. Many publications are available on the web site.

National Institute of Diabetes and Digestive and Kidney Diseases (NIDDKD)
National Institutes of Health
Center Drive, MSC 2560
Building 31, Room 9A-04
Bethesda, MD 20892
(301) 496-3583   www.niddk.nih.gov

Funds basic and clinical research in the causes, prevention, and treatment of diabetes. Free list of publications. The web site contains fact sheets and patient education materials. Publications available in English and Spanish.

National Kidney and Urologic Diseases Information Clearinghouse (NKUDIC)
3 Information Way
Bethesda, MD 20892
(800) 891-5390   (301) 654-4415   FAX (301) 907-8906
e-mail: nkudic@info.niddk.nih.gov www.niddk.nih.gov

Responds to individual requests from the public and professionals about diseases of the kidneys and the urologic system. Free list of publications. Also available on the web site. Publications available in English and Spanish.

National Kidney Foundation (NKF)
30 East 33rd Street
New York, NY 10016
(800) 622-9010   FAX (212) 779-0068   www.kidney.org

A professional membership organization that provides professional and public education; produces literature on kidney disease; and promotes kidney transplantation and organ donation. Information about kidney disease available on the web site.

Neuropathy Association
60 East 42nd Street, Suite 942
New York, NY 10165
(800) 247-6968   (212) 692-0662   FAX (212) 692-0668
e-mail: info@neuropathy.org   www.neuropathy.org

This organization serves individuals who experience neuropathy and their family members through the support of research into the causes and treatments of neuropathy, education, and dissemination of information. Membership, free, includes newsletter and informational materials.

The American Diabetes Association Complete Guide to Diabetes
American Diabetes Association
Order Fulfillment
PO Box 930850
Atlanta, GA 31193-0850
(800) 232-6733   FAX (404) 442-9742

This book includes information about type 1 and type 2 diabetes, including how to maintain good blood glucose levels, selecting health care providers, planning an exercise program, and enjoying sex. $23.95 plus $4.99 shipping and handling

Caring for Young Children Living with Diabetes: A Manual for Parents
Joslin Diabetes Center
Publications Department
One Joslin Place
Boston, MA 02215
(800) 344-4501   FAX (508) 285-8382   www.joslin.org

This book discusses how parents can successfully manage diabetes in children less than eight years old and how to interact with professional health care providers. $8.50 plus $4.00 shipping and handling

Coping with Limb Loss
by Ellen Winchell
Penguin Putnam, Inc.

Written by a woman who had a limb amputated, this book provides information about surgery, prosthetics, and rehabilitation as well as practical coping strategies. Out of print

Diabetes and the Kidneys
American Kidney Fund
6110 Executive Boulevard, Suite 1010
Rockville, MD 20852
(800) 638-8299   (301) 881-3052   FAX (301) 881-0898
e-mail: helpline@akfinc.org   www.kidneyfund.org

A booklet that describes how diabetes affects the kidneys' function and measures that may be taken to slow down the course of kidney disease. Single copy, free.

Diabetes and Vision Loss: Special Considerations
by Marla Bernbaum
in "Meeting the Needs of People with Vision Loss: A Multidisciplinary Perspective"
Resources for Rehabilitation
22 Bonad Road
Winchester, MA 01890
(781) 368-9094   FAX (781) 368-9096
e-mail: orders@rfr.org   www.rfr.org

Provides information on the psychosocial implications and special rehabilitation needs of individuals with vision loss due to diabetes. Available in standard print and audiocassette. $24.95 plus $5.00 shipping and handling. (See order form on last page of this book.)

The Diabetes Carbohydrate and Fat Gram Guide
by Lea Ann Holzmeister
American Dietetic Association (ADA)
PO Box 97215
Chicago, IL 60678-7215
(800) 877-1600, ext. 5000   (312) 899-0040, ext. 5000   FAX (312) 899-4899
www.eatright.org

This book lists the carbohydrate and fat content of foods, including packaged foods and foods purchased at fast food restaurants. $14.95 plus $4.99 shipping and handling

Diabetes: Caring for Your Emotions as Well as Your Health
by Jerry Edelwich and Archie Brodsky
Harper Collins
PO Box 588
Dunmore, PA 18512
(800) 242-7737   www.harpercollins.com

In addition to describing diabetes and its treatment, this book discusses the many effects diabetes has on social and psychological aspects of life. Practical suggestions for adaptation and relationships with medical personnel and family are provided. Information about sexual function, employment, technology, and support groups is also included. $15.00 plus $2.75 shipping and handling

The Diabetes Home Video Guide: Skills for Self Care
Joslin Diabetes Center
Publications Department
One Joslin Place
Boston, MA 02215
(800) 344-4501   FAX (508) 285-8382   www.joslin.org

This videotape covers exercise, blood glucose monitoring, nutrition, medications, lifestyle changes, and emotions. Uses people who have diabetes, not actors. 2 hours. Available in English and Spanish. $20.00 plus $4.00 shipping and handling

Diabetes Self-Management
PO Box 52890
Boulder, CO 80321-1125
(800) 234-0923   www.diabetes-self-mgmt.com

A bimonthly magazine that helps people with diabetes manage their disease. Tips on diet, foot care, medical news, etc. $18.00

Diabetes Type 2 & What to Do
by Virginia Valentine, June Biermann and Barbara Toohey
McGraw Hill, Order Services
PO Box 545
Blacklick, OH 43004
(800) 722-4726   FAX (614) 755-5645   www.mmhe.com

Written in question and answer format, this book addresses the effects of type 2 diabetes including information on diet and nutrition, exercise, emotional aspects, and paying for medical care. Many case examples are presented throughout the book. Includes reading list and Internet resources. Virginia Valentine and June Biermann have diabetes. $16.95 plus $5.00 shipping and handling

Diabetic Retinopathy: Information for Patients
National Eye Institute (NEI)
Building 31, Room 6A32
2020 Vision Place
Bethesda, MD 20892
(301) 496-5248   www.nei.nih.gov

This booklet discusses the symptoms of diabetic retinopathy; treatment; vitrectomy; and research. Available free in large print and on the web site from NEI and on audiocassette ($2.00) from VISION Community Services, 23A Elm Street, Watertown, MA 02472.

The Diabetic's Book
by June Biermann and Barbara Toohey
Penguin Putnam, Inc.
(800) 788-6262   www.penguinputnam.com

This book answers basic questions about diabetes, including diet, exercise, management of the disease, emotional responses, and other aspects of daily life. June Biermann has had type 2 diabetes since 1965. $13.95

Don't Lose Sight of Diabetic Eye Disease: Information for People at Risk
National Eye Institute (NEI)
Building 31, Room 6A32
2020 Vision Place
Bethesda, MD 20892
(301) 496-5248   www.nei.nih.gov

This booklet describes how diabetes affects the eyes and problems such as cataract, glaucoma, and diabetic retinopathy. Discusses symptoms, diagnosis, and treatment of diabetic retinopathy. Available free in large print and on the web site from NEI and on audiocassette ($2.00) from VISION Community Services, 23A Elm Street, Watertown, MA 02472.

Exchange Lists for Meal Planning
American Diabetes Association (ADA)
Order Fulfillment
PO Box 930850
Atlanta, GA 31193-0850
(800) 232-6733   FAX (404) 442-9742

This guide lists foods based on carbohydrate, protein, and fat content. $1.75 plus $4.99 shipping and handling. Discounts available on bulk orders.

Good Health with Diabetes through Exercise
Joslin Diabetes Center
Publications Department
One Joslin Place
Boston, MA 02215
(800) 344-4501   FAX (508) 285-8382   www.joslin.org

This booklet, written for those who use insulin and those who do not, tells how to get started on an exercise plan, what pitfalls to avoid, and how to integrate exercise with food and medications. $3.45 plus $4.00 shipping and handling

Guide to Raising a Child with Diabetes
by Linda Siminero and Jean Betschart
American Diabetes Association (ADA)
Order Fulfillment
PO Box 930850
Atlanta, GA 31193-0850
(800) 232-6733   FAX (404) 442-9742

This book provides advice that enables parents to help their child adjust to diabetes, insulin injection, and blood glucose testing while participating in normal childhood activities. $16.95 plus $4.99 shipping and handling

I Hate to Exercise
American Diabetes Association (ADA)
Order Fulfillment
PO Box 930850
Atlanta, GA 31193-0850
(800) 232-6733   FAX (404) 442-9742

This book promotes the value of 30 minutes of exercise a day to strengthen muscles, heart, and control diabetes. $14.95 plus $4.99 shipping and handling

The Johns Hopkins Guide to Diabetes for Today and Tomorrow
by Christopher D. Saudek, Richard R. Rubin, and Cynthia Shump
Johns Hopkins University Press
PO Box 50370
Baltimore, MD 21211-4370
(800) 537-5487   (410) 516-6989
FAX (410) 516-6998   www.press.jhu.edu

Written by a physician, a psychologist, and a nurse who specialize in treating individuals with diabetes, this book provides basic information on diabetes and its treatment, emotional and social aspects of the disease, complications, and sexuality and reproduction. $16.95; large print, $21.50; plus $5.00 shipping and handling.

Living with Diabetes $1.75 per copy
Living with Diabetic Retinopathy $1.75 per copy
Resources for Rehabilitation
22 Bonad Road
Winchester, MA 01890
(781) 368-9094   FAX (781) 368-9096
e-mail: orders@rfr.org   www.rfr.org

Designed for distribution by professionals to people with diabetes, these large print (18 point bold type) publications describe the condition, service providers, organizations, devices, and publications. Minimum purchase 25 copies. (See order form on last page of this book.)

Living with Diabetes: A Winning Formula
Info Vision
102 North Hazel Street
Glenwood, IA 51534
(800) 237-1808   FAX (888) 735-2622
e-mail: sales@4infovision.com   www.infovision.com

This videotape provides information about diet, weight loss, insulin, and self-monitoring of blood glucose and gives recipes. 35 minutes. $25.00 plus $5.00 shipping and handling

Living with Low Vision: A Resource Guide for People with Sight Loss
Resources for Rehabilitation
22 Bonad Road
Winchester, MA 01890
(781) 368-9094   FAX (781) 368-9096
e-mail: orders@rfr.org   www.rfr.org

A large print (18 point bold type) comprehensive directory that helps people with sight loss locate the services that they need to remain independent. Chapters describe products that enable people to keep reading, working, and carrying out their daily activities. Information about resources on the Internet is included. $46.95 plus $5.00 shipping and handling. (See order form on last page of this book.)

Managing Diabetes on a Budget
by Leslie Y. Dawson
American Diabetes Association (ADA)
Order Fulfillment
PO Box 930850
Atlanta, GA 31193-0850
(800) 232-6733   FAX (404) 442-9742

This book provides advice on finding the best buys on supplies and medications, cooking tips, and general diabetes management. $7.95 plus $4.99 shipping and handling

Managing Your Diabetes with Insulin
Joslin Diabetes Center
Publications Department
One Joslin Place
Boston, MA 02215
(800) 344-4501   FAX (508) 285-8382   www.joslin.org

Written for individuals with type 2 diabetes, this booklet provides information on how to use insulin in their treatment plan. $3.45 plus $4.00 shipping and handling

A Man's Guide to Coping with Disability
Resources for Rehabilitation
22 Bonad Road
Winchester, MA 01890
(781) 368-9094   FAX (781) 368-9096
e-mail: orders@rfr.org   www.rfr.org

This book includes information about men's responses to disability, with a special emphasis on the values men place on independence, occupational achievement, and physical activity.

Chapter on diabetes includes information about sexual functioning. $44.95 plus $5.00 shipping and handling (See last page of this book for order form.)

Mayo Clinic on Managing Diabetes
by Maria Collazo-Clavell (ed.)
Mayo Clinic Foundation
PO Box 609
Calverton, NY 11933
(800) 291-1128   FAX (631) 369-0615   www.mayo.com

This book provides a basic introduction for newly diagnosed patients and family members. Includes "20 Tasty Recipes for People with Diabetes." $14.95 plus $3.95 shipping and handling

Monitoring Your Blood Sugar
Juvenile Diabetes Research Foundation
120 Wall Street, 19th Floor
New York, NY 10005
(800) 223-1138   (212) 889-7575   FAX (212) 785-9595
e-mail: info@jdfcure.com   www.jdfcure.com

This brochure describes the process and benefits of blood glucose monitoring. Free

My Sister Rose Has Diabetes
by Monica Driscoll Beatty
Health Press
PO Box 37470
Albuquerque, NM 87176
(877) 411-0707   FAX (505) 888-1521
e-mail: goodbooks@healthpress.com
www.healthpress.com

Written for children ages seven to 12, this book describes diabetes as well as the reactions of Rose, her brother, and her parents. $8.95 plus $400 shipping and handling

National Diabetes Information Clearinghouse (NDIC)
1 Information Way
Bethesda, MD 20892
(301) 654-3327   FAX (301) 907-8906
e-mail: ndic@info.niddk.nih.gov   www.niddk.nih.gov/health/diabetes/ndic.htm

Sponsored by the federal government, this clearinghouse publishes a variety of booklets related to diabetes. Titles include "Diabetes Dictionary," a glossary of terms individuals with diabetes are likely to encounter; "Diabetes Overview;" "Medicines for People with Diabetes;"

"Diabetes and Periodontal Disease," a brochure describing the nature of periodontal disease, its relation to diabetes, and proper care of teeth and gums; and "Self-Monitoring of Blood Glucose." Free. Also available on the web site.

Resources for Elders with Disabilities
Resources for Rehabilitation
22 Bonad Road
Winchester, MA 01890
(781) 368-9094   FAX (781) 368-9096
e-mail: orders@rfr.org   www.rfr.org

This resource guide provides information about services and products that older individuals with disabilities and chronic conditions need to function independently. Includes chapters on diabetes, vision loss, hearing loss, Parkinson's disease, stroke, arthritis, and osteoporosis. Large print. $49.95 plus $5.00 shipping and handling. (See order form on last page of this book.)

The Role of Insulin
AIMS Media
9710 DeSoto Avenue
Chatsworth, CA 91311
(800) 367-2467   (818) 773-4300   FAX (818) 341-6700
www.aims-multimedia.com

This videotape describes how body cells use insulin and the causes and treatments for hypoglycemia and hyperglycemia. 18 minutes. $150.00 plus $9.95 shipping and handling

Take Charge of Your Diabetes
CDC Division of Diabetes Translation
PO Box 8728
Silver Spring, MD 20910
(877) 232-3422   FAX (301) 562-1050
e-mail: diabetes@cdc.gov   www.cdc.gov/diabetes

A book written in simple language and printed in large type to help people with diabetes manage their disease. Information on blood sugar, dental, foot, vision, and kidney problems, and nerve damage. Includes forms for keeping records of visits with health care providers and sick days. Free

A Touch of Diabetes: A Straightforward Guide for People Who Have Type 2, Non-Insulin Dependent Diabetes
by Lois Jovanovic-Peterson, Charles M. Peterson, and Morton Stone
John Wiley and Sons
1 Wiley Drive
Somerset, NJ 08875
(800) 225-5945   (908) 469-4400   FAX (908) 302-2300
www.wiley.com

This guide to help people with type 2 diabetes manage their condition includes information about preventing complications and dietary advice. $13.95 plus $5.00 shipping and handling

The Uncomplicated Guide to Diabetes Complications
by Marvin E. Levin and Michael A. Pfeifer
American Diabetes Association (ADA)
Order Fulfillment
PO Box 930850
Atlanta, GA 31193-0850
(800) 232-6733   FAX (404) 442-9742

This book covers the major complications that diabetes may cause, including nephropathy, heart disease, stroke, and neuropathy. Special issues such as obesity, pregnancy, and hypoglycemia are also discussed. $18.95 plus $4.99 shipping and handling

Weight Loss: A Winning Battle
Joslin Diabetes Center
Publications Department
One Joslin Place
Boston, MA 02215
(800) 344-4501   FAX (508) 285-8382   www.joslin.org

This booklet provides information that helps people control their weight and offers strategies for losing weight. $3.45 plus $4.00 shipping and handling

Weight Management for Type II Diabetes: An Action Plan
by Jackie Labat and Annette Maggi
John Wiley and Sons
1 Wiley Drive
Somerset, NJ 08875
(800) 225-5945   (908) 469-4400   FAX (908) 302-2300
www.wiley.com

This book provides recommendations for lifestyle changes for weight control and good diabetes management. $15.95 plus $5.00 shipping and handling

A Woman's Guide to Coping with Disability
Resources for Rehabilitation
22 Bonad Road
Winchester, MA 01890
(781) 368-9094   FAX (781) 368-9096
e-mail: orders@rfr.org   www.rfr.org

This book addresses the special needs of women with disabilities and chronic conditions, such as social relationships, sexual functioning, pregnancy, childrearing, caregiving, and employment. Written for women in all age categories, the book has chapters on the disabilities that are most prevalent in women or likely to affect the roles and physical functions unique to women including diabetes. $44.95 plus $5.00 shipping and handling (See last page of this book for order form.)

SPECIAL EQUIPMENT FOR PEOPLE WITH VISUAL IMPAIRMENT

Many types of equipment used by individuals with diabetes to monitor and manage their disease are made with large print or speech output. Major distributors of the most commonly used types of equipment are listed below.

Accu-Chek Voicemate
Roche Diagnostics
9115 Hague Road
Indianapolis, IN 46250
(800) 428-5074   e-mail: accu-chek.care@roche.com
www.accu-chek.com

This talking blood glucose monitor has a feature that identifies insulin vials. Instructions provided in large print and cassette. Available in English and Spanish.

Becton Dickinson Consumer Products
Becton Dickinson & Co.
One Becton Drive
Franklin Lakes, NJ 07417
(888) 232-2737
www.bd.com/diabetes

Sells Magni-Guide with magnification of 2X, that snaps onto Lilly, Nordisk, and Squibb-Novo insulin bottle caps. May be used with 1, .5, and .3 cc syringes.

Medicool, Inc.
23520 Telo Avenue, Suite 6
Torrance, CA 90505
(800) 433-2469   (310) 784-1200
e-mail: medicool@medicool.com   www.medicool.com

Sells Count-a-Dose, a device that measures insulin and is used with the Becton Dickinson .5 cc syringe; has tactile marking and audible clicks. Accommodates two insulin vials.

Meditec, Inc.
3322 South Oneida Way
Denver, CO 80224
(303) 758-6978

Sells the Holdease needle guide and syringe/vial holder and Insulgages, permanent, pre-calibrated for doses ranging from 2 to 85 units. May be marked with print, braille, or raised numbers.

Palco Labs
8030 Soquel Drive, #104
Santa Cruz, CA 95062
(800) 346-4488   In CA, (831) 476-3151   FAX (831) 476-1114
e-mail: palcodiab@aol.com   www.palcolabs.com

Manufactures Insul-eze, which magnifies the syringe calibrations, and Load-Matic, which allows users to set the dosage by touch. Sells the Insulcap, which attaches to an insulin vial, holding both vial and syringe, and guides insertion of syringe.

Whittier Medical, Inc.
865 Turnpike Street
North Andover, MA 01845
(800) 645-1115   (978) 688-5002

Manufactures the Truhand, a syringe and vial holder with 3x magnifier.

Chapter 7

EPILEPSY

Epilepsy is a condition in which the brain's cells undergo abnormal electrical activity, causing disturbances in the nervous system. An epileptic seizure occurs when there is an excessive discharge of electrical impulses from these nerve cells. To be classified as epilepsy, these seizures must be recurring events; individuals who have isolated incidents of seizures do not have epilepsy. Epilepsy is not a single disease or condition, nor is it contagious. It often develops in people whose families have no history of epilepsy, although children of individuals with epilepsy are thought to have a greater chance of developing this condition (Epilepsy Foundation of America: 1994).

Nearly 1.4 million American adults have epilepsy (Adams and Marano: 1995). About a third of the 125,000 new cases diagnosed each year occur in individuals under the age of 18 (Hauser and Hesdorffer: 1990). Children with cerebral palsy, autism, or mental retardation may also have epilepsy. Individuals with severe head trauma, stroke, and infections in the central nervous system are at the greatest risk for epilepsy. Nearly half (47%) of all individuals with epilepsy have activity limitations (National Center for Health Statistics: 1988).

Physicians must have accurate information about the patient's history in order to diagnose the type of epileptic seizures and epileptic syndromes. Patients are often asked to come to the physician's office with a family member or other individual who has witnessed their seizures. Patients, family members, or friends should provide the physician with a detailed description of the seizure activity, including onset, frequency, any changes in the seizures, duration, and medication usage.

The electroencephalograph (EEG) may help the physician determine whether an individual has epilepsy, and if so, where in the brain the seizure activity is taking place. Sometimes the EEG does not pick up the brain's electrical changes, or the individual may not experience any seizure activity while being monitored. In some instances, an individual may be hospitalized so that a 24 hour EEG recording may be made. Magnetic resonance imaging (MRI) is used to detect brain tumors, scar tissue, and blood clots.

Blood tests and tests of spinal fluid are conducted to determine if an infection has caused the seizure. Tests for lead poisoning and kidney or liver disease may be performed as well.

Some individuals with epilepsy who are candidates for surgery are participating in research to locate areas of abnormal brain metabolism. Positron emission tomography (PET) allows researchers to observe the brain's metabolic activity by measuring the brain's use of glucose, oxygen, and carbon dioxide. Positron emission tomography may also reveal the effects of antiepileptic drugs (National Institute of Neurological Disorders and Stroke: 1984).

TYPES OF SEIZURES

Generalized seizures affect both hemispheres of the brain and may lead to loss of consciousness, convulsions, and loss of memory. Two types of generalized seizures are the tonic-clonic and absence seizures.

A *tonic-clonic seizure* (previously called a grand mal seizure) is a generalized seizure with loss of consciousness. The individual may cry out, fall, and lie rigid. The body may jerk; bladder and bowel control may be lost; the individual may bite his or her tongue; and saliva may appear around the mouth. When the individual regains consciousness, he or she may feel sore or stiff and sleepy. The individual may or may not have any warning of the impending episode. The individual will not remember the seizure and may experience a headache and drowsiness, sometimes taking several days to return to normal functioning (Dichter: 1994).

An *absence seizure* (previously called a petit mal seizure) is characterized by sudden onset and a blank stare. These seizures last a short time but may occur many times a day, beginning and ending abruptly. The individual is unaware of his or her surroundings and may not respond when spoken to. Sometimes speaking to the individual will stop the absence seizure.

If only one hemisphere of the brain is affected, the seizure is called a *partial* (or *focal*) *seizure*. Symptoms of a partial seizure include an involuntary turning of the head, loss of speech, sweating, pallor, dilation of the pupils, and light flashes. Tingling or numbness in the face or fingers or hearing buzzing noises may also occur. Individuals do not lose consciousness during a partial seizure.

Complex partial seizures, which sometimes affect the temporal lobes (at the side of the brain near the ears), can also occur in several other areas of the brain. An individual having a complex partial seizure appears to be in a trance accompanied by involuntary motor activities, called *automatisms*. The individual loses consciousness and has no control over these movements, which may include lip and tongue smacking, mimicry, hand movements, or repetitive utterances.

The individual is conscious during a *simple partial seizure* but cannot control body movements. An arm or leg may jerk or tremble. Seizure activity occurs in the part of the brain which controls vision, hearing, sensation, or memory. The individual may feel disoriented, fearful, or experience odd sensations on one side of the body.

An *aura* is an unusual feeling experienced by many people with epilepsy prior to a seizure. The individual may feel sick or apprehensive, have aural or visual hallucinations, or notice a peculiar odor or taste. The individual retains memory of the sensation even if he or she loses consciousness. The aura often serves as a warning that a seizure is about to take place, allowing the individual to move away from potential hazards before the onset of a major seizure.

TREATMENT OF EPILEPSY

Most individuals with epilepsy use *anticonvulsant* or *antiepileptic medications* to control seizures. The choice of antiepileptic drug (AED) is determined by the type of seizure, other clinical aspects of the seizure, the drug's side effects, cost, and method of administration. Smith (1990) recommends that drug therapy begin with a single AED, although the individual experiencing more than one type of seizure may need more than one drug to gain control of the seizures. Drugs such as carbamazepine (Tegretol), phenobarbital (Luminal and others) and phenytoin (Dilantin) are used to treat tonic-clonic seizures; valproic acid (Depakene, Depakote) is effective in treating a variety of seizures (Brodie and Dichter: 1996).

After many years in which no new drugs were approved, the Food and Drug Administration (FDA) approved five new drugs for seizure control: gabapentin, lamotrigine, topiramate, felbamate, and fosphenytoin (Curry and Kulling: 1998). Gabapentin (Neurontin) and topiramate (Topamax), approved for adults with partial seizures, were reported to have side effects, such as dizziness, somnolence, and nausea. Users of lamotrigine (Lamictal), also approved for adults with partial seizures, experience more severe side effects, including a severe skin reaction. The risks increase when used with standard AEDs. Felbamate (Felbatol) has serious potential for aplastic anemia and hepatic failure; physicians are advised to use it only in patients in whom the risk is thought to be acceptable due to intractable seizures. Fosphenytoin (Cerebyx), administered intravenously, is used as a substitute for oral phenytoin, to prevent and control seizures during neurosurgery. On December 1, 1999, the Food and Drug Administration approved a new drug called levetiracetam (Keppra) for use in combination with other antiepileptic drugs to control partial seizures. Although dizziness and sleepiness are possible side effects, clinical trials did not disclose any harmful interaction with other medications or liver damage. Blood level tests are used to monitor the efficacy of the chosen drug and to detect toxicity.

It is important for individuals with epilepsy to maintain a fixed schedule for taking medication. Missing a dose, ceasing to take medication, or taking the wrong dosage may lead to seizure activity. Individuals taking antiepileptic medication should tell physicians treating them for other conditions about their epilepsy medicine and inquire about interactions with over-the-counter products and prescription drugs, such as antibiotics, birth control pills, pain medications, decongestants, and cimetidine (Tagament HB), used to treat stomach problems. Two-thirds of the individuals who are treated successfully with AEDs may be weaned off these medications (Brodie and Dichter: 1996).

Side effects of AEDs may include nausea, fatigue, slurring of words, staggering, or allergic reactions (a rash or hives). Some people experience emotional changes, while others may note memory, learning, or behavior problems. Effects on appearance are not uncommon, including alopecia (hair loss) and weight gain (McGuire: 1991). Individuals should ask the physician about each drug's side effects and what to do if a reaction occurs. Some believe that a *ketogenic diet*, which is high in fat and calories, may prevent seizures in children who experience multiple side effects from standard medication.

In a recent study of individuals with epilepsy in the U.S., 90% of the respondents used medications to control seizures (Fisher: 2000a). Slightly more than half of them used only one medication; a quarter used two drugs; and 6% and 2% used three and four medications respectively. Just a little more than two-thirds of these individuals were very satisfied with their AEDs. They cited concerns about seizure control, side effects, dosing schedules, and cost.

Individuals with epilepsy who cannot afford AEDs may receive assistance through the Pharmaceutical Research and Manufacturers Association, which publishes a list of members that offer certain drugs at low or no cost to uninsured or underinsured patients upon submission of a request from a physician (see "PUBLICATIONS AND TAPES" section below). The National Organization for Rare Disorders (NORD) sponsors a Medication

Assistance Program and Medical Equipment Exchange for its members (see Chapter 1, "ORGANIZATIONS" section).

Experimental drugs are available through special testing programs at medical comprehensive epilepsy centers. The Epilepsy Foundation will direct individuals to a local center (see "ORGANIZATIONS" section below).

Women with epilepsy who plan to become pregnant should discuss their medication with their physician, since some AEDs have been implicated in an increase in birth defects (Epilepsy Foundation of America: 1986). They should be carefully monitored during pregnancy and may expect to require some adjustment in antiepileptic medication.

Surgery may be considered when the seizures always originate in one part of the brain; if medication has been unsuccessful; or when surgery will not affect vision, speech, movement, or memory. In resective surgery, the portion of the brain that causes the seizures is removed. In a lobectomy, all or part of the temporal, frontal, parietal, or occipital lobe is removed in order to reduce partial seizures. Sixty-five to 85% of individuals who have temporal lobectomies are free of seizures (Epilepsy Foundation: 1998). Individuals who experience drop attacks (seizures that cause them to drop to the floor) may undergo surgery to interrupt the nerve pathways by cutting into the hemispheres of the brain in a procedure called a corpus callostomy (Gumnit: 1997). Individuals considering surgery must understand that although surgical procedures may reduce the number and frequency of drop attacks, most individuals will still require medication to bring remaining seizure activity under control (Gumnit: 1997). Individuals considering surgery must understand that although surgical procedures may reduce the number and frequency of seizures, most of them will still require medication to bring remaining seizure activity under control (Gumnit: 1997).

Tyler (1990) believes that surgery is not considered as often as it should be because the danger of such surgery is overestimated and the benefits underestimated. In addition, family physicians sometimes lack knowledge of specialized epilepsy surgery centers. The National Institute of Neurological Disorders and Stroke (1988) reports that more than 100,000 individuals with partial seizures who do not respond to medical therapy are candidates for surgery. Individuals should ask physicians about the risks and benefits of surgery in their own situation. If a physician cannot supply the information, individuals should ask for a referral to another specialist or contact the National Institute of Neurological Disorders and Stroke (NINDS) for information on surgical procedures. The National Institutes of Health Consensus Development Conference on Surgery for Epilepsy (1990) discussed selection of patients for surgery, diagnostic methods, choices of surgical procedures, and outcome measures. At that time, although controlled trials had not been conducted and investigations differed in their patient criteria and procedures, the panel agreed that surgery is an alternative option when seizures cannot be controlled by medication. A study found that nearly six years after individuals with epilepsy had undergone surgery, two-thirds had had no more than one seizure or experienced only auras compared with 11% of patients who had not had surgery (Vickrey et al.: 1995). The subjects who had surgery were also taking less medication than they had prior to surgery. In a recent study, Wiebe and colleagues (2001) conducted a randomized, controlled trial of temporal-lobe surgery and concluded that surgery was superior to medical treatment. Nearly 60% of the patients who had had surgery were free of seizures impairing awareness compared with only eight percent of those treated with AEDs.

Brain surgery should never be undertaken without serious investigation into the pros and cons. Talking with others who have chosen surgery and those who have not, consulting the medical literature, and getting advice from several neurosurgeons may help individuals make the best possible decision for their health.

In 1997, the Food and Drug Administration (FDA) approved the use of the NeuroCybernetic Prosthesis System, an implantable electronic nerve stimulator to control partial seizures. This vagus nerve stimulator (VNS) is implanted in the chest and is programmed to deliver short bursts of electrical energy to the brain via the vagus nerve. Typically, these bursts occur every five minutes for about 30 seconds. A magnet, worn on the wrist or belt, is used to activate the implant if a seizure seems imminent. For some users, passing the magnet over the implant halts the seizure, shortens its duration and severity, and may speed recovery. Hoarseness and changes in voice quality are common side effects. The Epilepsy Foundation (2001) reports that about a third of the individuals who use VNS have a major improvement in seizure control, about a third have some improvement, and the remainder experience no improvement. VNS is used in addition to medication.

Individuals whose seizures are under control have no restrictions on their recreational activities. However, it is important to take extra precautions with activities, such as swimming, waterskiing, scuba, and sky diving, since the occurrence of a seizure is very dangerous while engaged in these activities. It is a good idea for individuals to wear an identification bracelet or necklace or carry a wallet card which indicates that they have epilepsy. When traveling, it is wise to carry a letter from a physician describing the seizure disorder and medications currently used. A medication routine may need to be adjusted when travel affects sleep schedules.

Personal safety should be considered in everyday activities. Lowering the temperature of the water and sitting down to shower may prevent injury if a seizure occurs while bathing. Wall-to-wall carpeting and padding on sharp corners reduce the risk of injury in falls.

EPILEPSY IN CHILDREN

It is often difficult to determine the cause of seizures in children. The developmental stage of the brain, age of onset, and metabolic or genetic disorders all may influence the type of seizure.

Seizures are generally well controlled during youth, allowing medications to be withdrawn by early to middle age (Troupin and Johannessen: 1990). Epilepsy may actually disappear in some children who have experienced absence seizures only. Seizure frequency seems to decrease with age, unless there is a change in the underlying cause, such as tuberous sclerosis or a brain tumor (Epilepsy Foundation of America: 1994). Currently, it is not possible to predict the course of epilepsy in any one individual. A group of Finnish researchers followed 220 children who had been diagnosed with active epilepsy in the early 1960s for more than 30 years and found that those whose seizures were considered to be of genetic origin and who had responded quickly to therapy were more likely to be seizure free as adults (Sillanpaa et al.: 1998).

Unfortunately, children with epilepsy rarely receive adequate information about their condition. Physicians often discuss the child's diagnosis and treatment with the parents when the child is not present. Withholding information from children may be attributed to a belief that children will not understand; that they should be protected; or that parents, rather than physicians should inform their children about their condition (Schneider and Conrad: 1983). Masland (1985) reports that overprotection, overcompensation, and rejection are common reactions of parents to children with epilepsy. He believes that the attitude of the parents plays a major role in shaping the self-image of the child who develops epilepsy. He emphasizes that the physician must provide a thorough explanation of epilepsy and its ramifications to both parents and child. Patient and family education helps children, teenagers, and adults to cope better with everyday living with epilepsy.

Children with epilepsy may find that special recreation programs and summer camps help them to cope with seizures and medication and to deal with occasional discrimination. Peer support is especially important in adolescence.

Respite care programs offer families the opportunity for free time away from a child with a disability. Community agencies and affiliates of the Epilepsy Foundation (see "ORGANIZATIONS" section below) can provide information about these programs.

It is important for parents to inform their child's teacher about the child's condition; how epilepsy affects the child; and what to do if a seizure occurs. Medication may slow the child's functional level. Children who have both epilepsy and learning disabilities or mental retardation will require special education services. Teachers and administrators who are uninformed about epilepsy and its consequences may unnecessarily restrict activities and expect less of children with the condition, and, by these actions, influence interactions with peers (Leonard: 1984).

If a seizure should occur at school, classmates of the child with epilepsy should receive a brief explanation of what causes seizures. They should have an opportunity to ask questions and discuss their feelings.

EPILEPSY IN ELDERS

Seizures in elders may be the result of systemic illness; the use of medications such as analgesics and antihistamines; or the withdrawal of sedative drugs. It is crucial to identify any primary medical conditions that may precipitate seizures. Examples of systemic illnesses which may cause seizure activity include strokes (which may cause acute seizures followed by recurring seizure activity), head injury, and either primary or metastatic brain tumors. Once seizures symptomatic of systemic illness have been distinguished from epilepsy, they should be treated by managing the precipitating event without the use of anticonvulsant drugs (Troupin and Johannessen: 1990).

Tonic-clonic seizures pose additional problems for elders who also have heart disease, osteoporosis, or pulmonary disease. Stress on the heart, pain, fractures, or breathing problems are potential aftereffects of such seizures (Devinsky: 1994).

Individuals with chronic epilepsy may be affected by pharmacologic changes, such as changes in metabolism related to the aging process, and may require adjustment in their usual seizure therapy. Because elders often take drugs for a variety of conditions, elders with epilepsy must be concerned about the interaction of these drugs and AEDs. For example, cimetidine (Tagamet HB), used to treat stomach problems common in elders, is now available for over-the-counter purchase. However, cimetidine raises the levels of many antiepileptic drugs (Gumnit: 1997). Some antibiotics taken with antiepileptic drugs are also toxic. Individuals should be certain to ask their physicians about the possible interaction among the various drugs they are taking.

PSYCHOLOGICAL ASPECTS OF EPILEPSY

Various studies have concluded that depression is more common among people with epilepsy than among the general population. Although these studies have been conducted by psychiatrists, neurologists, and general practitioners, they are all remarkably consistent in reaching this conclusion (Robertson: 1991).

The diagnosis of epilepsy is difficult to accept:

> Some individuals are more disabled by the fact that they have epilepsy than by the seizures themselves and unduly restrict their activities or withdraw from social interactions (Dichter: 1994, 2233).

Depression in individuals with epilepsy may be due to the stresses of living with epilepsy; employment problems; or the inability to drive. Individuals may complain of fatigue or feeling sad; may sleep poorly; or may be unable to concentrate. These symptoms may be related to having epilepsy, or they may signal a problem with medication. In a community-based study, individuals with epilepsy said that the worse aspects of living with epilepsy were fear and the unpredictability of seizures (Fisher et al.: 2000b). They also cited limitations on their lifestyles, such as being unable to drive; the social stigma of having epilepsy; loss of confidence in their abilities; and cognitive problems.

Individuals with epilepsy often find that aspects of everyday life are affected by their physical condition. Masland (1985) found that disability in individuals with epilepsy was related to the disruption caused by the seizures; the effects of associated neurological impairments, including those caused by drugs; reactions of society; and the individual's self-concept. Upton and Thompson (1992) explored the use of coping strategies by people with chronic epilepsy. They found that "cognitive restructuring" reduces emotional distress when individuals accept the negative aspects of their condition and search for positive aspects of their experiences. Upton (1993) later found that perceived social support from family and friends had a positive effect on emotional adjustment, ameliorating the stresses of chronic illness.

Snyder's study (1990) of individuals age 18 or over who had had epilepsy for at least one year found that the need to take medications regularly and not knowing when a seizure would occur caused the greatest amount of stress. Ostracism, which has often been cited as a cause of stress, was not a high stressor for these subjects. Individuals who ranked their health as good were more likely to take measures to control their health than were subjects who ranked their health as poor; such measures included relaxation techniques and biofeedback, although the efficacy of these measures is not known.

Unemployment and underemployment are among the most serious social problems of individuals with epilepsy. Although unpredictable seizures are hazardous in certain environ-

199

ments, they are less significant than the ignorance and fear of employers and employees. Employers must understand that medications may reduce productivity. In addition, poor self-image may have a negative effect on the skills required to seek a job and interpersonal relationships. The combination of self-stigma, perceived and actual societal stigma, and the lack of social skills and confidence leads to a tendency to blame epilepsy for every failure in life.

The lack of a driver's license can be a significant barrier to employment, activities of everyday living, and social life for the individual with epilepsy. In most states, individuals must be free of seizures for six months to one year in order to be eligible for a driver's license. A letter from a physician which states that seizures are under control may be required. The Epilepsy Foundation's web site provides a state by state guide to driver licensing and reporting requirements and discusses physician reporting, liability, and immunity (www.epilepsyfoundation.org/answerplace/drivelaw/driving.html).

It is often difficult for individuals with epilepsy to purchase health, life, or automobile insurance. Even when insurance is available, the premiums may be very high or exclusions may be made for claims relating to epilepsy.

In the past, individuals with epilepsy were forbidden by law to marry, due to false beliefs about the role of heredity and mental function. Now that there is a better understanding of epilepsy, these laws no longer exist. Marriage and childbearing rates in women with epilepsy do not differ from those for women without epilepsy (Epilepsy Foundation of America: 1987).

In some individuals, epilepsy reduces libido and therefore sexual activity. Individuals with epilepsy may fear close relationships because they do not feel comfortable disclosing their condition. Some individuals may fear that sexual activity will cause seizures and that the seizures will be detrimental to their sexual relations. Although talking about epilepsy may be difficult at first, it is important to inform anyone who spends time with individuals with epilepsy, including sexual partners, about the condition and what to do if a seizure occurs.

Participating in a self-help group, discussing these feelings with the physician, and using stress reduction and relaxation techniques may be helpful.

PROFESSIONAL SERVICE PROVIDERS

Individuals who experience a seizure first see their *primary care physician*, either a family physician or a pediatrician. Hospitalization may be required to observe the individual for progressive symptoms or additional seizures. An outpatient visit may be sufficient if the seizure occurred more than a week before medical consultation and was an isolated event. The primary care physician may initiate treatment at this time.

If initial treatment does not achieve seizure control in about three months, the individual should be referred to a *neurologist* for a thorough evaluation. A neurologist is a physician who diagnoses and treats conditions involving the brain and nervous system, including epilepsy. A neurological assessment will include a patient history, physical examination, electroencephalogram (EEG), computerized tomography (CT) scan, magnetic resonance imaging (MRI), and other tests. If seizures are under control, the neurologist will follow the patient on an outpatient basis. A *neurosurgeon* performs any necessary brain surgery.

If seizures are not under control within nine months of treatment, referral to a comprehensive treatment center is recommended. The National Association of Epilepsy Centers has established guidelines for these specialized epilepsy treatment centers (Gumnit: 1990).

Rehabilitation counselors coordinate services such as vocational rehabilitation, education, and training for individuals with epilepsy. The rehabilitation counselor can serve as an advocate with prospective employers who may be uninformed or fearful about hiring an individual with epilepsy. Individuals with epilepsy who are unemployed or underemployed should apply to their state vocational rehabilitation agency for assistance with career planning, training, and placement.

WHERE TO FIND SERVICES

Physicians who treat people with epilepsy are often located in private practices. Individuals who live in metropolitan areas will find neurological clinics and comprehensive epilepsy centers available at major hospitals or universities. Comprehensive epilepsy centers and programs around the country provide medical care; conduct multidisciplinary research; train physicians, nurses and other caregivers; and help to organize community services. They are usually affiliated with university medical centers and serve a designated geographic area. The Epilepsy Foundation will refer individuals to local affiliates.

HOW TO RECOGNIZE A SEIZURE AND GIVE FIRST AID

Epileptic seizures have been mistakenly identified as heart attacks, drunkenness, and drug overdoses. It is important for all health professionals, rehabilitation professionals, and the general public to recognize epileptic seizures and to know simple first aid for epilepsy.

- Remove hard or sharp items that are in the vicinity.
- Loosen the individual's tie or collar to make breathing easier.
- Place a flat, soft cushion, folded jacket, or sweater under the individual's head.
- Gently turn the individual's head to the side to help keep the airway clear. Never try to place any object between the teeth of an individual experiencing a seizure.
- Do not try to stop the individual's jerking movements.
- Check to see if the individual is wearing an identification bracelet or necklace or carrying an identification card which states that he or she has epilepsy.
- Remain with the individual until the seizure ends and offer assistance.
- If the individual seems confused, offer to call a friend, family member, or taxi to help him/her get home.
- If the seizure continues for more than five minutes; if another seizure begins shortly after the first; or if the individual does not regain consciousness after the jerking movements have ceased, call an ambulance.

• If the individual is having an absence seizure, he or she may have a dazed appearance; stare into space; or exhibit automatic behavior such as shaking an arm or leg. Speak quietly and calmly and move the person away from any dangerous areas, such as a flight of stairs or a stove. Remain with the individual until consciousness returns.

References

Adams, P.F. and M.A. Marano
1995   Current Estimates from the National Health Interview Survey, 1994 National Center for Health Statistics, Vital Health Statistics 10(193)

Brodie, Martin J. and Marc A. Dichter
1996   "Antiepileptic Drugs" The New England Journal of Medicine 335:3(January):168-175

Curry, William J. and David L. Kulling
1998   "Newer Antiepileptic Drugs: Gabapentin, Lamotrigine, Felbamate, Topiramate and Fosphenytoin" American Family Physician 59(3):513-20

Devinsky, Orrin
1994   A Guide to Understanding and Living with Epilepsy Philadelphia, PA: F.A. Davis Company

Dichter, Mark A.
1994   "The Epilepsies and Convulsive Disorders" pp. 2223-2244 in Kurt J. Isselbacher et al. (eds.) Harrison's Principles of Internal Medicine New York, NY: McGraw Hill

Epilepsy Foundation
2001   VNS Therapy for Epilepsy Landover, MD: Epilepsy Foundation
1998   Surgery for Epilepsy Landover, MD: Epilepsy Foundation
1994   Epilepsy: Questions and Answers About Seizure Disorders Landover, MD: Epilepsy Foundation of America
1987   Epilepsy: Part of Your Life Landover, MD: Epilepsy Foundation of America
1986   A Patient's Guide to Medical Treatment of Childhood and Adult Seizure Disorders Landover, MD: Epilepsy Foundation of America

Fisher, Robert S. et al.
2000a "The Impact of Epilepsy from the Patient's Perspective II: Views about Therapy and Health Care" Epilepsy Research 41(2000):53-61
2000b "The Impact of Epilepsy from the Patient's Perspective I: Descriptions and Subjective Perceptions" Epilepsy Research 41(2000):39-51

Gumnit, Robert J.
1997   Living Well with Epilepsy New York, NY: Demos Vermande
1990   "Interplay of Economics, Politics, and Quality in the Care of Patients with Epilepsy: The Formation of the National Association of Epilepsy Centers" Appendix I in Dennis B. Smith (ed.) Epilepsy: Current Approaches to Diagnosis and Treatment New York, NY: Raven Press

Hauser, W. Allen and Dale C. Hesdorffer
1990   Facts About Epilepsy Landover, MD: Epilepsy Foundation of America

Leonard, Barbara J.

1984 "The Adolescent with Epilepsy" pp. 239-263 in Robert W. Blum (ed.) <u>Chronic Illness and Disabilities in Childhood and Adolescence</u> Orlando, FL: Grune & Stratton

Masland, R.L.

1985 "Psychosocial Aspects of Epilepsy" pp. 357-377 in Roger J. Porter (ed.) <u>The Epilepsies</u> Stoneham, MA: Butterworths

McGuire, A.M.

1991 "Quality of Life in Women with Epilepsy" pp. 13-30 in Michael R. Trimble (ed.) <u>Women and Epilepsy</u> Chichester, England: John Wiley & Sons

National Center for Health Statistics, Collins, John G.

1988 "Prevalence of Selected Chronic Conditions, United States, 1983-85" <u>Advance Data From Vital and Health Statistics</u> No. 155 DHHS Pub. No (PHS) 88-1250. Public Health Service. Hyattsville, MD

National Institute of Neurological Disorders and Stroke

1988 <u>The Surgical Management of Epilepsy</u> Bethesda, MD: National Institute of Neurological Disorders and Stroke

1984 <u>Positron Emission Tomography: Emerging Research Opportunities in the Neurosciences</u>

National Institutes of Health Consensus Development Conference on Surgery for Epilepsy

1990 <u>Surgery for Epilepsy NIH Consensus Statement</u> March 19-21

Robertson, Mary M.

1991 "Depression in Epilepsy" pp. 223-242 in Michael R. Trimble (ed.) <u>Women and Epilepsy</u> Chichester, England: John Wiley & Sons

Sillanpaa, Matti et al.

1998 "Long-Term Prognosis of Seizures with Onset in Childhood" <u>New England Journal of Medicine</u> 338:24(June 11):1715-1722

Smith, Dennis B.

1990 "Antiepileptic Drug Selection in Adults" pp. 111-138 in Dennis B. Smith (ed.) <u>Epilepsy: Current Approaches to Diagnosis and Treatment</u> New York, NY: Raven Press

Snyder, Mariah

1990 "Stressors, Coping Mechanisms, and Perceived Health in Persons with Epilepsy" <u>International Disability Studies</u> 12:3:100-103

Troupin, Alan S. and Svein I. Johannessen

1990 "Epilepsy in the Elderly" pp. 141-153 in Dennis B. Smith (ed.) <u>Epilepsy: Current Approaches to Diagnosis and Treatment</u> New York, NY: Raven Press

Tyler, Allen R.

1990 "The Role of Surgery in Therapy for Epilepsy" pp. 173-182 in Dennis B. Smith (ed.) <u>Epilepsy: Current Approaches to Diagnosis and Treatment</u> New York, NY: Raven Press

Upton, Dominic

1993 "Social Support and Emotional Adjustment in People with Chronic Epilepsy" <u>Journal of Epilepsy</u> 6:2:105-111

Upton, Dominic and Pamela J. Thompson

1992 "Effectiveness of Coping Strategies Employed by People with Chronic Epilepsy" <u>Journal of Epilepsy</u> 5:2:119-127

Vickrey, Barbara G. et al.

1995 "Outcomes in 248 Patients Who Had Diagnostic Evaluations for Epilepsy Surgery" The Lancet 346(December 2):1445-1449

Wiebe, Samuel et al.

2001 "A Randomized, Controlled Trial of Surgery for Temporal-Lobe Epilepsy" New England Journal of Medicine 345:5(August 2):311-318

ORGANIZATIONS

Antiepileptic Drug Pregnancy Registry
Massachusetts General Hospital
(888) 233-2334   www.aedpregnancyregistry.org

The AED Pregnancy Registry is seeking enrollees for its study of fetal risks of antiepileptic drugs in pregnancy. Requires three toll-free telephone interviews.

Brain Injury Association
105 North Alfred Street
Alexandria, VA 22314
Family Helpline (800) 444-6443   (703) 236-6000   FAX (703) 236-6001
e-mail: publicrelations@biausa.org www.biausa.org

A membership organization that provides information and support for individuals with head injury, their families, and professionals. (Seizures are often precipitated by a head injury.) Local affiliates. Membership, $35.00, includes newsletter, "TBI Challenge!" published six times a year, and discounts on publications, conferences, and seminars. Also publishes the "National Directory of Brain Injury Rehabilitation Services," $16.00, and "Catalogue of Educational Materials," free.

Epilepsy Foundation (EF)
4351 Garden City Drive, Suite 406
Landover, MD 20785
(800) 332-1000   (301) 459-3700   FAX (301) 577-9056
www.epilepsyfoundation.org

Provides information and education, advocacy, research support, and services to individuals with epilepsy, their family members, and professionals. Web site offers special interest chat rooms, a bulletin board, and special events with epilepsy experts. Local affiliates. Special resource materials for elementary and secondary school personnel include videotapes, a manual for school nurses, and comic books for classmates. Some publications and audio-visual materials are available in Spanish. Bimonthly newsletter, "EpilepsyUSA," $15.00.

Epilepsy-L
home.ease.lsoft.com/Archives/Epilepsy-L.html

This e-mail support group enables participants to "chat" with others who have seizure disorders and their family members.

Ketogenic Diet
www.stanford.edu/group/ketodiet

MEDLINEplus: Epilepsy
www.nlm.nih.gov/medlineplus/epilepsy.html

This web site provides links to sites for general information about epilepsy, symptoms and diagnosis, treatment, alternative therapy, clinical trials, disease management, nutrition, children with epilepsy, organizations, and research. Provides links to MEDLINE research articles and related MEDLINEplus pages.

National Association of Epilepsy Centers (NAEC)
5775 Wayzata Boulevard, Suite 225
Minneapolis, MN 55416
(763) 525-4526   FAX (763) 525-1560

An organization of epilepsy centers that helps to develop standards for medical and surgical treatment of epilepsy and for the facilities and programs that serve individuals with epilepsy. The NAEC also advises government and industry officials about the needs of people with epilepsy and offers technical assistance to the centers serving these individuals.

National Epilepsy Library
Epilepsy Foundation
4351 Garden City Drive
Landover, MD 20785
(800) 332-4050   (301) 459-3700, extension 684
FAX (301) 577-4941   e-mail: nel@epilepsyfoundation.org
www.epilepsyfoundation.org

A professional library for physicians and other health professionals. Maintains the Epilepsy and Seizure Disorders Information (ESDI) database of articles and publications on medical and psychosocial aspects of epilepsy.

National Institute of Neurological Disorders and Stroke (NINDS)
Building 31, Room 8A06
31 Center Drive, MSC 2540
Bethesda, MD 20892
(800) 352-9424   (301) 496-5751   FAX (301) 402-2186
e-mail: braininfo@ninds.nih.gov   www.ninds.nih.gov

Supports clinical and basic research, maintains national specimen banks for the study of brain and other tissue, and publishes professional and public education materials.

<u>National Stroke Association</u> (NSA)
9707 East Easter Lane
Englewood, CO 80112
(800) 787-6537   (303) 649-9299   FAX (303) 649-1328
e-mail: info@stroke.org   www.stroke.org

Assists individuals with stroke and educates their families, physicians, and the general public about stroke. Membership, $25.00. Publishes bimonthly newsletter, "Stroke Smart," $12.00. Publications are available on the web site.

The Brainstorms Companion: Epilepsy in Our View
by Steven C. Schachter
Lippincott Williams & Wilkins
PO Box 1580
Hagerstown, MD 21741
(800) 638-3030   FAX (301) 824-7390   www.lrpub.com

In this book, information about epilepsy is presented through the experiences of family members, friends, and associates of people with the condition. Information about types of seizures and living safely with epilepsy is also discussed. $35.00

Brainstorms: Epilepsy in Our Words
by Steven C. Schachter
Lippincott Williams & Wilkins
PO Box 1580
Hagerstown, MD 21741
(800) 638-3030   FAX (301) 824-7390   www.lrpub.com

In this book, people with epilepsy describe their seizures and their lives with this condition. Medical information about epilepsy and types of seizures is included. $35.00

The Brainstorms Family: Epilepsy on Our Terms
by Steven C. Schachter, Georgia D. Montouris, and John M. Pellock
Lippincott Williams & Wilkins
PO Box 1580
Hagerstown, MD 21741
(800) 638-3030   FAX (301) 824-7390   www.lrpub.com

This book is a collection of stories by children with seizures and their parents. $35.00

The Brainstorms Healer: Epilepsy in Our Experience
by Steven C. Schachter and A. James Rowan
Lippincott Williams & Wilins, Hagerstown, MD

In this book, professionals describe their interactions with individuals with epilepsy. Includes accounts of professionals who themselves have epilepsy. Out of print

Brothers and Sisters: A Guide for Families with Children with Epilepsy
Epilepsy Foundation (EF) (see "ORGANIZATIONS" above)
(800) 332-1000   (301) 459-3700   FAX (301) 577-9056
www.epilepsyfoundation.org

This guide examines the effects of epilepsy on family members, and it provides information based on age group. It also includes information for parents and other adult family members. $12.95 plus $6.00 shipping and handling

A Child's Guide to Seizure Disorders
Epilepsy Foundation (EF) (see "ORGANIZATIONS" above)
(800) 332-1000   (301) 459-3700   FAX (301) 577-9056
www.epilepsyfoundation.org

This pamphlet describes seizure disorders, medication, and first aid for seizures. $.68 plus $2.00 shipping and handling

Directory of Prescription Drug Patient Assistance Programs
Pharmaceutical Research and Manufacturers Association (PHRMA)
1100 15th Street, NW
Washington, DC 20005
(800) 762-4636   (202) 835-3400   www.phrma.org

A list of companies that offer certain drugs at low or no cost to uninsured or underinsured patients. Most programs require that a physician make the request. Free

Driving and Epilepsy: Information for People with Seizure Disorders
Epilepsy Foundation (EF) (see "ORGANIZATIONS" above)
(800) 332-1000   (301) 459-3700   FAX (301) 577-9056
www.epilepsyfoundation.org

This videotape describes how people whose seizures are under control may obtain a driver's license and offers practical advice to those who cannot drive due to uncontrolled seizures. $21.95 plus $6.00 shipping and handling

Epilepsy
Fanlight Productions
4196 Washington Street, Suite 2
Boston, MA 02131
(800) 937-4113   (617) 469-4999   FAX (617) 469-3379
e-mail: fanlight@fanlight.com   www.fanlight.com

This videotape looks at surgical treatment of epilepsy through the experience of an adult and a child. 28 minutes. $149.00 plus $9.00 shipping and handling

Epilepsy and the Family
by Richard Lechtenberg
Harvard University Press
79 Garden Street
Cambridge, MA 02138
(800) 448-2242   (617) 495-2600   FAX (800) 962-4983
www.hup.harvard.edu

In addition to basic information on epilepsy, this book includes chapters on children growing up with a parent who has epilepsy and on siblings and the extended family of individuals with epilepsy. $27.50 plus $4.50 shipping and handling

Epilepsy A to Z: A Glossary of Epilepsy Terminology
by Peter W. Kaplan et al.
Demos Medical Publishing
386 Park Avenue South, Suite 201
New York, NY 10016
(800) 532-8663   (212) 683-0072   FAX (212) 683-0118
e-mail: info@demospub.com   www.demosmedpub.com

This book provides definitions and discussions of terms used in epilepsy including diagnostic procedures and medical and surgical treatments. References to other source materials are also provided. $34.95 plus $4.00 shipping and handling. Orders made on the Demos web site receive a 15% discount.

Epilepsy: 199 Answers--A Doctor Responds to His Patients' Questions
by Andrew N. Wilner
Demos Medical Publishing
386 Park Avenue South, Suite 201
New York, NY 10016
(800) 532-8663   (212) 683-0072   FAX (212) 683-0118
e-mail: info@demospub.com   www.demosmedpub.com

This guide answers patients' questions about the condition, tests, medications, and research and provides information on driving, work, first aid, and safety. Includes a medical history form and seizure calendar. $19.95 plus $4.00 shipping and handling. Orders made on the Demos web site receive a 15% discount.

Epilepsy: Patient and Family Guide
by Orrin Devinsky
F.A. Davis Company
1915 Arch Street
Philadelphia, PA 19103
(800) 323-3555   FAX (215) 440-3016
e-mail: orders@fadavis.com   www.fadavis.com

This book discusses medical aspects of epilepsy and diagnosis and treatment. Also describes epilepsy in children and in adults and legal and financial issues. $24.95

Epilepsy: Seizures and Seniors
Epilepsy Foundation (EF) (see "ORGANIZATIONS" above)
(800) 332-1000   (301) 459-3700   FAX (301) 577-9056
www.epilepsyfoundation.org

This pamphlet provides basic information about epilepsy in older individuals. $1.15 plus $2.00 shipping and handling

Epilepsy: The Untold Stories
by Paul J. Joseph and Mark R. Brown
Fanlight Productions
4196 Washington Street, Suite 2
Boston, MA 02131
(800) 937-4113   (617) 469-4999   FAX (617) 469-3379
e-mail: fanlight@fanlight.com   www.fanlight.com

This videotape, featuring six individuals who have temporal lobe epilepsy, describes how complex partial seizures affect their lives. Also discusses clinical aspects, diagnosis, and treatment of epilepsy. 27 minutes. Purchase, $145.00; rental for one day, $50.00; rental for one week, $100.00; plus $9.00 shipping and handling.

Epilepsy: You and Your Child
Epilepsy Foundation (EF) (see "ORGANIZATIONS" above)
(800) 332-1000   (301) 459-3700   FAX (301) 577-9056
www.epilepsyfoundation.org

Designed to answer basic questions about epilepsy, this guide for parents also discusses psychosocial issues, such as parental expectations, family dynamics, and interpersonal relationships as well as practical advice about school, special care, and resources. $1.15 plus $2.00 shipping and handling

Family Video Library
Epilepsy Foundation (EF) (see "ORGANIZATIONS" above)
(800) 332-1000   (301) 459-3700   FAX (301) 577-9056
www.epilepsyfoundation.org

This collection of videotapes includes subjects such as "Understanding Seizure Disorders,"
"How Medicines Work," "Epilepsy and the Family," "Living with Epilepsy," "Understanding
Complex Partial Seizures," "Understanding Seizure Disorders," "Epilepsy in the Teen Years,"
and "The Rest of the Family." Each videotape is $16.95; discounts are available to members.
Many of the videotapes are also available in Spanish. Request catalogue, "Books, Videos,
Guides & Pamphlets," free.

First Aid for Seizures: (Complex Partial)
First Aid for Seizures: (Generalized Tonic-Clonic, Grand Mal)
Epilepsy Foundation (EF) (see "ORGANIZATIONS" above)
(800) 332-1000   (301) 459-3700   FAX (301) 577-9056
www.epilepsyfoundation.org

Printed in both English and Spanish, each poster gives simple first aid instruction for people
experiencing these types of seizures. $2.05 each plus $2.00 each shipping and handling

Issues and Answers: A Guide for Parents of Children with Seizures, Birth to Age Six
Issues and Answers: A Guide for Parents of Children with Seizures, Ages Six to Twelve
Issues and Answers: A Guide for Parents of Teens and Young Adults with Epilepsy
Issues and Answers: Exploring Your Possibilities -- A Guide for Teens and Young Adults with
Epilepsy
Epilepsy Foundation (EF) (see "ORGANIZATIONS" above)
(800) 332-1000   (301) 459-3700   FAX (301) 577-9056
www.epilepsyfoundation.org

The first two guides provide basic information about epilepsy and discuss family, child care,
and school issues. The second two guides focus on issues of specific concern to teens and
young adults, such as driving, dating, drinking, and marriage. They provide practical
solutions for dealing with social pressures, independent living, and transition to college and
work. $14.95 each plus $6.00 shipping and handling; discounts available to members.

The Ketogenic Diet: A Treatment for Epilepsy
by John M. Freeman, Jennifer B. Freeman, and Millicent T. Kelly
Demos Medical Publishing
386 Park Avenue South, Suite 201
New York, NY 10016
(800) 532-8663   (212) 683-0072   FAX (212) 683-0118
e-mail: info@demospub.com   www.demosmedpub.com

This book outlines a rigid high fat, low carbohydrate diet plan which the authors suggest as a possible treatment to improve seizure control in children with epilepsy. $24.95 plus $4.00 shipping and handling. Orders made on the Demos web site receive a 15% discount.

The Ketogenic Diet Video
Epilepsy Foundation (EF) (see "ORGANIZATIONS" above)
(800) 332-1000   (301) 459-3700   FAX (301) 577-9056
www.epilepsyfoundation.org

This videotape discusses the basics of the ketogenic diet. Includes interviews with physicians, dietitians, and parents of children with intractable seizures. Available in English and Spanish. $19.95 plus $6.00 shipping and handling

Lee, the Rabbit with Epilepsy
by Deborah Moss
Woodbine House
6510 Bells Mill Road
Bethesda, MD 20817
(800) 843-7323   FAX (301) 897-5838
e-mail: info@woodbinehouse.com   www.woodbinehouse.com

Written for children ages four to eight, this book helps the child with epilepsy, siblings, and friends to understand the condition and its treatment. $12.95 plus $4.50 shipping and handling

The Legal Rights of Persons with Epilepsy: An Overview of Legal Issues and Laws
Epilepsy Foundation (EF) (see "ORGANIZATIONS" above)
(800) 332-1000   (301) 459-3700   FAX (301) 577-9056
www.epilepsyfoundation.org

This manual discusses the legal issues and laws that affect individuals with epilepsy, such as health care, education, employment, driving, vocational rehabilitation, criminal justice, and housing. Includes information on the Americans with Disabilities Act of 1990. $14.95 plus $6.00 shipping and handling

Living Well with Epilepsy
by Robert J. Gumnit
Demos Medical Publishing
386 Park Avenue South, Suite 201
New York, NY 10016
(800) 532-8663   (212) 683-0072   FAX (212) 683-0118
e-mail: info@demospub.com   www.demosmedpub.com

Written for health professionals and individuals with epilepsy, this book discusses diagnosis and management of seizure disorders. $19.95 plus $4.00 shipping and handling. Orders made on the Demos web site receive a 15% discount.

Management by Common Sense
Epilepsy Foundation (EF) (see "ORGANIZATIONS" above)
(800) 332-1000   (301) 459-3700   FAX (301) 577-9056
www.epilepsyfoundation.org

This booklet, written for employers of individuals with epilepsy, describes the condition and discusses issues such as workers' compensation, effects of medication, and reactions of customers or clients. $1.95 plus $2.00 shipping and handling

Parenting and You: A Guide for Parents with Seizure Disorders
When Mom or Dad Has Seizures: A Guide for Young People
Epilepsy Foundation (EF) (see "ORGANIZATIONS" above)
(800) 332-1000   (301) 459-3700   FAX (301) 577-9056
www.epilepsyfoundation.org

"Parenting and You" discusses pregnancy, child care, and parenting issues. "When Mom or Dad Has Seizures" examines how children of various ages might feel about a parent's seizure disorder. $14.95 each plus $6.00 shipping and handling

Partial Seizure Disorders: Help for Patients and Families
by Mitzi Waltz
O'Reilly and Associates
101 Morris Street
Sebastopol, CA 95472
(800) 998-9938   (707) 829-0515
e-mail: order@oreilly.com   www.patientcenters.com

This book discusses the diagnosis and treatment of partial seizure disorders. Includes chapters on medical and alternative therapies, health care, insurance, and everyday living. $19.95 plus $4.50 shipping and handling

Safety and Seizures: Tips for Living with Seizure Disorders
Epilepsy Foundation (EF) (see "ORGANIZATIONS" above)
(800) 332-1000   (301) 459-3700   FAX (301) 577-9056
www.epilepsyfoundation.org

This brochure provides suggestions for seizure first aid and tips for personal, household, workplace, transportation, and recreation safety. $1.15 plus $2.00 shipping and handling

Seizure Free
by Leanne Chilton
English Press
PO Box 742945
Dallas, TX 75374
(888) 444-5603   (972) 239-5868   FAX (972) 980-9312
e-mail: englishpress@prodigy.net   www.englishpress.com

In this personal narrative, the author describes being diagnosed with epilepsy, her decision to undergo brain surgery, and recuperation. $12.95 plus $3.95 shipping and handling

Seizures and Epilepsy in Childhood: A Guide for Parents
by John M. Freeman, Eileen P.G. Vining, and Diana J. Pillas
Johns Hopkins University Press
PO Box 50370
Baltimore, MD 21211-4370
(800) 537-5487   FAX (410) 516-6998   www.press.jhu.edu/press

This book describes how seizures occur, diagnostic tests, medication, surgery, and social implications of epilepsy. $17.95 plus $4.00 shipping and handling

Seizures and Epilepsy Interactive Tutorial
www.nlm.nih.gov/medlineplus/tutorials/seizuresandepilepsy.html

This tutorial provides an overview of the condition, treatment options, and resources for everyday living.

Surgery for Epilepsy
National Institutes of Health Consensus Program
PO Box 2577
Kensington, MD 20891
(888) 644-2667   FAX (301) 816-2494
e-mail: consensus_statements@nih.gov
consensus.nih.gov

Published in 1990, this consensus statement concludes that brain surgery is an alternative treatment when medication fails to control seizures. Free. Also available on the web site.

VNS Therapy for Epilepsy
Epilepsy Foundation (EF) (see "ORGANIZATIONS" above)
(800) 332-1000   (301) 459-3700   FAX (301) 577-9056
www.epilepsyfoundation.org

This booklet discusses vagus nerve stimulation (VNS) therapy for partial onset seizures. It describes the implantation surgery, how the device is programmed and monitored, and its cost, and answers common questions. $.95 plus $2.00 shipping and handling

Voices from the Workplace
Epilepsy Foundation (EF) (see "ORGANIZATIONS" above)
(800) 332-1000   (301) 459-3700   FAX (301) 577-9056
www.epilepsyfoundation.org

In this videotape, individuals with epilepsy describe the coping strategies they use in the workplace. 14 minutes. $19.95 plus $6.00 shipping and handling

When the Brain Goes Wrong
by Jonathan David and Roberta Cooks
Fanlight Productions
4196 Washington Street, Suite 2
Boston, MA 02131
(800) 937-4113   (617) 469-4999   FAX (617) 469-3379
e-mail: fanlight@fanlight.com   www.fanlight.com

This videotape, which deals with seven types of brain dysfunctions, depicts the experiences of an individual with epilepsy. 45 minutes. Purchase, $195.00; rental for one day, $50.00; rental for one week, $100.00; plus $9.00 shipping and handling.

A Woman's Guide to Coping with Disability
Resources for Rehabilitation
22 Bonad Road
Winchester, MA 01890
(781) 368-9094   FAX (781) 368-9096
e-mail: orders@rfr.org   www.rfr.org

This book addresses the special needs of women with disabilities and chronic conditions, such as social relationships, sexual functioning, pregnancy, childrearing, caregiving, and employment. Written for women in all age categories, the book has chapters on the disabilities that are most prevalent in women or likely to affect the roles and physical functions unique to women, including epilepsy. $44.95 plus $5.00 shipping and handling (See last page of this book for order form.)

<u>Your Child and Epilepsy</u>
by Robert J. Gumnit
Demos Medical Publishing
386 Park Avenue South, Suite 201
New York, NY 10016
(800) 532-8663   (212) 683-0072   FAX (212) 683-0118
e-mail: info@demospub.com   www.demosmedpub.com

This book provides practical information for families of children with epilepsy. Includes chapters on diagnosis and treatment, infancy, childhood and adolescence. Also discusses issues such as driving, health insurance, and sexuality. $34.95 plus $4.00 shipping and handling. Orders made on the Demos web site receive a 15% discount.

Chapter 8

LOW BACK PAIN

Low back pain is one of the most prevalent debilitating conditions in North America. Back pain (both lower and upper) was the most common type of pain presented by patients whose primary reason for visiting physicians' offices was pain that lasted at least three months (National Center for Health Statistics: 1986). Low back pain occurs most frequently in people in the middle age range. Data from the National Health Interview Study (Hurwitz and Morgenstern: 1997) indicate that disabling back pain is most likely to occur among males, those older than 34, and among individuals whose weight ranks above the 50th percentile. Occupations that involve heavy lifting and other chronic repetitive movements have a clear relation with the incidence of low back pain (Vermont Rehabilitation Engineering Center: no date). People whose work requires that they sit in the same position for extended periods of time are also prone to low back pain; for example, it is known that truck drivers have a high rate of low back pain. Because low back pain is so common and can have severe effects upon daily functioning, it is not surprising that many new treatments, often unproven, have been developed.

THE BACK

The back has three main components, the *vertebrae*, the *disks*, and a *network of ligaments*. Each vertebra has two main parts, the anterior body consisting of bone, and the posterior arch, a thick bony hollow structure, through which the spinal cord passes. The 33 bony, interlocking vertebrae include seven cervical or neck vertebrae, 12 thoracic or high back vertebrae, five lumbar or low back vertebrae, five sacral vertebrae near the base of the spine, and four coccygeal vertebrae fused to form the coccyx. The higher vertebrae are larger than the lower vertebrae and therefore are stronger and able to withstand greater stress. Between each pair of vertebrae are disks, soft tissues made up largely of gelatinous substance and water. Intervertebral disks act as cushions to absorb the shock of motion. Cartilage and fiber between the disks, called nucleus pulposus, absorb shocks and strains. Joints lined with cartilage along the vertebral arch are called facets. The spinal cord, consisting of a narrow bundle of nerve cells and fibers, runs from the base of the brain through the hollow structure of the vertebrae. The brain's communication with the rest of the body is carried out through these nerve fibers. Smaller bundles of nerves branch out between each pair of vertebrae. These secondary nerve cells are called nerve roots (American Medical Association: 1982).

The lumbar, or lower region of the back, supports most of the torso and is susceptible to great stress. It is for this reason that most back problems occur in the lower or lumbar region. Low back pain may be caused by a variety of factors, including diseases such as osteoarthritis, osteoporosis, and gynecological disorders, and injuries incurred by twisting, bending, or lifting. Both too much exercise and too little exercise have been cited as causes of low back pain. Emotional stress, which causes muscle tension, has also been implicated as a causal factor. The normal aging process causes the disks to dry out and grow thinner;

however, older people are less likely to have back pain than younger people, probably because they are less likely to be engaged in occupations that require lifting or repetitive movements.

Because it is often not possible to identify the cause of low back pain, it is extremely important to understand the functional implications for the individual. As Press and his colleagues (1991) have noted, the medical history is especially important in determining the daily activities that have become problematic as a result of low back pain.

NONSPECIFIC LOW BACK PAIN

Most low back pain is "nonspecific," since the cause is not known; the usual diagnosis is a sprained or strained back. It is important to have back pain evaluated by a physician, since it is possible that there is a serious underlying cause, such as a tumor, a fracture, or neurological impairment. Although 90% of people with acute back pain (defined as activity intolerance due to back pain having a duration of three months or less) will recover spontaneously in one month or less (Bigos et al.: 1994), some people experience chronic, persistent back pain. For these individuals, chronic low back pain may alter their entire lifestyle, requiring time away from work and assistance with daily activities and household tasks.

In the first episode of nonspecific low back pain, the conventional treatment has been a combination of bed rest, aspirin, and perhaps the short term use of a muscle relaxant. The Agency for Health Care Policy Research (AHCPR) appointed a panel of specialists to review the research literature and suggest recommended treatments. The panel recommended that most people with acute low back pain do not need bed rest and, indeed, that extended bed rest (more than four days) may have a debilitating effect. In some cases of severe pain, two to three days of bed rest may be recommended. The panel recommended that individuals with low back pain curtail lifting heavy objects, avoid sitting for lengthy periods of time, and, within two weeks of the onset of pain, begin a gradually incremental program of aerobic exercise (Bigos et al.: 1994). Several years after the AHCPR published its treatment guidelines which claimed that there was no evidence that the conventional treatments were effective, a group of physicians who continued to provide these treatments challenged these recommendations. These physicians claimed that the lack of scientific evidence confirming the effectiveness of these treatments is not sufficient reason to stop offering such treatments when clinical experience suggests that they are effective (Frank: 1998).

In a review of treatments for low back pain, Deyo (1998) suggests that the traditional treatments of bed rest or exercise, still prescribed by many physicians, may in fact contribute to the high incidence of low back pain. According to Deyo, the use of x-rays for diagnosing the cause of low back pain is extremely common. However, x-rays not only expose sex organs to radiation, but radiologists often disagree on the interpretation of the x-rays; the x-rays rarely reveal any unexpected findings; and the abnormalities that are discovered may in fact have no relation to the pain. In another study, Atlas and Deyo (2001) recommended that imaging and laboratory tests not be routine and endorsed conservative care (minimal bed rest and activity as tolerated); time (referral for physical therapy only when symptoms have not improved over two to four weeks); and education (prevention of future pain).

Individuals who are overweight; whose occupations predispose them to back pain; or who do not exercise may be advised to lose weight and begin a program of exercise when the pain subsides (National Institute of Neurological Disorders and Stroke: 1989). A study of patients at a health maintenance organization visiting primary care physicians for back pain found that nonsteroidal anti-inflammatory drugs were the most commonly prescribed drug (59% of patients received them), sometimes in combination with muscle relaxants (Cherkin et al.: 1997). Analgesics are prescribed in just under half of all visits to physicians for back pain. Psychotropic drugs, defined as antianxiety agents, sedatives, antidepressants, and antipsychotic drugs, are prescribed in only 13% of all office visits for back pain (National Center for Health Statistics: 1986).

A variety of other treatments are prescribed for people with chronic back pain, although the benefit of many of these treatments is unproven. *Surgery* is considered in only a small proportion of all cases. Even in cases of chronic back pain, there is usually no evidence of a physical condition that can be remedied by surgery (Frymoyer: 1988).

Transcutaneous electric nerve stimulation (TENS) is a treatment method in which low level electric impulses are delivered to nerve endings under the skin near the source of pain. It is not known why TENS should alleviate pain, and research has found that patients with low back pain who received TENS treatment did not improve significantly more than the control group members, who received a "sham" treatment (Deyo et al.: 1990).

Traction, a treatment that involves the positioning of weights attached to pulleys, which are in turn tied to bandages on the legs, is another treatment that has not been proven effective (Bigos et al.: 1994).

Manipulation is a method of treatment that uses the hands to bend, twist, or stretch stiff joints and to relieve muscles spasms. It is not possible to manipulate bones, however (Hall: 1980). Although some studies suggest a temporary benefit of short term manipulation, there is little evidence to indicate that it has lasting benefits or that long term manipulation is effective (Frymoyer: 1988). Bigos et al. (1994) have stated that manipulation is effective only in the first month of acute low back pain without radiculopathy (disease of the nerve root); after the first month, its effectiveness is unproven.

Work hardening is an individualized rehabilitation plan in which the person performs tasks that are part of his or her occupation. The individual is taught to build up muscle strength and to carry out the work tasks in a safe and efficient way without causing damage to the body. Although the individual's capacity and endurance may be limited at first, the goal is to build up to the optimal capacity needed to perform the tasks without overloading the body.

Several studies have examined the various treatments for acute back pain and outcomes. Despite the care provider, whether physician, surgeon, or chiropractor, back pain recurred in more than 50% of patients (Carey et al.: 1999). Many individuals with low back pain see multiple providers; more than 50% of those who had not recovered after three months seek further care (Sundararajan et al.: 1998).

OTHER TYPES OF BACK PAIN

Prolapsed intervertebral disks are disks which have ruptured or burst (often incorrectly referred to as "slipped disks"). Disks may herniate or rupture because of weakening of the disks themselves or of intervertebral cartilage; excessive strain; or an injury. It is possible for any disk to burst, but ruptures occur most frequently in the lower back or the lumbar region, since this area is subject to the greatest stress. Disks that are likely to burst are those that have already degenerated or have cracks; when the stress is too great for these disks, they may burst or rupture. Although disks themselves have no nerves, when they burst, fragments of the disk may press on ligaments and nerves nearby, causing pain. The pain caused by the pressure of disk fragments on a nerve is often referred to as a pinched nerve.

According to Deyo (1998), surgery for herniated disks is valuable in only 10% of all cases. In most cases, the herniated disk will repair itself gradually by shrinking. Most specialists agree that surgery should be considered only when there is a definitive herniated disk that corresponds to the individual's pain, nerve root irritation is present, and the individual has not responded to nonsurgical treatment after six weeks. Despite these criteria and although herniated disks are not the most common cause of back pain, they are the most common cause of back surgery. In a recent study, 70% of patients who had had lumbar spine surgery for herniated disks reported improvement in leg or back pain after a five year follow-up compared to only 56% who initially received nonsurgical treatment (Atlas et al.: 2001).

The National Institutes of Health is currently conducting the Spine Patient Outcomes Research Trial, a multicenter, randomized, controlled trial testing the effectiveness of surgery or nonsurgical therapy for the three most commonly diagnosed conditions that cause low back pain. The conditions under study are lumbar intervertebral disk herniation, spinal stenosis, and spinal stenosis secondary to degenerative spondylolisthesis. The study is currently recruiting patients. (See ClinicalTrials.gov in "ORGANIZATIONS" section below.)

In some individuals, stiffness may precede the pain of a ruptured disk. In other cases, severe pain is very sudden, and the individual may be unable to stand erect. This pain is called *acute lumbago* (Jayson: 1981). Treatment for ruptured disks usually involves bed rest for several weeks on a firm bed with a board underneath to prevent the mattress from sagging. Bed rest is beneficial because it prevents movement and rubbing of the inflamed tissues, which exacerbate the pain. Surgery is usually not necessary; when surgery is performed, fragments of the ruptured disk and the remaining part of the disk that may potentially rupture are removed.

Sciatica involves pain along the sciatic nerve, which extends from the base of the spine to the thigh, with branches throughout the legs and feet. Sciatica may be caused by inflammation; toxicity such as lead or alcohol poisoning; injury to a disk; arthritis; or pressure on a nerve. Diagnosis of sciatica requires repeated physical examinations. Most patients recover from sciatica in six weeks or less, suggesting that surgery is warranted only in severe cases and in cases where a tumor, ruptured disk, or epidural abscess is present (Frymoyer: 1988; Jayson: 1981).

Ankylosing spondylitis is a stiffening of the spine that may be so severe that it results in the total loss of motion in the back. The person with ankylosing spondylitis may appear extremely round shouldered with a stoop in the upper back. Ankylosing spondylitis occurs most frequently in men age 15 to 25. Treatment includes physical therapy and correction of posture (Jayson: 1981).

Rheumatoid arthritis is a chronic condition which causes inflammation of the joints of the body, including those of the spine. Its onset is usually in midlife, although it may also occur in children and elders. Rheumatoid arthritis subsides and recurs and may cause severe disability. Rheumatoid arthritis can also cause general weakness, fatigue, and loss of appetite. Rheumatoid arthritis affects two million Americans and twice as many women as men (National Institute of Arthritis and Musculoskeletal and Skin Diseases: 1987).

Osteoarthritis is a noninflammatory condition in which the cartilage, the material that protects the end of bones and other joints, ulcerates, frays, or degenerates. It may occur in a single joint due to an injury or infection. Osteoarthritis is most common among elders. More than 16 million Americans are affected by osteoarthritis (National Institute of Arthritis and Musculoskeletal and Skin Diseases: 1987).

In an exception to their recommendations regarding x-rays in diagnosing the causes of low back pain in younger individuals, Deyo and Weinstein (2001) believe that it is useful in elders. For example, otherwise undetected osteoporotic or compression fractures may be seen on x-rays. Subsequent fractures may be prevented by the adoption of a regimen that includes better nutrition, exercise, calcium supplements, and hormonal or nonhormonal medications.

PSYCHOLOGICAL ASPECTS OF LOW BACK PAIN

Although many observers have suggested that psychological characteristics such as neurosis are related to low back pain, it is not clear whether the low back pain causes these psychological characteristics or vice versa. Certainly, individuals who experience unremitting pain are likely to have intense emotional responses. In some cases, pain may be so severe that it becomes the central aspect of an individual's life (Williams and Wood: 1988). Individuals with back pain find themselves unable to work and unable to carry out the minimal requirements of daily living; under these conditions, they may also feel socially isolated. When analgesics and sedatives are prescribed and used over a period of time, they can have effects on the individual's moods and behavior; therefore, most physicians prescribe these drugs for use on a short term basis only. Long and Rafii (1993) have stated that many patients visit a variety of specialists in order to find a cure for their pain; with none of the practitioners able to alleviate the pain, patients become frustrated and often are labeled as having psychological problems.

The inability to work causes financial problems for most individuals, resulting in increased tension and anxiety. Rehabilitation counselors can help individuals who are unable to continue with their usual work to seek out alternative employment and financial compensation to bridge the gap between positions.

Back pain also interferes with normal sexual activity, causing additional strain in marital relations. People who have experienced low back pain in the past may fear that sexual intercourse will precipitate another attack. Back schools (described below), pain clinics, and self-help groups teach individuals techniques that decrease stress on the back and concomitantly decrease anxiety associated with sexual intercourse.

Methods of alleviating tension, which may contribute to back pain in the form of tense muscles, may reduce anxiety and help people feel that they are in control of their own lives. Relaxation techniques and meditation are frequently used to help people with back pain to relieve tension. Behavior modification has the goal of changing the individual's lifestyle by increasing mobility and independence.

PROFESSIONAL SERVICE PROVIDERS

Most people who have back pain begin the search for treatment with their *family physician, general practitioner*, or *internist*. If a condition that requires special treatment is suspected, the family physician may refer the patient to a specialist.

Osteopaths are physicians whose training emphasizes the musculoskeletal system. *Orthopedists* or *orthopedic surgeons* specialize in diseases of the musculoskeletal system. When nerve involvement is suspected, *neurologists* will evaluate the patient to determine the exact location of the problem. *Rheumatologists* are physicians who specialize in rheumatic diseases such as osteoarthritis. *Physiatrists* are physicians who specialize in rehabilitation medicine and work closely with physical therapists. *Chiropractors* treat back problems through a procedure called manipulation, which involves exerting pressure on joints or muscles.

After examining patients with low back pain, physicians may refer patients to *physical therapists*, who evaluate the physical condition and the dysfunction it causes and prescribe remedies, such as manipulation, exercise, or massage.

Rehabilitation counselors assess the situation of individuals with low back pain; recommend training programs, if necessary; work with employers to arrange for modification of positions or job sharing; and help clients find appropriate positions.

WHERE TO FIND SERVICES

Pain clinics or centers are one source of help for people who experience chronic low back pain. More than 800 pain clinics or centers in the United States are settings where a multidisciplinary team of health care providers designs an individualized treatment plan for each patient. A variety of treatment modalities is used for each patient, including exercise, diet modification, individual or group psychotherapy, massage, and analgesic medications. Deyo and Weinstein (2001) suggest that optimizing daily functioning for individuals with chronic low back pain is a more achievable goal than complete pain relief.

Back school is a term that has been adopted to indicate a multifaceted treatment approach with an emphasis on patient education. Patients learn about anatomy; proper seating, posture, and lifting; and exercise regimens. In addition, many back schools offer psychological counseling and training in stress management (Carron and Tanenbaum: 1987). Back schools may be operated by physical therapists in private practice or in other medical settings. Some physical therapists work in hospitals or rehabilitation centers, while others are in private practice.

In some cases, it may be necessary for individuals with low back pain to be trained to obtain employment that is less physically demanding than their previous work. Both state and private rehabilitation agencies provide services that enable people with chronic back pain to obtain or retain employment (see the Appendix for a list of state vocational rehabilitation agencies). Many programs funded by the government are available to train people with disabilities for productive employment (see Meeting the Needs of Employees with Disabilities, described in "PUBLICATIONS AND TAPES" section below for a more detailed description of these programs). In some instances, insurance companies pay for the cost of these programs. Because back problems are frequently a result of injuries incurred on the job, some large employers also have in-house rehabilitation programs to enable employees to return to their previous position or to positions with modified work tasks.

Self-help groups enable people with low back pain to discuss their problems with others who may have similar situations; to share solutions to common problems; and to express their emotional responses to chronic pain. Several organizations (see "ORGANIZATIONS" section below) refer individuals to appropriate self-help groups in their own geographic area.

MODIFICATIONS IN DAILY LIVING

Suggestions for prevention of low back pain include the following:

• Modify the environment both in the home and the workplace so that chairs, work surfaces, beds, and driver's seats provide support for the back. For example, chairs should be well padded but not overly stuffed and should have a firm back. Beds should be firm, possibly shored up with a board underneath the mattress. Special back supports and cushions help some people feel more comfortable. These items are available in a number of health care product mail order catalogues (see Chapter 4, "Making Everyday Living Easier") as well as in retail stores.

• Long periods of sitting in one position should be avoided. If it is necessary to remain in one position for a prolonged period of time, there should be periodic breaks of moving around.

• Obesity causes an additional strain on the back; therefore, people who are overweight should strive to lose excess pounds.

• Many experts suggest regular exercise. Swimming, walking, and exercises such as sit-ups to strengthen the abdominal muscles are recommended. Individuals with specific back problems should consult the appropriate professional service provider to design a special exercise program to meet their needs.

• Heavy objects should be lifted by bending the legs and keeping the back straight.

• Poor posture, which is thought to be one possible cause of back pain, should be improved. Care should be taken to ensure that the buttocks do not protrude, as this causes the lower back to arch in an abnormal position.

No matter what the cause or condition, experts who treat people with low back pain all agree that early intervention is crucial. The longer that individuals with low back pain remain incapacitated and away from their work, the less likely it is that they will return.

References

American Medical Association
1982 Book of Back Care New York, NY: Random House

Atlas, Steven J. and Richard A. Deyo
2001 "Evaluating and Managing Acute Low Back Pain in the Primary Care Setting" Journal of Internal Medicine 16:2(February):120-131

Atlas, Steven J. et al.
2001 "Surgical and Nonsurgical Management of Sciatica Secondary to a Lumbar Disc Herniation" Spine 26:10(October):1179-1187

Bigos, Stanley J. et al.
1994 Acute Low Back Problems in Adults Clinical Practice Guidelines, Quick Reference Guide Number 14 Rockville, MD: U.S. Department of Health and Human Services, Public Health Service, Agency for Health Care Policy and Research, AHCPR Pub. No. 95-0643

Carron, Harold, and Richard L. Tanenbaum
1987 Rehabilitation of Persons with Chronic Low Back Pain Washington, DC: D:ATA Institute, Catholic University of America

Cherkin, Daniel C. et al.
1997 "Medication Use for Back Pain in Primary Care" Spine 223:5(March 1):507-614

Deyo, Richard A.
1998 "Low-Back Pain" Scientific American 279:2(August):48-53

Deyo, Richard A. and James N. Weinstein
2001 "Low Back Pain" New England Journal of Medicine 344:5(February 1):363-370

Deyo, Richard A. et al.
1990 "A Controlled Trial of Transcutaneous Electrical Nerve Stimulation (TENS) and Exercise for Chronic Low Back Pain" New England Journal of Medicine 322:23(June 7):1627-1634

Frank, John
1998 "The Nonsurgical Management of Acute Low Back Pain: Cutting Through the AHCPR Guidelines" New England Journal of Medicine 339:7(August 13):484

Frymoyer, John W.
1988 "Back Pain and Sciatica" New England Journal of Medicine 318:5(February 4):291-300

Hall, Hamilton
1980 The Back Doctor New York, NY: McGraw-Hill

Hurwitz, Eric L. and Hal Morgenstern
1997 "Correlates of Back Pain and Back-Related Disability in the United States" Journal of Clinical Epidemiology 50:6(June):669-681

Jayson, Malcolm
1981 Back Pain: The Facts New York, NY: Oxford University Press

Long, Stephen P. and Amir Rafii
1993 "The Multidisciplinary Management of the Chronic Pain Patient" Journal of Back and Musculoskeletal Rehabilitation 3(1):48-53

National Center for Health Statistics, Koch, H.

1986 "The Management of Chronic Pain in Office-Based Ambulatory Care: National Ambulatory Medical Care Survey" Advance Data from Vital and Health Statistics No. 123, DHHS Pub. No. (PHS) 86-1250 Public Health Service Hyattsville, MD

National Institute of Arthritis and Musculoskeletal and Skin Diseases

1987 Arthritis, Rheumatic Diseases, and Related Disorders Public Health Service

National Institute of Neurological Disorders and Stroke

1989 Chronic Pain: Hope through Research NIH Publication No. 90-2406

Press, Joel M., Michael Berkowitz, and Steven L. Wiesner

1991 "The Medical History and Low Back Pain" Journal of Back and Musculoskeletal Rehabilitation 1(1):7-22

Sundararajan, V. et al.

1998 "Patterns and Determinants of Multiple Provider Use in Patients with Acute Low Back Pain" Journal of General Internal Medicine 13:528-533

Vermont Rehabilitation Engineering Center

no "Biomechanics and Low Back Pain" REC Brief 1(1):1-10
date

Williams, Gareth H. and Philip H.N. Wood

1988 "Coming to Terms with Chronic Illness: The Negotiation of Autonomy in Rheumatoid Arthritis" International Disability Studies 10:3:128-133

ORGANIZATIONS

<u>American Academy of Orthopaedic Surgeons</u> (AAOS)
6300 North River Road
Rosemont, IL 60018
(800) 346-2267   (847) 223-7186   FAX (847) 823-8125
orthoinfo.aaos.org

A professional organization for orthopedic surgeons and allied health professionals. Web site offers a "Find a Surgeon" link. Click on "Spine" for fact sheets. A quarterly e-mail newsletter, "Your Orthopaedic Connection," is available upon request.

<u>American Back Society</u> (ABS)
St. Joseph's Professional Center
2647 International Boulevard, Suite 401
Oakland, CA 94601
(510) 536-9929   FAX (510) 536-1812
e-mail: info@americanbacksoc.org www.americanbacksoc.org

A membership organization dedicated to relieving the pain and impairment caused by back problems. Sponsors symposia for presenting research findings. Membership for licensed health care professionals, $225.00; for other interested individuals, $125.00. Publishes quarterly "ABS Newsletter," which is a benefit of membership, or it may be purchased for $62.50 a year.

<u>American Chronic Pain Association</u> (ACPA)
PO Box 850
Rocklin, CA 95677
(916) 632-0922   FAX (916) 632-3208
e-mail: acpa@pacbell.net   www.theacpa.org

Organizes groups throughout the U.S. to provide support and activities for people who experience chronic pain. $30.00 first year, $15.00 thereafter; includes quarterly newsletter, "ACPA Chronicle."

<u>American Pain Foundation</u> (APF)
201 North Charles Street, Suite 710
Baltimore, MD 2120
(888) 615-7246   FAX (410) 385-1832
e-mail: info@painfoundation.org www.painfoundation.org

This organization provides educational materials and advocates on behalf of people who are experiencing pain. It promotes research and advocates to remove barriers to treatment for pain. It distributes patient educational materials (free) and has information about the causes of pain and treatment as well as links to related sites on its web site.

American Pain Society (APS)
4700 West Lake Avenue
Glen View, IL 60025
(847) 375-4715   FAX (877) 734-8758
e-mail: info@ampainsoc.org   www.ampainsoc.org

The Society is a multidisciplinary membership organization that has the goals of advancing research, education, and professional services for people in pain. Membership dues for professionals vary by income level from $100.00 to $235.00. Individual membership, $125.00. Membership includes the quarterly publication "Pain Forum" and a newsletter, the "APS Bulletin." The Academy will provide a list of local physicians who specialize in treating pain.

The Arthritis Foundation
PO Box 7669
Atlanta, GA 30357-0669
(800) 283-7800   (404) 872-7100   FAX (404) 872-0457
www.arthritis.org

Supports research; offers referrals to physicians; provides public and professional education. Chapters throughout the U.S.; toll-free number connects to local chapter. Some chapters offer arthritis classes, clubs, and exercise programs. Membership, $20.00, includes chapter newsletter and magazine, "Arthritis Today;" also available by subscription, $12.95. Members receive discounts on purchases. Many brochures are available on the web site, including "Back Pain."

ClinicalTrials.gov
clinicaltrials.gov

This confidential web site has information on more than 4,000 Federal and private medical studies including the Spine Patient Outcomes Research Trial. Lists location of clinical trials, design and purpose, criteria for participation, information about the disease and treatment being studied, and links to personnel who are recruiting participants. Also available at www.nlm.nih.gov

Commission on Accreditation of Rehabilitation Facilities (CARF)
4891 East Grant Road
Tucson, AZ 85712
(520) 325-1044 (V/TTY)   FAX (520) 318-1129
e-mail: webmaster@carf.org   www.carf.org

Conducts site evaluations and accredits organizations that provide rehabilitation, pain management, adult day services, and assisted living. Provides a free list of accredited organizations in a specific state.

MEDLINEplus: Back Pain
www.nlm.nih.gov/medlineplus/backpain.html

This web site provides links to sites for general information about back pain, symptoms and diagnosis, treatment, specific aspects of the condition, clinical trials, statistics, organizations, and research. Provides links to MEDLINE research articles and related MEDLINEplus pages.

National Chronic Pain Outreach Association (NCPOA)
PO Box 274
Millboro, VA 24460-9606
(540) 862-9437   FAX (540) 862-9485
e-mail: ncpoa@cfw.com

A national clearinghouse for information about chronic pain. Refers individuals to support groups on chronic pain throughout the U.S. Produces publications and audiocassettes on a variety of topics related to chronic pain. Membership, individuals, $25.00; professionals, $50.00; includes quarterly newsletter, "Lifeline."

National Institute of Arthritis and Musculoskeletal and Skin Diseases (NIAMS)
Building 31, Room 4C05
31 Center Drive, MSC 2350
Bethesda, MD 20892
(301) 496-8190   FAX (301) 480-2814   www.nih.gov/niams

Sponsors specialized research centers in rheumatoid arthritis, osteoarthritis, and osteoporosis. These centers conduct basic and clinical research; provide professional, public, and patient education; and are involved in community activities. Also supports individual clinical and basic research.

National Institute of Arthritis and Musculoskeletal and Skin Diseases Information Clearinghouse (NAMSIC)
1 AMS Circle
Bethesda, MD 20892
(877) 226-4267   (301) 495-4484   (301) 565-2966 (TTY)
FAX (301) 718-6366   e-mail: niamsinfo@mail.nih.gov
www.nih.gov/niams

Distributes bibliographies, fact sheets, catalogues, and directories to the public and professionals. Free. Many of the fact sheets are available on the web site.

Spine-health.com
1840 Oak Avenue, Suite 112
Evanston, IL 60201
e-mail: admin@spine-health.com   www.spine-health.com

This web site provides information on coping with chronic back pain, treatment, pain management, and rehabilitation. Also offers a physician directory on the web site.

Back Pain
by David R. Goldmann and David A. Horowitz (eds.)
American College of Physicians
Dorling Kindersley Publishing, Inc.
95 Madison Avenue
New York, NY 10016
(877) 342-5357   (212) 213-4800   FAX (212) 213-5240
e-mail: customerservice@dk.com   www.dk.com

This book presents an overview of the spine, causes of back pain, and possible treatments. Includes strengthening exercises and information on conventional and alternative treatments. $6.95

The Back Pain Book
by Mike Hage
Peachtree Publishers
1700 Chattahoochee Avenue
Atlanta, GA 30318
(800) 241-0113   FAX (800) 875-8909   (404) 876-8761
www.peachtree-online.com

Written by a physical therapist, this book discusses how movement and posture may alleviate neck and back pain. $13.95 plus $3.25 shipping and handling

Back Pain Interactive Tutorial
www.nlm.nih.gov/medlineplus/tutorials/backpain.html

This tutorial provides an overview of the condition, treatment options, and resources for everyday living.

The Back Pain Sourcebook
by Stephanie Levin-Gervasi
McGraw Hill, Order Services
PO Box 545
Blacklick, OH 43004
(800) 722-4726   FAX (614) 755-5645   www.mmhe.com

This book describes the causes of back pain, conventional and alternative treatments, and recommends exercises and techniques to prevent further injury. $17.00

Back Sense
by Ronald D. Siegel, Michael H. Urdang, and Douglas R. Johnson
Random House, Order Department
400 Hahn Road, PO Box 100
Westminster, MD 21157
(800) 733-3000   (410) 848-1900   FAX (410) 386-7013
www.randomhouse.com

The authors of this book attribute most chronic back pain to stress and discuss a self-treatment method which includes stretching exercises and stress reduction techniques, such as meditation. $21.95 plus $5.50 shipping and handling

Low Back Pain Handbook
by Brian P. D'Orazio (ed.)
Elsevier Health Science
Attn: Order Department
11830 Westline Industrial Drive
St. Louis, MO 63146
(800) 545-2522   FAX (800) 545-2522   www.harcourthealth.com

Written by physical therapists, this book examines the anatomical and functional causes of low back pain and the diseases and disorders that may affect the back. Includes many photographs of exercises used in treating low back pain and describes rehabilitation after back surgery. $44.99 plus $7.00 shipping and handling

Low Back Pain Syndrome
by Rene Cailliet
F.A. Davis Company
1915 Arch Street
Philadelphia, PA 19103
(800) 323-3555   FAX (215) 440-3016
e-mail: orders@fadavis.com   www.fadavis.com

This book discusses the mechanism of low back pain, how it should be evaluated, and psychological aspects. $25.95

Managing Pain Before It Manages You
by Margaret A. Caudill
Guilford Publications
72 Spring Street
New York, NY 10012
(800) 365-7006   (212) 431-9800   FAX (212) 966-6708
e-mail: info@guilford.com   www.guilford.com

This book presents techniques for coping with chronic pain. It describes common pain disorders, pain medications, nutritional recommendations, and alternative medicine. Includes worksheets. $19.95 plus $4.50 shipping and handling

Meeting the Needs of Employees with Disabilities
Resources for Rehabilitation
22 Bonad Road
Winchester, MA 01890
(781) 368-9094   FAX (781) 368-9096
e-mail: orders@rfr.org   www.rfr.org

This resource guide provides information to help people with disabilities retain or obtain employment. Information on government programs and laws, supported employment, training programs, environmental adaptations, and the transition from school to work is included. Chapters on mobility, vision, and hearing and speech impairments include information on organizations, products, and services that enable employers to accommodate the needs of employees with disabilities. $44.95 plus $5.00 shipping and handling. (See order form on last page of this book.)

Musculoskeletal Disorders and the Workplace: Low Back and Upper Extremities
National Research Council
National Academy Press
2101 Constitution Avenue, NW
Lockbox 285
Washington, DC 20055
(888) 624-8373   (202) 334-3313   FAX (202) 334-2451
e-mail: zjones@nas.edu   www.nap.edu

In this book, a multidisciplinary panel examined the prevalence, incidence, and economic consequences of workplace injury and the effectiveness of various interventions. $59.95 plus $4.00 shipping and handling. A 20% discount is offered to individuals who purchase books through the National Academy's Web Bookstore.

Say Goodbye to Back Pain
Video Learning Library
15838 North 62nd Street
Scottsdale, AZ 85254
(800) 383-8811   e-mail: jspencer@videolearning.com
www.videolearning.com

A six week exercise program for individuals with back pain. 96 minutes. $39.95 plus $4.00 shipping and handling

<u>Sex and Back Pain</u>
The Saunders Group
4250 Norex Drive
Chaska, MN 55318
(800) 456-1289   FAX (800) 375-1119
www.thesaundersgroup.com

This booklet is a self-help manual that describes sexual techniques and activities to restore sexual function that has been lost due to back pain. $3.25 plus $4.00 shipping and handling. The videotape helps the couple to discuss the effects of back pain on sexual functioning as well as techniques for pain control. 25 minutes. $59.00 plus $6.00 shipping and handling

<u>Understand Your Backache: A Guide to Prevention, Treatment, and Relief</u>
by Rene Cailliet
F.A. Davis Company
1915 Arch Street
Philadelphia, PA 19103
(800) 323-3555   FAX (215) 440-3016
e-mail: orders@fadavis.com   www.fadavis.com

This book includes information about treatment and prevention of back pain as well as a description of the examinations performed by physicians and various types of surgery. $13.95

<u>Your Aching Back: A Doctor's Guide to Relief</u>
by Augustus A. White, III
Simon & Schuster
100 Front Street
Riverside, NJ 08075
(888) 866-6631   FAX (800) 943-9831   www.simonsays.com

This book discusses the basic mechanisms of the back, issues to consider when deciding whether to have surgery, how to take proper care of the back, and a section on commonly asked questions. $14.00 plus $4.98 shipping and handling

Chapter 9

MULTIPLE SCLEROSIS

Multiple sclerosis (MS) is a chronic central nervous system condition in which the nerve fibers of the brain and spinal cord are damaged. A fatty substance called myelin protects the nerve fibers and enables the smooth transmission of neurological impulses between the central nervous system and the rest of the body. If inflammation damages or destroys the myelin, it may heal with no loss of function. Later, however, scar (or plaque) may form and interfere with the transmission of neurological impulses. Function may be diminished or lost. The disease is called multiple sclerosis because there are multiple areas of scarring or sclerosis (Minden and Frankel: 1989).

Estimates of the number of individuals with multiple sclerosis vary from less than 200,000, based on hospital and physicians' records, to 500,000, based on public surveys and pathology records (National Institute of Neurological Disorders and Stroke: 1990). Multiple sclerosis affects twice as many women as men and twice as many whites as African-Americans (Scheinberg and Smith: 1989). Age of onset ranges from mid to late adolescence to middle age.

Over three-quarters (77%) of individuals with multiple sclerosis have activity limitations (National Center for Health Statistics: 1988). The broad economic and social implications of multiple sclerosis include medical expenses, unemployment or underemployment, the cost of special services, and the emotional and physical effects on the individual as well as the family. Cognitive problems such as memory loss, forgetfulness, and the inability to maintain a train of thought have been reported by many individuals with multiple sclerosis (Sullivan et al.: 1990).

Each person with multiple sclerosis has unique symptoms based on the location of the damage to the nervous system. These symptoms may include blurred or double vision, numbness in the extremities, balance or coordination problems, fatigue, muscle spasticity or stiffness, slurred speech, muscle weakness, or loss of bladder or bowel control.

The cause of multiple sclerosis is unknown. Scientists who believe that multiple sclerosis is an autoimmune disease are investigating the role of a variety of viruses in triggering damage to the immune system, which in turn may lead to the development of multiple sclerosis. Other investigators are studying the role of heredity. Their studies suggest that certain genetic factors may predispose some individuals to acquire multiple sclerosis, but there is no known pattern of direct inheritance.

DIAGNOSIS OF MULTIPLE SCLEROSIS

Unfortunately, there is no one symptom or test that can confirm a diagnosis of multiple sclerosis. In the past, positive diagnosis of multiple sclerosis often took months or years. Physicians would verify loss of function in more than one area of the central nervous system and confirm that these losses had occurred at least twice over an interval of at least a month. Individuals with multiple sclerosis were often frustrated by the length of time and the multiple procedures required to diagnose their symptoms. Since it is now recommended that treatment begin as soon as a positive diagnosis is confirmed (see "TREATMENT OF MULTIPLE SCLEROSIS" below), it is crucial that physicians follow the current diagnostic criteria.

The development of magnetic resonance imaging (MRI), which provides a recorded image of central nervous system lesions, has led to changes in diagnostic criteria. The MRI is now considered an essential key in making an MS diagnosis. In July 2000, in the first formal review since 1982, an International Panel on the Diagnosis of MS produced revised criteria, integrating the use of MRIs with cerebrospinal fluid (CSF) studies and visual evoked potentials (VEP) (McDonald et al.: 2001). Cerebrospinal fluid studies may detect certain immune system antibodies. Visual evoked potentials studies assess the visual pathway to the optic nerve. The diagnostic result is either "MS," "possible MS" (for individuals who are at risk but whose evaluations may not be complete or meet all criteria), or "not MS."

TYPES OF MULTIPLE SCLEROSIS

In 1996, an international panel of physicians who treat individuals with multiple sclerosis recommended that the following terms be used to describe the types of multiple sclerosis (Reingold: 1996). *Relapsing-remitting* describes a pattern of multiple sclerosis in which exacerbations are followed by either full recovery or partial recovery and lasting disability. Individuals with the *primary progressive* form experience steady disease progression. The *secondary progressive* form has a clear pattern of relapses and recovery, becoming progressively worse between acute exacerbations. *Progressive-relapsing* multiple sclerosis is progressive from onset with acute attacks.

These forms of multiple sclerosis are not exclusive; some individuals may experience progression of one form to another. Smith and Scheinberg (1985) report that there is a more favorable prognosis for individuals with early onset (before age 35); acute onset rather than gradual onset; complete remission after the first attack; and sensory rather than motor symptoms.

TREATMENT OF MULTIPLE SCLEROSIS

There is no cure for multiple sclerosis; however, physicians can treat the symptoms of multiple sclerosis and try to control its progress with anti-inflammatory medication.

Interferon beta-1b (Betaseron) is one of the medications used to treat ambulatory individuals ages 18 to 50 with relapsing-remitting multiple sclerosis. Clinical studies have shown that Betaseron reduces the frequency and severity of exacerbations. MRI studies have shown reduced number and size of brain lesions (Goodkin: 1995). Betaseron is injected by the individual subcutaneously every other day. The most common side effects reported are reactions at the injection site, such as swelling, redness, rashes, and flu-like symptoms, including chills, fatigue, fever, and muscle aches. Individuals using Betaseron must learn to inject the drug and determine an injection schedule that works best for them, minimizing side effects. Betaseron is expensive, nearly $10,000 a year. The Betaseron Foundation aids underinsured individuals to obtain the medication (see "ORGANIZATIONS" section below).

Interferon beta-1a (Avonex) has been shown to reduce disease activity in individuals with relapsing-remitting multiple sclerosis and to slow the progression of disability. Avonex is administered in a once-a-week intramuscular injection into the thigh, hip, or upper arm. Many individuals self-inject or receive treatments from a caregiver. In clinical trials, the major side effect was initial flu-like symptoms which diminished over the course of treatment. Women who are pregnant or who are trying to become pregnant should not use Avonex. Biogen, the manufacturer of Avonex, offers a toll-free support line and literature to individuals (see "ORGANIZATIONS" section below).

Glatiramer acetate (Copaxone) also slows the rate of relapse in individuals with relapsing-remitting multiple sclerosis. It is injected subcutaneously on a daily basis. It does not produce the flu-like symptoms or depression associated with Betaseron and Avonex but its benefits do not appear as soon.

In 1998, the Medical Advisory Board of the National Multiple Sclerosis Society released a consensus statement on the use of interferon beta-1a, interferon beta-1b, and glatiramer acetate therapy in the treatment of multiple sclerosis. The Board recommended that:
  • therapy be initiated as soon as possible following a definite diagnosis of multiple sclerosis and determination that the disease is the relapsing-remitting type
  • access to therapy not be limited by age, level of disability, or frequency of relapses
  • treatment should be continued unless there is a clear lack of benefit, intolerable side effects, new data which reveal other reasons for cessation, or better therapy is available
  • these drugs be covered by third party payers
  • the choice of drugs be decided upon jointly by the patient and physician
  • movement from one drug to another should be permitted (National Multiple Sclerosis Society: 1998)

Although Avonex, Betaseron, and Copaxone have been shown to reduce MS exacerbations, users may still have symptoms, such as spasticity, fatigue, and bladder control problems. These continuing symptoms may lead individuals to discontinue taking the medications, believing that if they don't feel better, the drugs are not working.

In 2000, the FDA approved the use of mitoxantrone (Novantrone), an immunosuppressive drug that is administered to individuals with relapsing-remitting MS intravenously every three months. Use of the drug resulted in diminished relapse rates and disability progression. Due to potential cardiac toxicity, dosage is carefully monitored. Its side effects may include low white blood cell counts, thinning of the hair, nausea, and menstrual irregularities. Mitoxantrone is the only drug approved in the U.S. to treat secondary progressive MS, although some European studies have shown benefits with interferon beta-1b.

Prednisone, adrenocorticotropic hormone (ACTH), prednisolone, and other anti-inflammatory drugs have been effective in reducing the severity and duration of multiple sclerosis flare-ups. These medications are not recommended for long term use because of side effects, such as nausea, drowsiness, changes in blood pressure and blood glucose levels, lowered resistance to infection, and thinning of bones (Lechtenberg: 1995). Medication may also be used to treat multiple sclerosis symptoms, such as spasticity, dizziness, fatigue, bladder problems, tremors, depression, and sensory problems (a "pins and needles" feeling). The individual with multiple sclerosis and the physician must carefully consider each medication and its possible side effects, which may appear to be symptoms of the disease itself.

Optic neuritis, *double vision*, and *nystagmus* are common visual symptoms of multiple sclerosis. Inflammation of the optic nerve (neuritis) causes loss of vision. If the muscles of the eye are weakened by nerve demyelination, the individual cannot focus and experiences double vision (diplopia). Double vision may occur during an exacerbation and disappear during remission of multiple sclerosis symptoms. Cortisone is often used to treat optic neuritis and double vision. Nystagmus is an involuntary rapid eye movement; it interferes with focusing and may cause dizziness.

Fatigue is the most common symptom experienced by individuals with multiple sclerosis (Multiple Sclerosis Council: 1998). The lack of physical and/or mental energy interferes with activities of daily living, increasing individuals' feelings of powerlessness or lack of control over their lives. Since 1986 the Social Security Administration has recognized fatigue as a major determinant in evaluating individuals with multiple sclerosis for disability benefits (Taylor: 1998). The Multiple Sclerosis Council (1998) differentiates between chronic persistent fatigue, which is present for half the time for more than six weeks, and acute fatigue, new or significant increase of feelings of fatigue. The Council developed self-report tools for individuals with multiple sclerosis that measure sleep habits, fatigue symptoms, and the effects of fatigue on everyday living (see "PUBLICATIONS AND TAPES" section below). Occupational therapists may recommend energy conservation techniques that may help reduce fatigue, including moderate exercise, using assistive devices, and rest. Heat-induced fatigue may be treated with cooling devices, such as ice packs and vests, air conditioning, and cool showers. Medications used to treat fatigue include amantadine (Symmetrel), an antiviral drug; stimulants; and antidepressants.

Some individuals with multiple sclerosis experience *problems with gait* including weakness, spasticity, and lack of coordination (ataxia). Antispastic medications, stretching exercises, and swimming relieve symptoms, such as a stiff gait, foot drop, and toe dragging. Tizanidine (Zanaflex) was approved by the FDA in 1997 for the treatment of spasticity (Kalb et al.: 1997). It may be used alone or in combination with baclofen, another antispastic drug. Orthoses are assistive devices used to support weakened areas, provide proper alignment, and improve function. An ankle foot orthosis worn inside the shoe may relieve the symptoms of spasticity. Ataxia is treated with a sequential exercise program in which the individual performs repetitive movements, often watching himself or herself in a mirror, to increase sensory feedback and restore coordination.

About 80% of individuals with multiple sclerosis experience *urinary dysfunction* (Holland: 1996). Urinary tract infections, formation of bladder stones, and kidney damage may occur if the bladder is not completely emptied during voiding. Symptoms of urinary dysfunction include urgency, frequency, hesitancy, nocturia, and incontinence. Although some individuals with occasional incontinence rely on absorbent undergarments, medications and catheterization are used when symptoms are more severe. Anticholinergic drugs may be used to control bladder dysfunction by regulating bladder contractions (Lechtenberg: 1995). Oxybutynin chloride (Ditropan XL), an antispasmodic, is often prescribed to decrease bladder muscle spasms and the urge to urinate. Taken once a day, the only major side effect is dry mouth. Tolterodine tartrate (Detrol) reduces contractions of the bladder muscle and increases the volume of urine voided. It, too, may cause dry mouth. In intermittent self-catheterization, a flexible catheter is inserted in the urethra, urine is emptied from the bladder, and the catheter is removed. Many individuals find that self-catheterization allows the bladder to regain normal function (Holland: 1996).

238

Constipation is the most common bowel problem and may be caused by inadequate fluid and fiber consumption, medication, lack of physical activity, and decreased sensation in the rectal area. Eating high fiber foods, drinking eight to 12 cups of liquid daily, increasing physical activity, and using stool softeners or bulk formers (if necessary), are important in a bowel management program that will reduce symptoms and discomfort. To avoid constipation, individuals should develop a regular schedule for bowel movements, ideally about 30 minutes after eating. Holland and Frames (1996) also recommend changing the angle between the rectum and anus by using a footstool or altering the height of the toilet seat. Other bowel dysfunctions include diarrhea, caused by loss of sphincter control, medications, or viruses; fecal impaction, caused by weakened abdominal muscles; and flatulence.

Weakness of upper extremities and *speech problems* (dysarthria) are other disabling symptoms of multiple sclerosis. Individuals with severe multiple sclerosis may also have difficulty swallowing. Treatment options for these symptoms include medication, exercise, adaptations in everyday living, and counseling.

PSYCHOLOGICAL ASPECTS OF MULTIPLE SCLEROSIS

From the onset of symptoms of multiple sclerosis, the course of the disease is fraught with uncertainty and unpredictability. Individuals with the disease have a near normal life expectancy (Scheinberg: 1983) and must continually adjust to the exacerbations that may occur at any time.

Individuals must plan their daily living and work schedules to accommodate the effects of the condition. For example, exacerbations often cause fatigue, which interferes with normal activities, including employment. Individuals must find a balance between activity and rest periods. Not surprisingly, individuals who are experiencing exacerbations express higher levels of emotional disturbances than individuals who are in remission (Warren et al.: 1991).

Fears about the future are to be expected, given the unpredictable course of the disease and the serious consequences that may ensue. Family members may often find that they are taking on additional responsibilities for running the household and making important decisions. Role reversal is not an uncommon phenomenon. Individuals in well adjusted marital relationships often find the relationship a source of strength and support to help them cope with the condition (Rodgers and Calder: 1990). At the same time, multiple sclerosis may add a strain to the relationship, including sexual problems. Counseling for both the person with multiple sclerosis and other family members is often beneficial. Often ignored by health care professionals, the caregiving partner should receive advice on respite care and supportive counseling (White et al.: 1993). However, professional counselors themselves sometimes have fears about the disease that must be addressed in order to provide counseling that meets their clients' psychological needs (Segal: 1991).

In addition to the many physical adaptations that individuals with multiple sclerosis make, about half of all individuals with multiple sclerosis experience cognitive problems (Mahler: 1992; Rao et al.: 1991) and must take measures to overcome these difficulties. Among these difficulties are memory problems, concept formation, and depression. Rao and colleagues (1991) found that individuals with multiple sclerosis who had cognitive problems were less likely to be employed and to engage in social activities than individuals without cognitive impairments, even though the severity of physical problems and the duration of the disease were similar for both groups. A study by Sullivan and his colleagues (1990) found that most individuals who experienced memory loss and forgetfulness used simple aids, such as notepads or daily agendas to enable them to keep abreast of their daily needs and schedules. If there are vision problems, large print or a tape recorder may be used to record information.

Symptoms such as stumbling, dropping items, incontinence, and slurred speech may lead to self-consciousness, anxiety, and depression. The individual's personal coping mechanisms and the support provided by family, friends, and the community are crucial to the active problem solving required in living with multiple sclerosis (Shuman and Schwartz: 1988). Individuals who exhibit these symptoms may also benefit from antidepressants and individual or group counseling or a combination of these therapies.

PROFESSIONAL SERVICE PROVIDERS

The unique symptoms of each individual with multiple sclerosis require individualized treatment plans. The physical and emotional needs of each individual are best served through a team approach involving medical, allied health, and rehabilitation professionals.

Neurologists, who specialize in diseases and conditions of the brain and central nervous system, conduct neurological examinations and interpret the results of tests, such as MRIs to diagnose multiple sclerosis and to rule out other possible conditions. *Physiatrists*, or rehabilitation physicians, design an individual treatment plan for the patient with multiple sclerosis.

Physical therapists teach individuals with multiple sclerosis how to perform a range of exercises which help build endurance and strength. Physical therapists also prescribe therapeutic exercises to diminish or eliminate weakness, spasticity, and lack of coordination. Physical therapists provide training in the use of assistive devices, such as canes, crutches, and orthoses. *Occupational therapists* assess functioning in activities of everyday living and teach simplified techniques of accomplishing them. They may recommend adaptations to the home and work environments. Occupational therapists also suggest adaptive recreation equipment and programs.

Orthotists make and fit assistive devices (orthoses) for improving gait in individuals with multiple sclerosis. Orthotists, physical therapists, or occupational therapists provide instruction in the use of these devices, such as ankle or foot braces.

Psychologists provide therapy for individuals and families living with multiple sclerosis. Depression and burnout, for example, may be reduced through marital therapy, helping the couple to balance each other's needs.

Social workers offer practical and emotional support to individuals adjusting to a disability or chronic condition and to their families. Social workers provide information about financial and medical benefits, housing, and community resources. They conduct individual, family, or group counseling and may refer individuals to self-help or peer counseling groups.

Rehabilitation counselors help individuals with multiple sclerosis develop a plan that will enable them to continue functioning and working. Some individuals will need assistance in returning to their previous position or retraining to obtain a different type of position.

Rehabilitation counselors help make the contacts and placements necessary to attain these goals.

Low vision specialists may be ophthalmologists, optometrists, opticians, or other professionals trained to help individuals with vision loss use their remaining vision to the greatest extent possible with the assistance of optical and nonoptical aids.

WHERE TO FIND SERVICES

Neurologists work in private practices, acute care hospitals, and specialty clinics. Neurologists and other members of the multidisciplinary team may also work in transitional or independent living programs and in rehabilitation hospitals. In addition to medical services, MS Comprehensive Care Centers provide services such as physical and occupational therapy, counseling, and patient and family education. A list of these centers is available from the National Multiple Sclerosis Society (see "ORGANIZATIONS" section below). Individuals who have mobility problems and difficulty traveling to professional service providers' offices often may obtain services in their homes from physical and occupational therapists. Low vision services are often available in ophthalmologists' or optometrists' offices, in private or public agencies that serve individuals who are visually impaired or blind, or in independent practices (see Chapter 11, "Vision Impairment and Blindness," for more information about these services).

ENVIRONMENTAL ADAPTATIONS

Individuals with multiple sclerosis use a combination of environmental adaptations and assistive devices to make everyday routines easier. When making plans for living arrangements or for travel, individuals with multiple sclerosis must consider a variety of alternatives in the event that their functional abilities deteriorate. For instance, in purchasing a home, it is wise to determine if there is room for a wheelchair ramp or a chair lift.

Some individuals with gait problems use a cane, crutches, walker, wheelchair, scooter, or a combination of these mobility aids. An individual who usually uses a cane or crutches may prefer to use a wheelchair or scooter when traveling long distances. Special controls installed on cars with automatic transmissions enable many individuals with multiple sclerosis to continue driving. The gas and brake pedals are operated by hand. These attachments do not interfere with the foot pedals used by other family members. Rehabilitation hospitals and centers offer driver evaluation services, such as clinical testing and observation to determine an individual's need for adaptive equipment or training. Major automobile manufacturers offer reimbursement for adaptive equipment installed on new vehicles. (See Chapter 4 "TRAVEL AND TRANSPORTATION ORGANIZATIONS" section for a listing of programs that offer adaptive equipment for automobiles.)

Heat and humidity affect many individuals with multiple sclerosis. Air conditioning helps to reduce fatigue and weakness. Physicians, rehabilitation counselors, or tax advisers may provide advice on whether the purchase of an air conditioner is a tax deductible expense.

A referral to a low vision rehabilitation center offers individuals with vision problems the opportunity to improve visual function with low vision aids. An eye patch may reduce double vision. Prisms, mounted on the eyeglasses lens, will expand the visual field of the eye that is not patched. Sunglasses reduce glare and improve contrast for individuals with optic neuritis. Nonoptical aids, such as large print, tape recorders, and high contrast markings are also useful (see Chapter 11, "Visual Impairment and Blindness").

Bathtub rails, elevated toilet seats, and grab bars are useful bathroom safety devices. A stall shower is safer and easier to use than a combination tub/shower. A shower chair or tub seat provides additional safety.

Some individuals use assistive devices for dressing, including elastic shoelaces, velcro closures, and buttoning aids. Velcro, the hook and loop material, may be substituted for buttons or zippers for ease in dressing. National mail order companies offer clothes that open in front and have reinforced seams, elastic waistbands, and buttons sewn with elastic thread. Formerly these items were limited to leisure and hospital wear, but manufacturers are now designing suits, outerwear, and dressy items for working men and women who have disabilities. Loops of Velcro, attached to a brush or razor handle, slip around the hand, providing control for the user. Foam hair rollers, water pipe foam insulation, or layers of tape are used to build up the handles of items as varied as toothbrushes, pens, pencils, eating utensils, paint brushes, and crochet hooks. Weighted utensils, clamps, and suction cups assist individuals who experience impaired coordination or tremor. Dycem, a nonslip plastic, may be used as a pad under items such as mixing bowls, cups, or dinner plates to hold them in place. Remote controls turn on and off lights and televisions and open and close garage doors. Voice dialer telephones permit the storage of frequently called telephone numbers and automatic dialing. A speaker phone allows the individual with poor motor control or tremors to carry on a telephone conversation comfortably. Many mail order catalogues offer a wide selection of assistive devices for individuals with disabilities and chronic conditions (see Chapter 4, "RESOURCES FOR ASSISTIVE DEVICES" section, for sources of these devices).

Computer technology can enable individuals with multiple sclerosis to continue working and living independently. Screen readers or large print software, keyguards used to prevent unwanted keystrokes, and specially designed keyboards and word prediction software for individuals with limited dexterity are useful adaptations.

Individuals with multiple sclerosis can save time and energy by reorganizing the kitchen and changing food preparation routines. Many individuals learn valuable tips and techniques from peers in multiple sclerosis support groups or from occupational therapists.

References

Goodkin, Donald E.
1994 "Interferon Beta-Ib" The Lancet 344:8929:1057
Holland, Nancy
1996 "For Urinary Problems: Get A Diagnosis First!" Inside MS New York, NY: National Multiple Sclerosis Society 14:1:19-20
Holland, Nancy and Robin Frames
1996 Understanding Bowel Problems in MS New York, NY: National Multiple Sclerosis Society

Kalb, Rosalind et al.

1997 "Multiple Sclerosis: The Questions You Have, The Answers You Need, 1997 Update" Multiple Sclerosis Quarterly Report 16:3

Lechtenberg, Richard

1995 Multiple Sclerosis Fact Book Philadelphia, PA: F.A. Davis Company

Mahler, M.E.

1992 "Behavioral Manifestations Associated with Multiple Sclerosis: Psychiatric Clinics of North America 15:2(June):425-438

McDonald, W. Ian et al.

2001 "Recommended Diagnostic Criteria for Multiple Sclerosis: Guidelines from the International Panel on the Diagnosis of Multiple Sclerosis" Annals of Neurology 50:1(July):121-127

Minden, Sarah L. and Debra Frankel

1989 PLAINTALK: A Booklet About Multiple Sclerosis For Family Members New York, NY: National Multiple Sclerosis Society

Multiple Sclerosis Council for Clinical Practice Guidelines

1998 Fatigue and Multiple Sclerosis Washington, DC: Paralyzed Veterans of America

National Center for Health Statistics, Collins, John G.

1988 "Prevalence of Selected Chronic Conditions, United States, 1983-85" Advance Data From Vital and Health Statistics No. 155 DHHS Pub. No (PHS) 88-1250. Hyattsville, MD: Public Health Service

National Institute of Neurological Disorders and Stroke

1990 Multiple Sclerosis: 1990 Research Program Bethesda, MD: National Institutes of Health

National Multiple Sclerosis Society

1998 National Multiple Sclerosis Society Disease Management Consensus Statement New York, NY: National Multiple Sclerosis Society

Rao, S.M. et al.

1991 "Cognitive Dysfunction in Multiple Sclerosis II. Impact on Employment and Social Functioning" Neurology 41:5(May):692-696

Reingold, Stephen C.

1996 "New Terms for MS Types" Inside MS Fall

Rodgers, Jennifer and Peter Calder

1990 "Marital Adjustment: A Valuable Resource for the Emotional Health of Individuals with Multiple Sclerosis" Rehabilitation Counseling Bulletin 34:1(September):24-32

Scheinberg, Labe

1983 "Signs, Symptoms, and Course of MS" pp. 35-43 in Lab C. Scheinberg (ed.) Multiple Sclerosis: A Guide for Patients and Their Families New York, NY: Raven Press

Scheinberg, Labe and Charles R. Smith

1989 Rehabilitation of Patients with Multiple Sclerosis New York, NY: National Multiple Sclerosis Society

Segal, Julia

1991 "Counselling People with Multiple Sclerosis and Their Families" pp.147-160 in Hilton Davis and Lesley Fallowfield (eds.) Counselling and Communication in Health Care London: John Wiley and Sons

Shuman, Robert and Janice Schwartz

1988 Understanding Multiple Sclerosis Riverside, NJ: MacMillan Publishing Company

Smith, Charles R. and Labe Scheinberg

1990 "Symptomatic Treatment and Rehabilitation in Multiple Sclerosis" pp. 327-350 in Stuart D. Cook (ed.) Handbook of Multiple Sclerosis New York, NY: Marcel Dekker, Inc.

1985 "Clinical Features of Multiple Sclerosis" Seminars in Neurology 5(June)2:85-93

Sullivan, Michael J., L. Krista Edgley, and Eric Dehoux

1990 "A Survey of Multiple Sclerosis Part 1: Perceived Cognitive Problems and Compensatory Strategy Use" Canadian Journal of Rehabilitation 4:2:99-105

Taylor, Ronald S.

1998 "Multiple Sclerosis Potpourri: Paroxysmal Symptoms, Seizures, Fatigue, Pregnancy, and More" pp. 551-559 in George H. Kraft and Ronald S. Taylor (eds.) Multiple Sclerosis: A Rehabilitative Approach Philadelphia, PA: W.B. Saunders Company

Warren, S., K.G. Warren, and R. Cockrill

1991 "Emotional Stress and Coping in Multiple Sclerosis Exacerbations" Journal of Psychosomatic Research 35:1:37-47

White, David M., Marci L. Catanzaro, and George H. Kraft

1991 "An Approach to the Psychological Aspects of Multiple Sclerosis: A Coping Guide for Healthcare Providers and Families" Journal of Neurological Rehabilitation 7:2:43-52

American Autoimmune Related Diseases Association (AARDA)
22100 Gratiot Avenue
Detroit, MI 48205
(586) 776-3900   www.aarda.org

Provides information on autoimmune diseases including multiple sclerosis, lupus, type 1 diabetes, Sjogren's syndrome, and rheumatoid arthritis. Web site offers brief explanations of conditions. Additional information is available for a donation of any size.

Avonex Alliance
Avonex Start Assistance Program
(800) 456-2255   www.avonex.com

Provides information on Avonex, a drug used in treating relapsing forms of multiple sclerosis, distribution options, insurance reimbursement counseling, and/or training for self-administration of the drug. Phone lines open Monday through Friday, 8:30 a.m. to 8:00 p.m., E.S.T. Publishes quarterly newsletter, "The Alliance Exchange;" free. Also available on the web site.

Betaseron Foundation
4828 Parkway Plaza Boulevard, Suite 220
Charlotte, NC 28217
(800) 948-5777   FAX (704) 357-0036
www.betaseronfoundation.org

Provides Betaseron to qualified underinsured patients. Requirements include a confirmed diagnosis of multiple sclerosis, prescription for Betaseron, inadequate medical insurance, and U.S. residence. Patient financial contribution is required (up to $25.00 per month). Uninsured patients will be referred to Berlex, the manufacturer of Betaseron, for assistance [(800) 788-1467].

Brain Resources and Information Network (BRAIN)
National Institute of Neurological Disorders and Stroke (NINDS)
PO Box 5801
Bethesda, MD 20824
(800) 352-9424   FAX (301) 402-2186
e-mail: braininfo@ninds.nh.gov   www.ninds.nih.gov

This clearinghouse distributes fact sheets and brochures about neurological disorders such as multiple sclerosis to individuals and their families. Free

Consortium of Multiple Sclerosis Centers/North American Research Committee on Multiple Sclerosis (CMSC/NARCOMS)
Yale Neuroimmunology Program
PO Box 208018
New Haven, CT 06520-8018
(800) 253-7884   (203) 764-4285
e-mail: narcoms@mscare.org   www.mscares.org

Multidisciplinary organization of health care professionals who specialize in the care of individuals with multiple sclerosis. Participates in partnerships with Multiple Sclerosis Societies for education and outreach and with the Paralyzed Veterans Association (PVA) and Eastern Paralyzed Veterans Association (EPVA) to support research for veterans with multiple sclerosis. Maintains the CMSC/NARCOMS Registry, which recruits individuals with multiple sclerosis for clinical trials and surveys MS patients. Individuals may enroll on the web site or by calling the telephone numbers listed above. Publishes a quarterly newsletter that reports on advances in the diagnosis and treatment of multiple sclerosis. Available on the web site. To receive a print version, individuals must be enrolled in the NARCOMS Patient Registry.

Functional Electrical Stimulation Information Center
11000 Cedar Avenue, Suite 230
Cleveland, OH 44106
(800) 666-2353   (216) 231-3257 (V/TTY)   FAX (216) 231-3258
e-mail: info@fesc.org   feswww.fes.cwru.edu

The center provides information to consumers and professionals about research on functional electrical stimulation to help individuals with multiple sclerosis and spinal cord injuries. The web site provides information on resources, references, and referrals.

MEDLINEplus: Multiple Sclerosis
www.nlm.nih.gov/medlineplus/multiplesclerosis.html

This web site provides links to sites for general information about multiple sclerosis, symptoms and diagnosis, treatment, alternative therapy, clinical trials, disease management, organizations, and research. Provides links to MEDLINE research articles and related MEDLINEplus pages.

MSActiveSource.com
(800) 456-2255   www.msactivesource.com

Sponsored by Biogen, maker of Avonex, this web site offers educational modules, information, "Ask the Expert," and real life stories. Those who do not have access to the Internet may call the toll-free number, Monday through Friday, 8:30 am to 8 pm, E.S.T.

MS Pathways
Betaseron
PO Box 52171
Phoenix, AZ 85072-2171
(800) 788-1467   www.betaseron.com

Sponsored by Berlex, the manufacturer of Betaseron, this program provides information on Betaseron, a drug used in treating relapsing-remitting multiple sclerosis, self-administration training, insurance reimbursement, community support groups, and online services. Publishes quarterly newsletter, "MessageS," free. Also available on the web site.

MSWatch
www.mswatch.com

Sponsored by Teva Neuroscience, the manufacturer of Copaxone, this site offers multiple sclerosis and health news, discussion boards and chat, journal, library, and "Ask An Expert."

National Association for Continence (NAFC)
PO Box 8310
Spartanburg, SC 29305-8310
(800) 252-3337   FAX (864) 579-7902   www.nafc.org

An information clearinghouse for consumers, family members, and medical professionals. Answers individual questions if self-addressed stamped envelope is enclosed with letter. Membership, $25.00, includes a quarterly newsletter, "Quality Care," a "Resource Guide: Products and Services for Continence" (nonmembers, $10.00), and a continence resource service. Free publications list.

National Easter Seal Society
230 West Monroe Street, Suite 1800
Chicago, IL 60606
(800) 221-6827   (312) 726-6200   (312) 726-4258 (TTY)
FAX (312) 726-1494   e-mail: info@easter-seals.org   www.easter-seals.org

Offers rehabilitation programs and support groups for individuals with multiple sclerosis. Services at local affiliates may vary.

National Institute of Neurological Disorders and Stroke (NINDS)
Building 31, Room 8A06
31 Center Drive, MSC 2540
Bethesda, MD 20892
(800) 352-9424   (301) 496-5751   FAX (301) 402-2186
e-mail: braininfo@ninds.nih.gov www.ninds.nih.gov

A federal agency which conducts basic and clinical research on the causes and treatment of multiple sclerosis.

National Multiple Sclerosis Society
733 Third Avenue
New York, NY 10017
(212) 986-3240   FAX (212) 986-7981
(800) 344-4867 Information Resource Center and Library
e-mail: Nat@nmss.org   www.nationalmssociety.org

Provides professional and public education and information and referral; supports research. Offers counseling services, physician referrals, advocacy, discount prescription and health care products program, and assistance in obtaining adaptive equipment. Regional affiliates throughout the U.S. Information Resource Center and Library answers telephone inquiries from 11:00 a.m. to 5:00 p.m. E.S.T., Monday through Thursday. Membership, $20.00, includes large print magazine, "Inside MS," published three times a year. Individuals with multiple sclerosis may receive a courtesy membership if they are unable to pay.

Shared Solutions
Teva Marion Partners
2800 Rock Creek Parkway
Kansas City, MO 64117
(800) 887-8100   www.tevamarionpartners.com

This program, sponsored by Teva Marion Partners pharmaceutical company, provides information about Copaxone, a drug used to reduce the frequency of relapses in individuals with the relapsing-remitting form of multiple sclerosis, treatment reimbursement programs, and local resources. The web site provides a medication diary, discussion groups, chat rooms, and advice from professionals.

Simon Foundation for Continence
PO Box 835
Wilmette, IL 60091
(800) 237-4666   (847) 864-3913   FAX (847) 864-9758
e-mail: simoninfo@simonfoundation.org
www.simonfoundation.org

Provides information and assistance to people who are incontinent. Organizes self-help groups. Web site offers discussion groups. Membership, individuals, $15.00; professionals, $35.00; includes quarterly newsletter, "The Informer." Also available on the web site.

ADA and People with MS
by Laura Cooper and Nancy Law with Jane Sarnoff
National Multiple Sclerosis Society (see "ORGANIZATIONS" above)
(800) 344-4867   www.nationalmssociety.org

This booklet explains how the Americans with Disabilities Act applies to individuals with multiple sclerosis. Large print. Also available on the web site.

Aqua Exercise for Multiple Sclerosis
National Multiple Sclerosis Society (see "ORGANIZATIONS" above)
(800) 344-4867   www.nationalmssociety.org

This videotape presents exercises for building strength and endurance as well as reducing spasticity. Includes print reference card. 15 minutes. $15.00

At Home with MS: Adapting Your Environment
National Multiple Sclerosis Society (see "ORGANIZATIONS" above)
(800) 344-4867   www.nationalmssociety.org

This booklet suggests modifications that can be made to the home to compensate for mobility or visual impairment. Also available on the web site.

dirty details, the days and nights of a well spouse
by Marion Deutsche Cohen
Temple University Press
11030 South Langley Avenue
Chicago, IL 60628
(800) 621-2736   FAX (800) 621-8476
e-mail: kh@press.uchicago.edu   www.press.chicago.edu

A frank, personal account, written by a woman whose husband has multiple sclerosis, this book describes her caregiving experiences. Hardcover, $49.95; softcover, $18.95; plus $4.00 shipping and handling.

Disease Modifying Therapies in Multiple Sclerosis
Multiple Sclerosis Council for Clinical Practice Guidelines
PVA Distribution Center
PO Box 753
Waldorf, MD 20604-0753
(888) 860-7244   (301) 932-7834   FAX (301) 843-0159
www.pva.org

These guidelines present the evidence for treating multiple sclerosis with anti-inflammatory, immunomodulatory, and immunosuppressive agents. Free plus $3.00 shipping and handling

Employment Issues and Multiple Sclerosis
by Phillip D. Rumrill
Demos Medical Publishing
386 Park Avenue South, Suite 201
New York, NY 10016
(800) 532-8663   (212) 683-0072   FAX (212) 683-0118
e-mail: info@demospub.com www.demosmedpub.com

This book discuss how employment may be affected by multiple sclerosis. Includes information about vocational rehabilitation, job placement and retention, the Americans with Disabilities Act, and other legal issues. $29.95 plus $4.00 shipping and handling. Orders made on the Demos web site receive a 15% discount.

Enabling Romance: A Guide to Love, Sex, and Relationships for People with Disabilities
by Ken Kroll and Erica Levy Klein
Nine Lives Press
PO Box 220
Horsham, PA 19044
(888) 850-0344, extension 109 (215) 675-9133, extension 109
FAX (215) 675-9376   e-mail: kim@leonardmediagroup.com
www.newmobility.com

Written by a man who has a disability and his wife who does not, this book provides examples of how people with a variety of disabilities have established fulfilling relationships. $15.95 plus $3.00 shipping and handling

Fatigue: What You Should Know
PVA Distribution Center
PO Box 753
Waldorf, MD 20604-0753
(888) 860-7244   (301) 932-7834   FAX (301) 843-0159
www.pva.org

This consumer guide describes the types of fatigue associated with multiple sclerosis, their diagnosis, and treatment. Free plus $3.00 shipping and handling

Gentle Fitness
732 Lake Shore Drive
Rhinelander, WI 54501
(800) 566-7780   (715) 362-9260   FAX (715) 362-0304
www.gentlefitness.com

This videotape offers six exercise routines. Most may be done from a seated position. Includes "Guide to Exercise" booklet. $29.95 plus $4.80 shipping and handling. Orders placed on the web site receive a 20% discount.

Keep S'myelin
National Multiple Sclerosis Society (see "ORGANIZATIONS" above)
(800) 344-4867   www.nationalmssociety.org

Quarterly publication for children ages five to 10 years and their relatives who have MS.

Knowledge is Power
National Multiple Sclerosis Society (see "ORGANIZATIONS" above)
(800) 344-4867   e-mail: KIP@nmss.org
www.nationalmssociety.org

This home study course provides information about multiple sclerosis including a medical overview, emotional aspects, legal issues, fatigue, sexuality, job accommodation under the Americans with Disabilities Act, family issues, and more. Once individuals are registered for the program, one article per week is mailed to them. Free

Living Well with Multiple Sclerosis: A Guide for Patient, Caregiver, and Family
by David L. Carroll and Jon Dudley Dorman
Harper Collins Publishers
PO Box 588
Scranton, PA 18512
(800) 242-7737   www.harpercollins.com

In addition to information on multiple sclerosis and diagnosis, prognosis, and treatment, this book discusses emotional and sexual functioning. $13.00 plus $2.75 shipping and handling

Living with Low Vision: A Resource Guide for People with Sight Loss
Resources for Rehabilitation
22 Bonad Road
Winchester, MA 01890
(781) 368-9094   FAX (781) 368-9096
e-mail: orders@rfr.org   www.rfr.org

A large print (18 point bold type) comprehensive directory that helps people with sight loss locate the services that they need to remain independent. Chapters describe products that enable people to keep reading, working, and carrying out their daily activities. Information about Internet resources is included. $46.95 plus $5.00 shipping and handling. (See order form on last page of this book.)

Living with Multiple Sclerosis: A Wellness Approach
by George H. Kraft and Marci Catanzaro
Demos Medical Publishing
386 Park Avenue South, Suite 201
New York, NY 10016
(800) 532-8663   (212) 683-0072   FAX (212) 683-0118
e-mail: info@demospub.com   www.demosmedpub.com

This book suggests strategies for everyday living with multiple sclerosis. Includes information on diet, nutrition, and exercise. $18.95 plus $4.00 shipping and handling. Orders made on the Demos web site receive a 15% discount.

Mainstay: For the Well Spouse of the Chronically Ill
by Maggie Strong
Bradford Books
45 Lyman Road
Northampton, MA 01060
(413) 586-5207

Written by a woman whose husband was diagnosed with multiple sclerosis at age 46, this book provides her personal account and others' stories, practical suggestions, and advice from health care professionals. $15.00 plus $3.00 shipping and handling

Managing Incontinence
by Cheryle B. Gartley, (ed.)
Simon Foundation for Continence
PO Box 835
Wilmette, IL 60091
(800) 237-4666   (847) 864-3913   FAX (847) 864-9758
e-mail: simoninfo@simonfoundation.org
www.simonfoundation.org

This book provides medical advice, information on products, interviews with individuals who are incontinent, and advice on sexuality. $12.95

A Man's Guide to Coping with Disability
Resources for Rehabilitation
22 Bonad Road
Winchester, MA 01890
(781) 368-9094   FAX (781) 368-9096
e-mail: orders@rfr.org   www.rfr.org

This book includes information about men's responses to disability, with a special emphasis on the values men place on independence, occupational achievement, and physical activity.

A chapter on multiple sclerosis includes information about sexual functioning. $44.95 plus $5.00 shipping and handling (See last page of this book for order form.)

<u>Meeting the Challenge of Progressive Multiple Sclerosis</u>
by Patricia K. Coyle and June Halper
Demos Medical Publishing
386 Park Avenue South, Suite 201
New York, NY 10016
(800) 532-8663   (212) 683-0072   FAX (212) 683-0118
e-mail: info@demospub.com   www.demosmedpub.com

This book describes the diagnosis and treatments for this form of multiple sclerosis. Includes strategies for management of symptoms, everyday living, and coping. A chapter discusses gender-related issues and sexuality. $19.95 plus $4.00 shipping and handling. Orders made on the Demos web site receive a 15% discount.

<u>Multiple Sclerosis: A Guide for Families</u>
by Rosalind C. Kalb (ed.)
Demos Medical Publishing
386 Park Avenue South, Suite 201
New York, NY 10016
(800) 532-8663   (212) 683-0072   FAX (212) 683-0118
e-mail: info@demospub.com   www.demosmedpub.com

This book discusses issues such as caregiving, adults with MS and their parents, cognitive problems, financial planning, sexuality, and reproduction. Includes bibliography and resources. $24.95 plus $4.00 shipping and handling. Orders made on the Demos web site receive a 15% discount.

<u>Multiple Sclerosis: A Guide for the Newly Diagnosed</u>
by Nancy Holland, T. Jock Murray, and Stephen Reingold
Demos Medical Publishing
386 Park Avenue South, Suite 201
New York, NY 10016
(800) 532-8663   (212) 683-0072   FAX (212) 683-0118
e-mail: info@demospub.com   www.demosmedpub.com

This book provides information about multiple sclerosis and medical treatments as well as its effect on the individual and the family. $21.95 plus $4.00 shipping and handling. Orders made on the Demos web site receive a 15% discount.

Multiple Sclerosis: A Self-Care Guide to Wellness
by Nancy Holland and June Halper
PVA Distribution Center
PO Box 753
Waldorf, MD 20604-0753
(888) 860-7244   (301) 932-7834   FAX (301) 843-0159
www.pva.org

This book discusses how MS affects the lives of both those with the disease and those who provide care, emphasizing strategies to promote independence, well-being, and productivity. $17.95 plus $3.00 shipping and handling

Multiple Sclerosis in Clinical Practice
by Stanley van den Noort and Nancy J. Holland (eds.)
Demos Medical Publishing
386 Park Avenue South, Suite 201
New York, NY 10016
(800) 532-8663   (212) 683-0072   FAX (212) 683-0118
e-mail: info@demospub.com   www.demosmedpub.com

This book provides an overview of the disease, diagnosis, and treatments. Includes chapters on mobility, bowel, and bladder dysfunction, pain, cognitive loss, emotional issues, and community resources. $34.95 plus $4.00 shipping and handling. Orders made on the Demos web site receive a 15% discount.

Multiple Sclerosis: The Guide to Treatment and Management
by Chris H. Polman, Alan J. Thompson, T. Jock Murray, and W. Ian McDonald
Demos Medical Publishing
386 Park Avenue South, Suite 201
New York, NY 10016
(800) 532-8663   (212) 683-0072   FAX (212) 683-0118
e-mail: info@demospub.com   www.demosmedpub.com

This book describes current therapies. Includes sections on acute exacerbations, disease-modifying therapies, symptom management, and alternative therapies. $24.95 plus $4.00 shipping and handling. Orders made on the Demos web site receive a 15% discount.

Multiple Sclerosis: The Questions You Have, The Answers You Need
by Rosalind Kalb (ed.)
Demos Medical Publishing
386 Park Avenue South, Suite 201
New York, NY 10016
(800) 532-8663   (212) 683-0072   FAX (212) 683-0118
e-mail: info@demospub.com   www.demosmedpub.com

Written by professionals who care for individuals with multiple sclerosis, this book provides information about living with the condition and answers questions most commonly asked. Topics include neurology, treatment, employment, legal issues, physical and occupational therapy, psychosocial issues, sexuality, and reproductive health. $21.95 plus $4.00 shipping and handling. Orders made on the Demos web site receive a 15% discount.

Multiple Sclerosis: Your Legal Rights
by Lanny E. Perkins
Demos Medical Publishing
386 Park Avenue South, Suite 201
New York, NY 10016
(800) 532-8663   (212) 683-0072   FAX (212) 683-0118
e-mail: info@demospub.com   www.demosmedpub.com

This book discusses the legal problems that individuals with multiple sclerosis face and suggests possible solutions. Includes explanations of the Americans with Disabilities Act (ADA), Health Insurance Portability and Availability Act (HIPAA), and the Family and Medical Leave Act (FMLA). $21.95 plus $4.00 shipping and handling. Orders made on the Demos web site receive a 15% discount.

The Other Victim - Caregivers Share Their Coping Strategies
by Alan Drattell
Seven Locks Press
PO Box 25689
Santa Ana, CA 92799
(800) 354-5348   e-mail: sevenlocks@aol.com

This book is a collection of personal accounts of nine caregivers of individuals with multiple sclerosis. Also includes a resource list of organizations and suggestions for coping. $17.95 plus $4.50 shipping and handling

PLAINTALK: A Booklet about Multiple Sclerosis for Family Members
by Sarah L. Minden and Debra Frankel
National Multiple Sclerosis Society (see "ORGANIZATIONS" above)
(800) 344-4867   www.nationalmssociety.org

This booklet simulates a support group meeting for families of individuals with multiple sclerosis. Discusses diagnosis, everyday living, talking with children, and the well parent. Large print. Also available on the web site.

Someone You Know Has MS: A Book for Families
by Cyrisse Jaffee, Debra Frankel, Barbara LaRoche, and Patricia Dick
When a Parent Has MS: A Teenager's Guide
by Pamela Cavallo with Martha Jablow
National Multiple Sclerosis Society (see "ORGANIZATIONS" above)
(800) 344-4867   www.nationalmssociety.org

These two booklets, one written for children age 6 to 12 and the other for teenagers, help youngsters understand their parent's condition and discuss the youngsters' concerns and fears. Large print.   Free

Surviving Your Spouse's Chronic Illness
by Chris McGonigle
Von Holtzbrinck Publishing Services, Gordonsville, VA

Building on her own background as the well spouse of a man with multiple sclerosis, the author interviewed more than 40 spouses of women and men with chronic conditions and describes the emotional and psychological aspects of their experiences.   Out of print

Symptom Management in Multiple Sclerosis
by Randall T. Schapiro
Demos Medical Publishing
386 Park Avenue South, Suite 201
New York, NY 10016
(800) 532-8663   (212) 683-0072   FAX (212) 683-0118
e-mail: info@demospub.com   www.demosmedpub.com

A multidisciplinary guide for health care professionals and individuals with multiple sclerosis which suggests management strategies for treating multiple sclerosis and minimizing and controlling its symptoms. $19.95 plus $4.00 shipping and handling.   Orders made on the Demos web site receive a 15% discount.

Talking Books for People with Physical Disabilities
National Library Service for the Blind and Physically Handicapped (NLS)
1291 Taylor Street, NW
Washington, DC 20542
(800) 424-8567 or 8572 (Reference Section)
(800) 424-9100 (to receive application)
(202) 707-5100   (202) 707-0744 (TTY)   FAX (202) 707-0712
e-mail: nls@loc.gov   www.loc.gov/nls

This brochure describes a free program which provides books and magazines recorded on discs and audiocassettes for individuals with multiple sclerosis and other disabling conditions. Application forms are available from the NLS, public libraries, or local affiliates of the

National Multiple Sclerosis Society. A health professional must certify that the individual is unable to hold a book or turn pages; has blurred or double vision; extreme weakness or excessive fatigue; or other physical limitations which prevent the individual from reading standard print.

300 Tips for Making Life with Multiple Sclerosis Easier
by Shelley Peterman Schwarz
Demos Medical Publishing
386 Park Avenue South, Suite 201
New York, NY 10016
(800) 532-8663   (212) 683-0072   FAX (212) 683-011
e-mail: info@demospub.com   www.demosmedpub.co

Writing from personal experience, the author shares basic tips for conserving time and energy and provides practical information on everyday living. $16.95 plus $4.00 shipping and handling. Orders made on the Demos web site receive a 15% discount.

Understanding Bowel Problems in MS
by Nancy J. Holland and Robin Frames
National Multiple Sclerosis Society (see "ORGANIZATIONS" above)
(800) 344-4867   www.nationalmssociety.org

This booklet describes common bowel problems and suggests coping strategies. Large print. Free. Also available on the web site.

Wheelchairs: Your Options and Rights Guide to Obtaining Wheelchairs from the Department of Veterans Affairs
PVA Distribution Center
PO Box 753
Waldorf, MD 20604-0753
(888) 860-7244   (301) 932-7834   FAX (301) 843-0159
www.pva.org

This booklet provides information on eligibility criteria, lists the types of wheelchairs available, and describes VA procedures. Available in English and Spanish. Free plus $3.00 shipping and handling

A Woman's Guide to Coping with Disability
Resources for Rehabilitation
22 Bonad Road
Winchester, MA 01890
(781) 368-9094   FAX (781) 368-9096
e-mail: orders@rfr.org   www.rfr.org

This book addresses the special needs of women with disabilities and chronic conditions, such as social relationships, sexual functioning, pregnancy, childrearing, caregiving, and employment. Written for women in all age categories, the book has chapters on the disabilities that are most prevalent in women or likely to affect the roles and physical functions unique to women including multiple sclerosis. $44.95 plus $5.00 shipping and handling (See last page of this book for order form.)

Women Living with Multiple Sclerosis
by Judith Lynn Nichols and Her Online Group of MS Sisters
Hunter House
PO Box 2914
Alameda, CA 94501-0914
(800) 266-5592   (510) 865-5282   FAX (510) 865-4295
e-mail: ordering@hunterhouse.com www.hunterhouse.com

This book presents the results of two years of online "conversations" between women with multiple sclerosis. Topics discusses include the search for a diagnosis, family reactions, sexuality, spirituality, depression, and employment issues. $13.95 plus $4.50 shipping and handling

Yes, You Can!
MS Awareness Foundation
PO Box 1193
Venice, FL 34284
(888) 336-6723   FAX (949) 733-3211
e-mail: info@MSAwareness.org   www.msawareness.org

This videotape demonstrates exercises for individuals living with multiple sclerosis. $19.95 plus $4.00 shipping and handling

You Are Not Your Illness
by Linda Noble Topf
Simon & Schuster
100 Front Street
Riverside, NJ 08075
(888) 866-6631   FAX (800) 943-9831   www.simonsays.com

In this book, the author, who has multiple sclerosis, shares her personal perspectives on living with chronic illness. She describes a step-by-step process for dealing with loss and maintaining feelings of self-worth. $12.00 plus $4.98 shipping and handling

Chapter 10

SPINAL CORD INJURY

The spinal cord is responsible for transmitting the brain's electrical impulses that control other organs of the body. Therefore, when the spinal cord is injured, there are effects on many of the body's systems, requiring modifications of activities of everyday living and of the home and workplace environments.

Tumors and diseases such as *poliomyelitis*, *arthritis*, *spina bifida*, and *multiple sclerosis* may cause spinal cord injuries; however, spinal cord injuries occur most frequently as a result of *accidents*. Young males who have been in an automobile accident account for the greatest proportion of spinal cord injuries. Because it is often the case that individuals with spinal cord injury were extremely physically active prior to their injury, the effects of the injury may seem overwhelming to them at first. However, rehabilitation opportunities and the development of a wide variety of special assistive devices have enabled thousands of individuals with spinal cord injuries to live productive lives and to continue to participate in many recreational activities, albeit in modified forms.

It has been estimated that there are between 183,000 and 230,000 living Americans who have experienced spinal cord injuries, the majority of whom were injured during or after World War II. The annual incidence of accidents that cause spinal cord injury where the injured individual survives is 40 per million population or approximately 11,000 a year (National Spinal Cord Injury Statistical Center: 2001). Prior to World War II and the development of penicillin and of sulfa drugs that prevented death from urinary tract infections, it was unusual for those who had a spinal cord injury to survive (DeVivo et al.: 1987). Today, due to the development of these drugs and improved emergency medical care at the scene of accidents, the vast majority of individuals with spinal cord injuries live for many years.

Studies of patients admitted to the Model Spinal Cord Injury Care Systems have yielded demographic characteristics about the population. The average age at onset is 32.1 years, and 81.6% of individuals with spinal cord injuries are males. Automobile accidents account for 38.5% of spinal cord injuries. Violence as a cause of spinal cord injury has increased in recent years; it now accounts for 24.5% of all spinal cord injuries. Sports accidents (frequently diving accidents) account for 7.2% of all spinal cord injuries and are a major cause of spinal cord injuries among the younger population, while falls, which account for 21.8% of all spinal cord injuries, are a major cause among the older population (National Spinal Cord Injury Statistical Center: 2001).

A study by DeVivo and colleagues (1992) investigated the characteristics of individuals who had received treatment for spinal cord injuries at six federally supported model treatment centers between 1973 and 1986. The study found several significant differences between the population who had been injured in the period 1973-77 and those who had been injured in the period 1984-86; the mean age at the time of injury increased over time as did the proportion of individuals who were not white and the proportion with quadriplegia. Although the mean length of stays in hospitals for rehabilitation decreased, the cost of the rehabilitation increased. For those who entered the centers within the first 24 hours of injury, the probability of dying in the first two years following injury decreased by two-thirds for the latter group. While virtually all of the subjects were discharged to live in the community during the entire study period, only a small percentage of the subjects were employed two years post-injury, ranging from a low of 12.5% in the 1978-80 period to a high of 14.7% for those who had been injured from 1984-86. While a substantial proportion were students and small proportions were either homemakers or retired two years post-injury, over half of the subjects were unemployed throughout the study period.

THE SPINAL CORD

The spine has 33 bony, hollow, interlocking vertebrae including seven cervical or neck vertebrae, 12 thoracic or high back vertebrae, five lumbar or low back vertebrae, five sacral vertebrae near the base of the spine, and four coccygeal vertebrae fused to form the coccyx. The spinal cord, consisting of a narrow bundle of nerve cells and fibers, runs from the base of the brain through the hollow structure of the vertebrae. The brain's communication with the rest of the body is carried out through these nerve fibers.

Paralysis, the loss or impairment of motor function, occurs below the site of the injury or fracture. Not all injuries are complete, meaning that sometimes the individual may retain some sensation or movement below the site of the injury. *Paraplegia*, or paralysis of the legs and often the lower part of the body, occurs when the spinal cord is injured at the thoracic, lumbar, or sacral level of the spine. When injuries are complete, individuals also lose their sense of touch, pain, and temperature in the affected region.

Quadriplegia (or tetraplegia) is paralysis of all four limbs and the part of the body beneath the site of the spinal cord injury. Quadriplegia occurs when the injury to the spinal cord is at the level of the cervical vertebrae or the neck region. The lower the lesion within the cervical area, the greater amount of function that remains. Some individuals with cervical spinal cord injuries retain some function of the shoulders, biceps, upper arms, and the wrists. In general, the higher the site of the injury, the less function the individual retains. Individuals whose injuries are complete and at the chin level require respirators in order to breathe. These individuals require assistance with their everyday activities, although the use of mouthsticks and sip-and-puff mechanisms enables them to operate wheelchairs, computers, and other devices (Trieschmann: 1988).

According to Young and his associates (1982), there is a higher prevalence of quadriplegia (53%) than paraplegia (47%), but the injuries are more likely to be complete in paraplegia (60%) than for quadriplegia (52%).

TREATMENT AND COMPLICATIONS OF SPINAL CORD INJURY

Acute medical care following an accident that has caused spinal cord injury includes x-rays, possible treatment for shock, and immobilization of the patient. Patients are often placed in a Stryker frame, which is used to immobilize the spine and prevent further injury. A catheter to control bladder function is inserted and urine output is monitored. In some cases, surgery may be performed to stabilize or fuse the spine, free nerve roots, or remove bony fragments. Immediately following the injury, swelling and bruising near the site of the fracture may be present, preventing the determination of the extent of neurological damage (Trieschmann: 1988). Patients are positioned and turned frequently in an effort to prevent pressure sores (see below). Other injuries that often accompany spinal cord injury, such as fractures and lung injuries, must also be treated. Pain may also be a major problem in the first weeks following injury.

Studies on the use of drugs immediately following spinal cord injury have found some positive benefits. Administration of methylprednisolone within eight hours following the injury resulted in the recovery of an average of 20% of the motor and sensory function lost as a result of the injury (Hingley: 1993).

Although treatments have been developed for many of the complications of spinal cord injury, it is still necessary to constantly be aware of the development of these complications and to take measures to prevent them. *Pressure sores* or *decubitus ulcers* are lesions on the skin that usually occur over a bony surface and result from lack of motion. Because the individual may have no sensation at the site where the sores begin to develop, they may become deep before they are discovered. In an effort to prevent pressure sores, individuals who are confined to bed immediately following the injury should be moved frequently and great attention should be paid to cleansing the skin regularly. Special flotation pads and sheepskins are sometimes used to relieve pressure and distribute body weight. Because of their restricted mobility, individuals with spinal cord injury must take precautions to prevent pressure sores for the rest of their lives.

Despite the loss of sensation to temperature and touch below the site of the lesion, *pain* and unusual sensations may be a problem for people with spinal cord injuries. According to Trieschmann (1988), until recently it was assumed that pain was not a problem, and little attention was paid to the subject. However, Trieschmann states that many individuals experience a tingling or pins and needles sensation as well as other types of pain, such as shooting or burning sensations.

Transcutaneous electric nerve stimulation (TENS) is a treatment method for pain in which low level electric impulses are delivered to nerve endings under the skin near the source of pain. It is not known why TENS should be effective in relieving pain or if it is really effective.

Loss of bladder and bowel control is another complication of spinal cord injury. One study (Kuhlemeier et al.: 1985) concluded that patients with spinal cord injuries are likely to maintain good renal output ten years after injury. Those individuals who have indwelling catheters are prone to develop bladder infections. When the extent of nerve damage permits, it is preferable to have the individual learn how to control his or her bladder through an individualized training program. When urinary tract infections become symptomatic, they are treated with antibiotics for a period of 7 to 14 days (National Institute on Disability and Rehabilitation Research: 1992). Programs for bowel control enable the individual to empty the bowel on a regular schedule, thereby avoiding gastrointestinal complications, such as distention and impaction. Attention to diet and the use of rectal suppositories may also contribute to control of bowel movements.

Spasticity (involuntary jerky motions) is common in individuals with spinal cord injuries. These spasms are caused by random stimulation of the nerves leading to the muscles.

Severe spasms may interfere with some activities and in some cases may be strong enough to throw the individual from the bed or chair.

Sexual function may be affected in both men and women, although the effects are greater for men. Women will resume menstruating and may conceive and bear children. Because of the loss of motor function, a man's ability to have an erection may be impaired. As with all other effects of spinal cord injury, the extent of the impairment is determined by the level and completeness of the injury. Rehabilitation programs for people with spinal cord injuries should include counseling in the area of sexual functioning; however, a national survey of individuals with spinal cord injuries concluded that over half of the subjects could not remember having received education or counseling related to sexual function (Tepper: 1992).

Functional electrical stimulation (FES) is an experimental method that uses electrical stimulation to evoke skeletal muscle responses in areas that do not function normally because injury or disease has cut off the pathway for central nervous system communication from the brain. A functional electrical stimulation system consists of a control unit, a stimulator unit, and electrodes. In some instances, the goal of functional electrical stimulation is to restore movement or function and in other cases to strengthen muscles. A study by Petrofsky (1992) found that subjects with spinal cord injuries who participated in a two year experiment using functional electrical stimulation to exercise muscles had a reduction in the incidence of pressure sores and urinary tract infections. Another experiment (Granat et al.: 1992) that used functional electrical stimulation to restore movement in six subjects with incomplete spinal cord injuries found that all subjects were able to stand and walk using an FES system, but half of the subjects found that the system was not practical for their lifestyles.

A number of research projects are working on potential cures for spinal cord injury through nerve regeneration and drug therapy. Other projects have the goal of re-training individuals to walk (Huelskamp: 1998). Electrical stimulation devices implanted in the body utilize the control that remains in individuals with incomplete injuries to enable them to regain some motor function, improve bowel and bladder control, and enable individuals with paraplegia to walk (Finn: 1998).

SPINAL CORD INJURY IN YOUTHS

Since automobile accidents and accidents that occur during sports activities are major causes of spinal cord injuries, it is not surprising that a substantial number of these injuries occur during adolescence and the teenage years. The most common age at which spinal cord injury occurs is 19, with a third of the injuries occurring between the ages of 17 and 23 (Stover: 1996). The physical impact of the injury is compounded by a variety of factors, including the interruption of education, the inability to fulfill career aspirations, and the value that the peer culture places on body image and physical activities. In some instances, the youths had played sports seriously and hoped to continue with this endeavor as a career; spinal cord injuries make this impossible. In addition, some youths with spinal cord injuries are sexually inexperienced, and they fear they will never be able to be sexually active. Both youths who are sexually inexperienced and those who have been sexually active must learn new ways of experiencing sexual pleasure. Rehabilitation professionals and counselors must help youths with spinal cord injuries plan to complete their education using assistive technology, reassess their career goals, and help them and those with whom they have sexual relationships to learn how to fulfill themselves.

Spinal cord injury that occurs in adolescence interferes with the development of independence that normally occurs at this stage. At a time when peers are becoming more independent from their parents, youths with spinal cord injuries become more dependent. Anderson (1997) suggests that these youths should have the opportunity to participate in peer support groups, adapted recreation activities, and adapted driving as well as sexuality and career counseling. The risk of drug abuse must also be addressed.

LeBaron and associates (1984) have suggested that adolescents be given the opportunity to express their anger and despair at their situation. Those who are able to express their feelings adjust better than those who do not. Youths with spinal cord injuries who are unwilling or unable to express their feelings are at higher risk for depression and possibly suicide.

Once youths with spinal cord injuries have completed their rehabilitation program, they return to school where they must overcome both attitudinal and physical barriers. Both faculty and students need to be educated about the needs of a student with a spinal cord injury. The student may feel socially isolated as many of the social interactions of youths center around physical activities that are no longer feasible. It is wise for a health care provider, a social worker, and the student's parents to visit the school prior to the student's return to check on physical accessibility and to discuss the student's special needs with faculty members.

AGING AND SPINAL CORD INJURY

As more individuals with spinal cord injuries survive longer, they are also experiencing the physiological processes that accompany aging. There is little information on how these processes affect people with spinal cord injuries who have been disabled for many years. However, preliminary indications are that physiological changes associated with aging have a greater impact on people with spinal cord injuries. Menter (1990) calls this phase "decline," noting that there is a decrease in muscle strength, range of motion, and respiratory and cardiovascular capacity and an increase in the breakdown of the skin.

One study (Gerhart et al.: 1993) of individuals who had lived with spinal cord injuries from 20 to 47 years found that the need for physical assistance increased over time for 22% of the subjects. Older age was significantly related to the need for greater assistance with transfers, dressing, mobility, and toileting. Another study (Pentland et al.: 1995) found that as subjects lived longer with spinal cord injuries, they experienced less financial security and more illness.

PSYCHOLOGICAL ASPECTS OF SPINAL CORD INJURY

Individuals who experience spinal cord injuries have changed in an instant from able-bodied individuals into individuals with severe physical limitations. The suddenness with which this change takes place and the wide ranging effects are likely to cause great anguish to the individuals as well as to their families and friends. The more severe the disability, the greater the loss of independence. For many individuals, these circumstances result in a loss of self-esteem and fear of re-entering the larger community. It is essential that individuals with spinal cord injuries receive help with their emotional adjustment, through individual or group counseling from professionals, self-help groups, or role models of individuals who have adjusted successfully to spinal cord injuries.

Indeed, survival itself has been found to be positively related to good emotional adjustment following spinal cord injury. Krause and Crewe (1987) compared survivors of spinal cord injuries and those who had died several years after their injuries on a number of variables that measured adjustment. Those who were better adjusted in terms of vocational and social activity were more likely to survive regardless of their age. Krause and Crewe suggest that the frequent neglect of counseling in social skills and sexual functioning during the rehabilitation process contributes to poor adjustment. A study by Krause (1991) that builds upon the earlier study confirmed the findings that social, psychological, and vocational maladjustment was higher among deceased subjects than among the survivors. A study by McColl and Rosenthal (1994) found that emotional support continues to be crucial many years after the injury occurred. In a sample of men age 45 or over who had experienced spinal cord injuries at least 15 years before, emotional support was the only variable that predicted life satisfaction, adjustment to disability, and lack of depression. Other investigations have found relationships between social support and well being (Rintala et al.: 1992) and employment and self-perception of both physical and psychological adjustment (Krause: 1992).

Some individuals may never lose the anger or guilt they feel about the circumstances surrounding the accident that caused the injury. In the period immediately following the accident, they may feel overpowered by the many professionals who have begun to make major decisions for them. In many cases, the accident that caused spinal cord injury involved the use of alcohol while driving. These factors, combined with inadequate counseling and the inability to cope with the effects of the injury, may cause some individuals to abuse alcohol or other drugs. Bozzacco (1990) suggests that all patients in rehabilitation units be assessed for their vulnerability to alcohol and drug abuse. She further suggests that patients become part of the decision-making process for their own treatment and rehabilitation plans as soon as possible and that alcohol and drug treatment programs be an integral part of rehabilitation.

Because most of the individuals who experience spinal cord injuries are males, women who have spinal cord injuries may feel isolated and without accessible peers or role models. They may need counseling about the physical aspects of becoming pregnant; about handling the responsibilities of motherhood; and other physical and emotional issues that affect women.

The need to modify the activities of everyday living as well as the physical environment; the impairment of sexual function; and the financial aspects of living with a spinal cord injury may place a great strain on marital and family relationships. In cases where attendant care is necessary, the spouse often becomes a caretaker by default when financial resources do not permit hiring an attendant. In these instances, it is not uncommon for the able-bodied spouse and offspring to feel both overburdened and guilty. DeVivo and his colleagues (1995) found that individuals with spinal cord injuries who married post-injury had higher divorce rates than the general public. Both education and severity of injury were related to divorce rates. Individuals without a college education had higher divorce rates than those with a college education; those with lumbosacral injuries had lower divorce rates than individuals with higher injuries. Divorce rates were higher for men than for women and for African-Americans than for whites.

Other issues that affect marriages where one partner has a spinal cord injury include the spouse's feelings of guilt. A study (Gerhart: 1995) of Britons who had survived spinal cord injuries at least 20 years and their spouses found that spouses often feel guilty about leaving their mate alone and about participating in activities that are not possible for their spouse. Participants indicated that it was important for each spouse to develop his or her own special interests and to adapt activities that they had enjoyed prior to the injury so that both spouses could participate. Furthermore, spouses who were caregivers for their injured mates experienced more depression, physical and emotional stress, fatigue, anger, and resentment than spouses who did not act as caregivers.

Social workers should work with the family where spouses and children feel psychologically, physically, and financially overburdened and socially isolated. Arranging for respite care, financial assistance, and other services may alleviate some of the burden. According to Young and his associates (1982), over half (54%) of all individuals with spinal cord injuries were single when their injury occurred; these individuals may benefit from counseling in order to develop satisfactory relationships and marriage.

PROFESSIONAL SERVICE PROVIDERS

In most cases, the physician in charge serves as the case manager or coordinator for the person with spinal cord injury. The physician in charge may be a *physiatrist* (a specialist trained in rehabilitation medicine); an *orthopedist* (a specialist in treatment of the skeletal system); or a *neurologist* or *neurosurgeon* (a specialist in disorders of the nervous system). All of these physicians receive training in treatment of spinal cord injury. Also on the multidisciplinary team are *urologists*, who specialize in treatment of kidneys, the bladder, the ureter, and the urethra.

Rehabilitation nurses receive special training available at schools throughout the country and may receive certification in this specialty after working two years in a rehabilitation setting (Livingston: 1991). They work closely with the physicians and in some instances may serve as case managers. In inpatient settings, rehabilitation nurses work with other health care and rehabilitation professionals to develop and implement medical and rehabilitation plans for patients. They may act as consultants in planning for discharge and may evaluate the individual's home to ensure that appropriate environmental modifications have been made. They are often the professionals in charge of following up on the individual's needs after discharge from the rehabilitation unit.

Orthotists specialize in the design of braces and other devices that help with mobility, support, and prevention of further injury. They also fit the devices and provide instruction in their use. *Rehabilitation engineers* specialize in the design of devices that enable people with disabilities to function at their maximum level of independence. Their research includes the development of robotic devices and other computer driven devices that serve as substitutes for the function that was lost as a result of injury or disease. In some instances, they may consult on individual cases to adapt wheelchairs or other devices for specific needs.

Physical therapists design exercise programs to maintain and strengthen residual motor function. They also teach transfer skills to and from the bed and how to use wheelchairs and orthotic devices, such as canes, braces, and walkers. They develop exercise programs to help individuals who are able to use crutches to build up muscles in their arms and shoulders.

Occupational therapists teach individuals with spinal cord injuries how to re-learn the activities of daily living. Included are eating, dressing, grooming, and the use of "high tech" devices that contribute to increased independence.

Psychologists provide individual or group counseling to people with spinal cord injuries and to their family members. They may also provide special help in the area of sexual functioning. *Social workers* help to make the arrangements that enable individuals to return to the community. They also ensure that individuals with spinal cord injuries receive the financial assistance that they are entitled to. Social workers may also provide counseling for individuals and their families.

Rehabilitation counselors help individuals with spinal cord injuries develop a plan that will enable them to continue functioning and working. Many individuals with spinal cord injuries will need assistance in returning to their previous position or retraining to obtain a different type of position. Rehabilitation counselors help make the contacts and placements necessary to attain these goals.

Employment after spinal cord injury is more likely for people who have higher education and who work in office jobs that do not require physical effort. Individuals who were employed in office or clerical work prior to their spinal cord injuries are most likely to be able to perform the same type of work, with or without modifications in the office environment. Individuals whose work involved physical skills will in most instances need to be trained to carry out the requirements of more sedentary occupations (for a more detailed discussion of this topic, see Meeting the Needs of Employees with Disabilities described in "PUBLICATIONS AND TAPES" section below).

WHERE TO FIND SERVICES

The federal government sponsors the "Model System of Spinal Cord Injury Care" in order to provide coordinated comprehensive care and to conduct research related to spinal cord injury. Administered by the National Institute on Disability and Rehabilitation Research (NIDRR) within the U.S. Department of Education, this model system encompasses treatment centers throughout the country that participate in research and data collection efforts. The major components of the model system include early access to care through rapid, effective transportation; an acute level one traumatology setting; a comprehensive acute rehabilitation program; psychosocial and vocational services that begin in the hospital and continue through discharge; and follow-up to ascertain that medical and psychosocial needs are met once patients have re-entered the community (Thomas: 1990).

Another federal system that offers special treatment for individuals with spinal cord injuries is the U.S. Department of Veterans Affairs (VA). Spinal cord units are located at 23 regional VA Medical Centers across the country. About two-thirds of the veterans treated at these centers have a service-connected disability; however, even if their injuries are not service-connected, veterans may receive SCI care at VA medical centers.

Many rehabilitation hospitals have spinal cord injury units. One of the advantage of obtaining treatment in these settings is that other patients serve as role models. Some acute care hospitals also have rehabilitation units, and outpatient rehabilitation facilities offer services to people with spinal cord injuries. Many long term care facilities provide services to people with spinal cord injuries. The Commission on Accreditation of Rehabilitation Facilities (CARF) provides accreditation for these facilities (see "ORGANIZATIONS" section below). Independent living centers offer services and referrals to people with spinal cord injuries.

MODIFICATIONS IN EVERYDAY LIVING

In order to remain living in the community, many individuals with spinal cord injuries, especially those with quadriplegia, require personal assistance services (PAS). Personal assistance services may be provided by a family member, friend, or a person specifically employed for this purpose. Personal assistants perform tasks that enable the person with a disability to carry out his or her activities of daily living. Health care providers have observed that personal assistance services contribute not only to the improved physical well-being of individuals with spinal cord injuries and other disabilities, but also to their mental well-being (Nosek: 1993).

The major source of funding for the employment of personal assistants is Medicaid, although other state, local, and federal programs as well as private agencies often contribute. According to Nosek (1991), most individuals with disabilities rely on family members and have had no contacts with formal programs that provide personal assistants. Furthermore, those interested in hiring personal assistants often have difficulty locating qualified individuals. A number of consumer advocacy organizations, research organizations, and the federal government are paying increased attention to the issue of personal assistance services in an attempt to improve the provision of these services.

Most individuals with spinal cord injuries use wheelchairs for mobility. A wide variety of wheelchairs designed for different purposes and different types of impairments is available. Individuals whose injury prohibits them from using manually operated wheelchairs may use battery operated wheelchairs. Sip-and-puff controls, tubes that respond to changes in pressure caused by inhaling and exhaling, enable people with more severe impairments to control the movement of their wheelchairs. Wheelchairs are prescribed by physicians and must accommodate the individual's body size, disability, and functional criteria.

Individuals whose injury has resulted in paraplegia sometimes use braces as an alternative to wheelchairs. One study (Heinemann et al.: 1987) found that only about a quarter of those individuals who had braces continued to use them, while the remainder preferred using wheelchairs. Those who continued to use braces were less likely to have complete lesions than those who stopped using braces. Those who stopped using braces said that they preferred wheelchairs because they were safer, required less energy, and were less likely to fail.

Modification of the home environment requires the installation of ramps; wide doorways with doors that open easily; the removal of thresholds between rooms; and lifts for getting from one level of the home to the other. The kitchen should have accessible appliances, shelves, and working space, and pulls and knobs that are easy to use. The bathroom should be large enough to accommodate a wheelchair; the sink must be at an accessible level; showers should be the roll-in variety with grab bars; and toilets should have grab bars.

Many individuals with paraplegia learn to drive with special hand controls, locks, steering mechanisms, and wheelchair lifts. Major automobile manufacturers offer programs to purchase adapted vehicles with special controls and wheelchair lifts; some individuals may be eligible for reimbursement of the cost of this equipment from the automobile manufacturer (see Chapter 4, "TRAVEL AND TRANSPORTATION ORGANIZATIONS" section for a listing of these programs). Parking must be arranged so that there is enough space for entering and exiting the vehicle.

Special feeding devices are available for individuals with quadriplegia who do not have the use of their upper limbs. Devices may be installed that move people around a room. Use of these specialized devices increases the independence of individuals with quadriplegia.

References

Anderson, Caroline J.
1997 "Unique Management Needs of Pediatric Spinal Cord Injury Patients" Journal of Spinal Cord Medicine 20:1(January):21-24

Bozzacco, Victoria
1990 "Vulnerability and Alcohol and Substance Abuse in Spinal Cord Injury" Rehabilitation Nursing 15:2(March-April):70-72

DeVivo, Michael J. et al.
1995 "Outcomes of Post-Spinal Cord Injury Marriages" Archives of Physical Medicine and Rehabilitation 76(February):130-138

DeVivo, Michael J. et al.
1992 "Trends in Spinal Cord Injury Demographics and Treatment Outcomes Between 1973 and 1986" Archives of Physical Medicine and Rehabilitation 73(May):424-430

DeVivo, Michael J. et al.
1987 "Seven-Year Survival Following Spinal Cord Injury" Archives of Neurology 44(August):872-875

Finn, Robert
1998 "Neural Prosthetics Come of Age as Research Continues" FES Update 8:1(Summer):1-2

Gerhart, Kenneth A.
1995 "Marriage to a Spinal Cord Injury Survivor" Spinal Cord Injury Life Fall 24-27

Gerhart, Kenneth A. et al.
1993 "Long-Term Spinal Cord Injury: Functional Changes over Time" Archives of Physical Medicine and Rehabilitation 74(October):1030-1034

Granat, M. et al.
1992 "The Use of Functional Electrical Stimulation to Assist Gait in Patients with Incomplete Spinal Cord Injury" Disability and Rehabilitation 14(2):93-97

Heinemann, Allen W. et al.
1987 "Mobility for Persons with Spinal Cord Injury: An Evaluation of Two Systems" Archives of Physical Medicine and Rehabilitation 68(February):90-93

Hingley, Audrey T.

1993 "Spinal Cord Injuries: Science Meets Challenge" <u>FDA Consumer</u> July/August:15-19

Huelskamp, Scott

1998 "When Will We Cure Spinal Cord Injuries? <u>Advance for Occupational Therapy Practitioners</u> 14:31(August 3):28-30

Krause, James S.

1992 "Adjustment to Life after Spinal Cord Injury: A Comparison among Three Participant Groups Based on Employment Status" <u>Rehabilitation Counseling Bulletin</u> 35:4(June):218-229

1991 "Survival Following Spinal Cord Injury: A Fifteen-Year Prospective Study" <u>Rehabilitation Psychology</u> 36:2:89-98

Krause, James S. and Nancy M. Crewe

1987 "Prediction of Long-Term Survival of Persons with Spinal Cord Injury: An 11-Year Prospective Study" <u>Rehabilitation Psychology</u> 32:4:205-213

Kuhlemeier, K.V., L.K. Lloyd, and S.L. Stover

1985 "Urological Neurology and Urodynamics" <u>Journal of Urology</u> 134(September):510-513

LeBaron, Samuel, Donald Currie, and Lonnie Zeltzer

1984 "Coping with Spinal Cord Injury in Adolescents" pp. 277-297 in Robert William Blum (ed.) <u>Chronic Illness and Disabilities in Childhood and Adolescence</u> Orlando, FL: Grune and Stratton

Livingston, Carolyn

1991 "Opportunities in Rehabilitation Nursing" <u>American Journal of Nursing</u> 91:2 (February):90-95

McColl, M.A. and C. Rosenthal

1994 "A Model of Resource Needs of Aging Spinal Cord Injured Men" <u>Paraplegia</u> 32:261-70

Menter, Robert R.

1990 "Aging and Spinal Cord Injury: Implications for Existing Model Systems and Future Federal, State, and Local Health Care Policy" pp. 72-80 in David F. Apple and Lesley M. Hudson (eds.) <u>Spinal Cord Injury: The Model</u> Atlanta, GA: Spinal Cord Injury Care System, Sheperd Center for the Treatment of Spinal Injuries

National Institute on Disability and Rehabilitation Research

1992 <u>The Prevention and Management of Urinary Tract Infection among People with Spinal Cord Injuries</u> Washington, D.C.: U.S. Department of Education

National Spinal Cord Injury Statistical Center

2001 <u>Spinal Cord Injury: Facts and Figures at a Glance</u> University of Alabama at Birmingham May

Nosek, Margaret A.

1993 "Personal Assistance: Its Effect on the Long-Term Health of a Rehabilitation Hospital Population" <u>Archives of Physical Medicine and Rehabilitation</u> 74(February):127-132

1991 "Personal Assistance Services: A Review of the Literature and Analysis of Policy Implications" <u>Journal of Disability Policy Studies</u> 2(2):1-17

Pentland, W., M. McColl, and C. Rosenthal
1995 "The Effect of Aging and Duration of Disability on Long Term Health Outcomes following Spinal Cord Injury" Paraplegia 33:367-373

Petrofsky, Jerrold S.
1992 "Functional Electrical Stimulation, a Two-Year Study," Journal of Rehabilitation July/August/September 29-34

Rintala, Diana H. et al.
1992 "Social Support and the Well-Being of Persons with Spinal Cord Injury Living in the Community" Rehabilitation Psychology 37:3:155-163

Stover, Samuel L.
1996 "Facts, Figures, and Trends on Spinal Cord Injury" American Rehabilitation Autumn

Tepper, Mitchell S.
1992 "Sexual Education in Spinal Cord Injury Rehabilitation: Current Trends and Recommendations" Sexuality and Disability 10(1):15-31

Thomas, J. Paul
1990 "Definition of the Model System of Spinal Cord Injury Care" pp. 7-9 in David F. Apple and Lesley M. Hudson (eds.) Spinal Cord Injury: The Model Atlanta, GA: Spinal Cord Injury Care System, Sheperd Center for the Treatment of Spinal Injuries

Trieschmann, Roberta B.
1988 Spinal Cord Injuries: Psychological, Social and Vocational Rehabilitation New York: Demos Publications

Young, John S. et al.
1982 Spinal Cord Injury Statistics Phoenix, AZ: Good Samaritan Medical Center

American Association of Spinal Cord Injury Nurses (AASCIN)
75-20 Astoria Boulevard
Jackson Heights, NY 11370
(718) 803-3782   FAX (718) 803-0414   e-mail: aascin@epva.org
www.aascin.org

A professional membership organization that encourages and improves nursing care of individuals with spinal cord injuries and sponsors research. Membership, $90.00, includes quarterly journal, "SCI Nursing."

American Paraplegia Society (APS)
75-20 Astoria Boulevard
Jackson Heights, NY 11370
(718) 803-3782   FAX (718) 803-0414   e-mail: aps@epva.org
www.apssci.org

A professional membership organization for physicians, scientists, and allied health care professionals. Holds an annual meeting for the presentation of scientific research related to spinal cord injury. Membership, $125.00, includes quarterly journal, "Journal of Spinal Cord Medicine."

American Spinal Injury Association (ASIA)
Rehabilitation Institute of Chicago
345 East Superior, Room 1436
Chicago, IL 60611
(312) 238-1242   FAX (312) 238-0869
e-mail: mars@northwestern.edu
www.asia-spinalinjury.org

A professional membership organization for health care providers dedicated to improving the care of individuals with spinal cord injury through research, education, and development of regional spinal cord injury care systems. Holds an annual meeting with presentation of scientific papers. Membership ranges from $75.00 to $300.00 depending on category; includes newsletter "ASIA Bulletin."

Brain Resources and Information Network (BRAIN)
National Institute of Neurological Disorders and Stroke (NINDS)
PO Box 5801
Bethesda, MD 20824
(800) 352-9424   FAX (301) 402-2186
e-mail: braininfo@ninds.nh.gov   www.ninds.nih.gov

This clearinghouse distributes fact sheets and brochures about neurological disorders such as spinal cord injury to individuals and their families.

Christopher Reeve Paralysis Foundation (CRPF)
500 Morris Avenue
Springfield, NJ 07081
(800) 225-0292   (973) 379-2690   FAX (973) 912-9433
e-mail: info@crpf.org   www.paralysis.org

Supports research to find a cure for paralysis caused by spinal cord injury and other central nervous system disorders. Publishes "Walking Tomorrow," a newsletter about the organization's activities, and "Progress in Research," a newsletter about spinal cord injury research. Free. Also available on the web site. Operates the Christopher and Dana Reeve Resource Center, a federally funded center that enables consumers to obtain information on a wide variety of topics related to spinal cord injury.

Commission on Accreditation of Rehabilitation Facilities (CARF)
4891 East Grant Road
Tucson, AZ 85712
(520) 325-1044 (V/TTY)   FAX (520) 318-1129
e-mail: webmaster@carf.org   www.carf.org

Conducts site evaluations and accredits organizations that provide rehabilitation, pain management, adult day services, and assisted living. Provides a free list of accredited organizations in a specific state.

Craig Hospital Aging with Spinal Cord Injury
Craig Hospital
3425 South Clarkson
Englewood, CO 80110
(303) 789-8202   FAX (303) 789-8441
e-mail: HealthResources@craighospital.org
www.craighospital.org (click on "Research Information")

A federally funded center that studies the physiological and psychological effects of changes brought about by aging on individuals with spinal cord injuries. The center has been following individuals with spinal cord injuries for 25 years. Produces consumer information brochures in English and Spanish. Many publications available on the web site.

Foundation for Spinal Cord Injury Prevention, Care and Cure (FSCIPCC)
19223 Roscommon
Harper Wood, MI 48225
(800) 342-0330   FAX (313) 245-0812   e-mail: ron@fscip.org
www.fscip.org

This organization supports research to find a cure for spinal cord injury, provides referrals to individuals and their families, and conducts a program to prevent spinal cord injury. The web site provides information about spinal cord injury as well as links to other resources.

Functional Electrical Stimulation Information Center
11000 Cedar Avenue, Suite 230
Cleveland, OH 44106
(800) 666-2353   (216) 231-3257 (V/TTY)   FAX (216) 231-3258
e-mail: info@fesc.org   feswww.fes.cwru.edu

The center provides information to consumers and professionals about research on functional electrical stimulation to help individuals with spinal cord injuries and multiple sclerosis. The web site provides information on resources, references, and referrals.

MEDLINEplus: Spinal Cord Injuries
www.nlm.nih.gov/medlineplus/spinalcordinjuries.html

This web site provides links to sites for general information about spinal cord injuries, symptoms and diagnosis, treatment, specific aspects of the condition, clinical trials, statistics, organizations, and research. Includes an interactive tutorial on myelograms. Some information is available in Spanish. Provides links to MEDLINE research articles and related MEDLINEplus pages.

Miami Project to Cure Paralysis
PO Box 0169 (R-48)
Miami, FL 33101-6960
(305) 243-6001   FAX (305) 243-6017
Automated Information Line: (800) 782-6387
e-mail: mpinfo@miamiproj.med.miami.edu
www.miamiproject.miami.edu

A research organization dedicated to finding a cure for spinal cord injury.

National Association for Continence (NAFC)
PO Box 8310
Spartanburg, SC 29305-8310
(800) 252-3337   FAX (864) 579-7902   www.nafc.org

An information clearinghouse for consumers, family members, and medical professionals. Will answer individual questions if self-addressed stamped envelope is enclosed with letter. Membership, $25.00, includes a quarterly newsletter, "Quality Care," a "Resource Guide: Products and Services for Continence" (nonmembers, $10.00), discount on publications, and a continence resource service. Free publications list.

National Association on Alcohol, Drugs, and Disability, Inc. (NAADD)
2165 Bunker Hill Drive
San Mateo, CA 94402
(650) 578-8047 (V/TTY)   FAX (650) 286-9205
e-mail: jdem@aimnet.com   www.naadd.org

Promotes awareness and education about substance abuse in individuals with disabilities. Newsletters and other publications are available on the web site.

National Easter Seal Society
230 West Monroe Street, Suite 1800
Chicago, IL 60606
(800) 221-6827   (312) 726-6200   (312) 726-4258 (TTY)
FAX (312) 726-1494   e-mail: info@easter-seals.org   www.easter-seals.org

Offers rehabilitation programs and support groups for individuals with spinal cord injury. Services provided by local affiliates may vary.

National Institute on Disability and Rehabilitation Research (NIDRR)
U.S. Department of Education
400 Maryland Avenue, SW
Washington, DC 20202-2572
(202) 205-8134   (202) 205-4475 (TTY)   FAX (202) 205-8515
www.ed.gov/offices/OSERS/NIDRR

A federal agency that supports research into various aspects of disability and rehabilitation, including demographic analyses, social science research, and the development of assistive devices. Supports a nationwide system of model spinal cord injury centers.

National Spinal Cord Injury Association (NSCIA)
6701 Democracy Boulevard, Suite 300-9
Bethesda, MD 20817
(800) 962-9629   (301) 588-6959   FAX (301) 588-9414
www.spinalcord.org

A membership organization with chapters throughout the U.S. Disseminates information to people with spinal cord injuries and to their families; provides counseling; and advocates for the removal of barriers to independent living. Participates in the development of standards of care for regional spinal cord injury care. NSCIA will perform a customized database search; call for details. Holds annual meeting and educational seminars. Membership, individuals with a disability or family members, $25.00; allied health professionals, $50.00; attorneys or physicians, $100.00; organizations, $250.00 to $1000.00; includes quarterly magazine, "SCI Life" (nonmember price, $30.00), fact sheets, and discounts on other publications, medical products, and pharmaceutical supplies.

Paralyzed Veterans of America (PVA)
801 18th Street, NW
Washington, DC 20006
(800) 424-8200   (800) 795-4327 (TTY)   (202) 872-1300
FAX (202) 785-4452   e-mail: info@pva.org   www.pva.org

A membership organization for veterans with spinal cord injury. Advocates and lobbies for the rights of paralyzed veterans and sponsors research. Membership fees are set by state chapters. The national office refers callers to the nearest chapter. The PVA Spinal Cord Injury Education and Training Foundation accepts applications to fund continuing education, post-professional specialty training, and patient/client and family education. The PVA Spinal Cord Research Foundation accepts applications to fund basic and clinical research, the design of assistive devices, and conferences that foster interaction among scientists and health care providers. Some publications are available on the web site.

Rehabilitation Research and Training Center on Secondary Complications of Spinal Cord Injury
Spain Rehabilitation Center
University of Alabama at Birmingham
619 19th Street South, SRC 529
Birmingham, AL 35249
(205) 934-3283   (205) 934-4642 (TTY)   FAX (205) 975-4691
e-mail: rtc@uab.edu   www.spinalcord.uab.edu

A federally funded center that conducts research and holds educational conferences for people with spinal cord injuries, their families, and professionals. The National Spinal Cord Injury Statistical Center collects data from spinal cord injury centers throughout the country. Produces a variety of audio-visual materials and books for professional care providers and consumers, as well as a series of information sheets. A list of articles documenting some of the center's research findings is also available. Information sheets are available on the web site. Newsletter, "Pushin' On," is published twice a year; free. Also available on the web site. Also administers the Spinal Cord Injury Information Network.

Simon Foundation for Continence
PO Box 835
Wilmette, IL 60091
(800) 237-4666   (847) 864-3913   FAX (847) 864-9758
e-mail: simoninfo@simonfoundation.org
www.simonfoundation.org

Provides information and assistance to people who are incontinent. Organizes self-help groups. Offers discussion groups on the web site. Membership, individuals, $15.00; professionals, $35.00; includes quarterly newsletter, "The Informer." Also available on the web site.

Substance Abuse Resources & Disability Issues (SARDI)
Rehabilitation Research and Training Center on Drugs and Disability
School of Medicine, Wright State University
PO Box 927
Dayton, OH 45401-0927
(937) 775-1484 (V/TTY)   FAX (937) 775-1495
www.med.wright.edu/som/sardi

A federally funded research center that investigates the relationship between drug use and disabilities. Free newsletter, "SARDI Online."

Vocational Rehabilitation and Employment
Veterans Benefits Administration
U.S. Department of Veterans Affairs (VA)
(800) 827-1000 (connects with regional office)
www.vba.va.gov/bln/vre/index.htm

Provides education and rehabilitation assistance and independent living services to veterans with service related disabilities through offices located in every state as well as regional centers, medical centers, and insurance centers. Medical services are provided at VA Medical Centers, Outpatient Clinics, Domiciliaries, and Nursing Homes. Veterans may apply for benefits on the web site.

WheelchairNet
e-mail: wheelchairnet@shrs.pitt.edu www.wheelchairnet.org

This virtual community of wheelchair users enables participants to exchange information about wheelchair technology. The web site includes resources, articles, and a discussion area.

Aging with Spinal Cord Injury
by Gale G. Whiteneck et al.
Demos Medical Publishing
386 Park Avenue South, Suite 201
New York, NY 10016
(800) 532-8663   (212) 683-0072   FAX (212) 683-0118
e-mail: info@demospub.com   www.demosmedpub.co

This book is an anthology of articles by a multidisciplinary group of experts in the field of spinal cord injury. Topics include research in the area of aging with a spinal cord injury, physiological and psychological aspects of the aging process, and societal perspectives. $99.95 plus $4.00 shipping and handling. Orders made on the Demos web site receive a 15% discount.

Alcohol, Disabilities, and Rehabilitation
by Susan A. Storti
Thomson Learning, Florence, KY

This book discusses alcohol abuse in individuals with disabilities and chronic conditions. Includes treatment and rehabilitation strategies. Out of print

The Challenged Life: Spinal Cord Injury
Rehabilitation Institute of Chicago
Education and Training Center
345 East Superior Street, Suite 1641
Chicago, IL 60611
(312) 238-2859   FAX (312) 238-4451   e-mail: ric-lrc@nwu.edu
www.rehabchicago.org

A videotape in which a young man with a spinal cord injury discusses his feelings and his need to relearn how to carry out functional activities. The staff members who treated him discuss the function of the spinal cord, mobility skills, and social skills that individuals with spinal cord injuries need to learn. 22 minutes. $25.00 plus $3.00 shipping and handling

A Change in Perspective
Synergem
115 Newfield Avenue
Edison, NJ 08837
(800) 867-5432   FAX (732) 225-7555

Produced by the Eastern Paralyzed Veterans Association [EPVA, (718) 803-3782], this videotape shows five individuals with spinal cord injury during the course of their everyday life. 30 minutes. $29.95 plus $4.95 shipping and handling

A Consumer's Guide to Home Adaptation
Adaptive Environments Center
374 Congress Street, Suite 301
Boston, MA 02210
(617) 695-1225 (V/TTY)   FAX (617) 482-8099
e-mail: adaptive@adaptenvironments.org
www.adaptenvironments.org

A workbook that enables people with mobility impairments to plan the modifications necessary to adapt their homes. Includes descriptions of widening doorways, lowering countertops, etc. $12.00

Depression: What You Should Know
PVA Distribution Center
PO Box 753
Waldorf, MD 20604-0753
(888) 860-7244   (301) 932-7834   FAX (301) 843-0159
www.pva.org

This consumer guide discusses the signs of depression, its causes, and treatments available. $9.95 plus $3.00 shipping and handling

Enabling Romance: A Guide to Love, Sex, and Relationships for People with Disabilities
by Ken Kroll and Erica Levy Klein
Nine Lives Press
PO Box 220
Horsham, PA 19044
(888) 850-0344, extension 109   (215) 675-9133, extension 109
FAX (215) 675-9376   e-mail: kim@leonardmediagroup.com
www.newmobility.com

Written by a man who has a disability and his wife who does not, this book provides examples of how people with a variety of disabilities have established fulfilling relationships. $15.95 plus $3.00 shipping and handling

Family Adjustment in Spinal Cord Injury
Spain Rehabilitation Center
University of Alabama at Birmingham
619 19th Street South, SRC 529
Birmingham, AL 35249
(205) 934-3283   (205) 934-4642 (TTY)   FAX (205) 975-4691
e-mail: rtc@uab.edu   www.spinalcord.uab.edu

This booklet provides support for family members, discussing their concerns and feelings. $2.00. Also available on the web site.

A Guide to Wheelchair Selection: How to Use the ANSI/RESNA Wheelchair Standards to Buy a Wheelchair
PVA Distribution Center
PO Box 753
Waldorf, MD 20604-0753
(888) 860-7244   (301) 932-7834   FAX (301) 843-0159
www.pva.org

This book enables wheelchair users to make informed choices when purchasing a wheelchair. $19.95 plus $3.00 shipping and handling

Journal of Rehabilitation Research and Development (JRRD)
Scientific and Technical Publications Section
Rehabilitation Research and Development Service
103 South Gay Street, 5th floor
Baltimore, MD 21202
(410) 962-1800   FAX (410) 962-9670   e-mail: pubs@vard.org
www.vard.org

A journal that includes articles on disability, rehabilitation, sensory aids, gerontology, and disabling conditions. Annual supplements provide research progress reports. Clinical supplements report on specific topics. Published six times a year. Available in standard print and on the web site. Free

Journal of Spinal Cord Medicine
American Paraplegia Society
75-20 Astoria Boulevard
Jackson Heights, NY 11370
(718) 803-3782   FAX (718) 803-0414   e-mail: aps@epva.org
www.apssci.org

A quarterly journal that covers a wide range of topics related to treatment of the physical and psychological aspects of spinal cord injury. Free

Living with Spinal Cord Injury
by Barry Corbet
Fanlight Productions
4196 Washington Street, Suite 2
Boston, MA 02131
(800) 937-4113   (617) 469-4999   FAX (617) 469-3379
e-mail: fanlight@fanlight.com   www.fanlight.com

A series of three videotapes produced by an individual who has experienced spinal cord injury himself. "Changes" is about the consequences of spinal cord injury and the process of rehabilitation. "Outside" emphasizes the life-long aspect of rehabilitation for people with spinal cord injuries. "Survivors" interviews 23 men and women who have lived at least 24 years with spinal cord injuries. Purchase of single videotape, $99.00; rental for one day, $50.00; rental for one week, $100.00; $9.00 shipping and handling. Purchase of series, $250.00; call for shipping and handling.

Managing Incontinence
by Cheryle B. Gartley, (ed.)
Simon Foundation for Continence
PO Box 835
Wilmette, IL 60091
(800) 237-4666   (847) 864-3913   FAX (847) 864-9758
e-mail: simoninfo@simonfoundation.org
www.simonfoundation.org

This book provides medical advice, information on products, interviews with individuals who are incontinent, and advice on sexuality. $12.95

Managing Personal Assistants: A Consumer Guide
PVA Distribution Center
PO Box 753
Waldorf, MD 20604-0753
(888) 860-7244   (301) 932-7834   FAX (301) 843-0159
www.pva.org

This book provides information on recruiting, hiring, training, retaining and firing personal care assistants. Describes funding sources and discusses tax issues. $15.95 plus $3.00 shipping and handling

<u>A Man's Guide to Coping with Disability</u>
Resources for Rehabilitation
22 Bonad Road
Winchester, MA 01890
(781) 368-9094   FAX (781) 368-9096
e-mail: orders@rfr.org   www.rfr.org

This book includes information about men's responses to disability, with a special emphasis on the values men place on independence, occupational achievement, and physical activity. Chapter on spinal cord injury includes information about sexual functioning. $44.95 plus $5.00 shipping and handling (See last page of this book for order form.)

<u>Moving Violations: War Zones, Wheelchairs, and Declarations of Independence</u>
by John Hockenberry
AOL-Time-Warner Trade Publishing
Attn: Order Department
3 Center Plaza
Boston, MA 02108
(800) 759-0190   FAX (800) 286-9471

Written by a television reporter who became a paraplegic at the age of 19 as a result of an automobile accident, this book describes his adjustment to disability, rehabilitation, jobs in radio and television, and the stories of other family members with disabilities. $14.45

<u>National Database of Educational Resources on Spinal Cord Injury</u>
The Institute for Rehabilitation and Research (TIRR)
Division of Education, B 107
1333 Moursund
Houston, TX 77030
(800) 732-8124   (713) 797-5971   (713) 797-5970 (TTY)
FAX (713) 797-5982   e-mail: mgordon@bcm.tmc.edu   www.tirr.org

This database of publications, audiocassettes, and videotapes on spinal cord injury covers topics such as environmental modifications and accessibility, adaptive equipment and aids, vocational management, and recreation and leisure. Printouts for up to two subject areas are free. Complete database of both audio-visual materials and unpublished written materials, $55.00 plus $5.00 shipping and handling.

<u>Neurogenic Bowel: What You Should Know</u>
PVA Distribution Center
PO Box 753
Waldorf, MD 20604-0753
(888) 860-7244   (301) 932-7834   FAX (301) 843-0159
www.pva.org

This guide describes the effects of spinal cord injury on bowel function and how to deal with these changes. $9.95 plus $3.00 shipping and handling

Neurological Disorders
Brain Resources and Information Network (BRAIN)
National Institute of Neurological Disorders and Stroke (NINDS)
PO Box 5801
Bethesda, MD 20824
(800) 352-9424   (301) 496-5751
e-mail: braininfo@ninds.nih.gov   www.ninds.nih.gov

This directory lists voluntary health agencies and other patient resources. Free

New Mobility
PO Box 220
Horsham, PA 19044
(888) 850-0344, extension 109   (215) 675-9133, extension 109
FAX (215) 675-9376   e-mail: kim@jvleonard.com
www.newmobility.com

This monthly magazine provides information for individuals with spinal cord injury on topics such as recreation, travel, and everyday living. $27.95

PN/Paraplegia News
2111 East Highland Avenue, Suite 180
Phoenix, AZ 85016
(888) 888-2201   FAX (602) 224-0507   www.pn-magazine.com

A monthly magazine sponsored by the Paralyzed Veterans of America. Features information for paralyzed veterans and civilians, articles about everyday living, new legislation, employment, and research. $23.00

Silent Storm
c/o United Cerebral Palsy of America/New Jersey
354 South Broad Street
Trenton, NJ 08608
(888) 322-1918   (609) 392-4004   (609) 392-7044 (TTY)

This videotape explores substance abuse among individuals with disabilities and describes programs designed to meet their needs. Open or closed captioned. 10 minutes. Accompanying brochure available in English and Spanish. $45.00 plus $5.00 shipping and handling

Spinal Cord Injury Desk Reference
by Terry L. Blackwell et al.
Demos Medical Publishing
386 Park Avenue South, Suite 201
New York, NY 10016
(800) 532-8663   (212) 683-0072   FAX (212) 683-011
e-mail: info@demospub.com   www.demosmedpub.com

This reference book provides basic concepts about spinal cord injury, including epidemiology, potential complications, long term management, and life care planning guidelines. $59.95 plus $4.00 shipping and handling

Spinal Network
by Barry Corbet et al. (eds.)
PO Box 220
Horsham, PA 19044
(215) 675-9133, extension 108   FAX (215) 675-9376
e-mail: kim@jvleonard.com   www.spinalnetwork.net

This book describes the medical aspects of spinal cord injury and the wide variety of effects on functioning. Presents biographical accounts of people who have lived with spinal cord injuries. Discusses issues of everyday living, including recreation and sports, travel, and legal and financial concerns. $49.95 plus $7.50 shipping and handling

Sports 'N Spokes
2111 East Highland Avenue, Suite 180
Phoenix, AZ 85016
(888) 888-2201   FAX (602) 224-0507   www.pva.org

A magazine that features articles about sports activities for people who use wheelchairs. Eight issues, $21.00.

Wheelchairs: Your Options & Rights - Guide to Obtaining Wheelchairs from the Department of Veterans Affairs
PVA Distribution Center
PO Box 753
Waldorf, MD 20604-0753
(888) 860-7244   (301) 932-7834   FAX (301) 843-0159
www.pva.org

This booklet describes the eligibility criteria for obtaining wheelchairs from the U.S. Department of Veterans Affairs, as well as different type of wheelchairs. Available in English and Spanish. Free plus $3.00 shipping and handling

A Woman's Guide to Coping with Disability
Resources for Rehabilitation
22 Bonad Road
Winchester, MA 01890
(781) 368-9094   FAX (781) 368-9096
e-mail: orders@rfr.org   www.rfr.org

This book addresses the special needs of women with disabilities and chronic conditions, such as social relationships, sexual functioning, pregnancy, childrearing, caregiving, and employment. Written for women in all age categories, the book has chapters on the disabilities that are most prevalent in women or likely to affect the roles and physical functions unique to women including spinal cord injury. $44.95 plus $5.00 shipping and handling (See last page of this book for order form.)

Yes, You Can! A Guide to Self-Care for Persons with Spinal Cord Injury
PVA Distribution Center
PO Box 753
Waldorf, MD 20604-0753
(888) 860-7244   (301) 932-7834
FAX (301) 843-0159   www.pva.org

This manual offers practical information and resources, including chapters on substance abuse, pain, exercise, alternative medicine, equipment, and staying healthy. $15.00 plus $3.00 shipping and handling

Chapter 11

VISUAL IMPAIRMENT AND BLINDNESS

According to the U.S. Bureau of the Census, about 7.7 million Americans age 15 or older have reported that they have difficulty seeing; 1.8 million could not see at all (McNeil: 2001). The number of people with visual impairments has increased in recent years. Two major factors have contributed to the increase in visual impairment. First, advances in technology have enabled very low birth weight babies to survive, often with serious disabilities including visual impairment. Second, the number of older people, who account for a large portion of the population with visual impairment, has increased rapidly. It is projected that the older population will continue to grow and that by the year 2030, there will be 65.6 million Americans 65 years or older (Fowles: 1991).

A study of individuals age 40 or over living in East Baltimore, Maryland suggests that less than normal visual acuity is often attributable to improper refraction. Proper refraction improved visual acuity by at least one line on the Snellen acuity chart in 54% of the population and by three or more lines for 7.5% of the population (Tielsch et al.: 1991). The same study also found that African-Americans were less likely than whites to have had surgery for glaucoma and senile cataracts. These findings indicate that African-Americans were more likely than whites to experience blindness that could have been prevented (Sommer et al.: 1991).

MAJOR TYPES AND CAUSES OF VISUAL IMPAIRMENT AND BLINDNESS

Low vision is the term that is commonly used to refer to visual impairments that leave the individual with some residual vision. Although there are no standard definitions of low vision, professionals usually consider an acuity of 20/70 or worse to be low vision. In the United States, individuals are considered *legally blind* if they have a visual acuity of 20/200 or worse in the better eye with all possible correction or a field restriction of 20 degrees diameter or less in the better eye. Most individuals who are legally blind retain some useful vision and should be encouraged to use it to the maximum extent possible. The classification of legal blindness entitles American citizens to tax benefits and to rehabilitation services provided by state governments. Definitions of legal blindness vary in other countries. A relatively small proportion of the population that is visually impaired or blind has only light perception or is totally blind.

Central vision loss and peripheral field loss are two major types of visual impairment. *Central vision* enables people to read, to recognize faces, and to do close work. The retina is the layer at the back of the eye that acts as the eye's camera. The macula is the small central part of the retina that is responsible for acute vision. When the macula is destroyed or damaged, central vision is affected. Although individuals with macular diseases have difficulty reading or may not be able to read at all, they usually have useful peripheral vision. A person with macular disease may sometimes appear to be looking at another person's face out of the side of his or her eyes.

Individuals use *peripheral vision* for mobility and to see the full scope of the scene they are facing. Diminished peripheral vision is often referred to as tunnel vision. This impairment affects mobility, although the central vision may still be intact. Some progressive diseases, such as glaucoma, begin with loss of peripheral vision but may progress to total loss of vision, including central vision.

The leading causes of visual impairment or blindness are macular degeneration, glaucoma, diabetic retinopathy, and cataract. Other conditions which may lead to vision loss are corneal diseases, retinitis pigmentosa, stroke, retinal detachment, trauma, and tumors. Blindness or vision loss in children may be caused by congenital deficits, hereditary conditions, or diseases, such as retinoblastoma, a cancer of the eye.

Macular degeneration describes a variety of diseases that cause the macula to deteriorate. The most common form of macular degeneration is age-related macular degeneration (AMD). As its name implies, this form of the disease occurs most frequently among the population age 50 or older. It is the leading cause of vision loss among Americans age 65 or older. The disease causes loss of central vision, but some useful central vision may remain. Initial symptoms of macular degeneration include distortion of straight lines or a loss of clarity in the central field of vision. For some forms of macular degeneration, laser treatment temporarily halts the progressive vision loss.

Currently there is no treatment for the drusenoid or dry form of AMD. The neovascular or wet form involves the development of abnormal blood vessels and usually causes more severe impairment than the dry form. In April, 2000, the Food and Drug Administration (FDA) approved the use of photodynamic therapy with a light-activating drug called verteporfin (Visudyne) in individuals with the wet form of AMD. However, this treatment is not able to restore vision that has already been lost. In 2001, the National Eye Institute reported the results of the Age-Related Eye Disease Study (AREDS). In this major clinical trial, the risk of developing the more serious wet form of AMD in those who have dry AMD was reduced in participants who took antioxidants and zinc supplements (Age-Related Eye Disease Study: 2001). AMD is not cured nor is vision restored by taking the supplements. Optical and nonoptical aids (described below) enable many individuals with macular degeneration to use their remaining vision to continue reading, working, and living independently.

Glaucoma encompasses a group of eye diseases in which increased intraocular pressure, caused by improper drainage of the fluid in the eye, results in damage to the optic nerve. Glaucoma is often not diagnosed until the late stages of the disease, because symptoms are not present in the early stages. When symptoms do appear, they are in the form of peripheral field defects and blurred vision. Routine ophthalmological examinations are recommended in order to detect asymptomatic diseases such as glaucoma. In addition to measuring intraocular pressure, the ophthalmologist should examine the optic nerve through dilated pupils. Progression of glaucoma can be prevented, but sight that has been lost as a result of glaucoma cannot be restored. The most common form of treatment is medication used to decrease the intraocular pressure. Medication is sometimes administered orally and sometimes applied topically as drops for the eyes. In some cases, laser treatment or microsurgery is necessary to decrease intraocular pressure.

A *cataract* is an opacity or clouding of the lens of the eye which causes decreased visual acuity. A cataract may develop in one eye only or in both eyes at different rates. Symptoms of cataracts include blurred vision, reduced contrast sensitivity, reduced color perception, and difficulty with reading and night driving. Cataracts may be removed by surgery, which has a high success rate. When the cataract is removed, the function of the lens is usually replaced by an intraocular lens (IOL), which is placed in the eye surgically. In some individuals, the lens capsule becomes cloudy a year or more after cataract surgery (posterior capsular opacification). This condition can be treated by laser surgery, usually on an outpatient basis. Cataracts may be present with other eye diseases that cause reduced vision; thus removing a cataract does not always restore vision to normal.

The major cause of visual impairment in young adults is *diabetic retinopathy*. Complications of diabetes that cause vision loss include macular edema, or a build-up of fluid in the central part of the retina, and proliferative retinopathy, the growth of abnormal blood cells which may rupture and then form scar tissue. Blood from damaged blood vessels in the eye may seep into the vitreous, blocking the passage of light to the retina. Diabetic retinopathy is often treated with laser photocoagulation. Sometimes it is necessary to perform a vitrectomy, or surgical removal of blood and scar tissue from the vitreous, in the attempt to restore useful vision. The vitreous or gel which fills the eye between the lens and the retina is replaced with a saline solution.

VISUAL IMPAIRMENT AND BLINDNESS IN CHILDREN

A study by Kirchner (1990) reports an increase in the rates of congenital blindness since 1970 and evidence that there are many more children who are visually impaired or blind being served in schools. *Retinopathy of prematurity* (formerly known as retrolental fibroplasia) is one cause of the increase in congenital blindness. Retinopathy of prematurity (ROP) is an eye condition in which there is a growth of abnormal blood vessels and scar tissue in the eyes of some low birth weight premature infants. First observed in the 1940s, this condition was formerly attributed to the use of excessive oxygen in the incubators. Research no longer supports this single cause (Zierler: 1988). Other factors which have been implicated are vitamin A and E deficiencies; low oxygen and high carbon dioxide blood levels; and other metabolic factors (Repka: 1989). Most researchers agree that prematurity itself and low birth weight are primary contributors to retinopathy of prematurity. Long term complications observed in older children and young adults include retinal detachment and narrow-angle glaucoma (Repka: 1989). Therefore, individuals with retinopathy of prematurity should receive regular ophthalmological examinations throughout their lives.

Macular degeneration, described above as a major cause of visual impairment in adults, may also be present in infants, children, and adolescents. The hereditary form of macular degeneration is called "juvenile macular degeneration." Reduced visual acuity is the primary symptom. Although there is no treatment for this condition, special glasses and low vision aids enable individuals to function independently.

Other conditions which cause vision loss or blindness in children are *congenital cataracts, retinoblastoma* (a cancer of the eye), *congenital glaucoma, aniridia* (a partial or

287

complete absence of the iris), and *albinism*. Some of these conditions may lead to further visual loss as children grow older.

VISUAL IMPAIRMENT AND BLINDNESS IN ELDERS

Visual impairment is one of the most common impairments among the population age 65 years or older. A survey found that 17% of adults age 65 to 74, or 3.1 million individuals, report a visual impairment. Visual impairment is reported by one-quarter of those age 75 years and older, or 3.5 million people (Louis Harris and Associates, Inc.: 1995).

Visual impairment increases elders' awareness of the decline of their physical powers and makes them intimately familiar with the incapacities of old age (Ainlay: 1989). It is difficult for a person to mobilize strengths and compensate for the loss of vision by sharpening the use of other senses when those other senses are also deteriorating and strengths are diminishing (Associated Services for the Blind: 1988).

The individual's personal and social independence is affected, influencing attitudes and emotional status, as well as the ability to adapt to loss. In addition, vision loss is responsible for many of the falls experienced by elders; the misuse of medication when labels cannot be read; and driving accidents (Wright: 1987). (For a more detailed discussion of the ways in which vision loss affects elders and services available to help them, see Resources for Elders with Disabilities, described in "PUBLICATIONS AND TAPES" section below.)

PSYCHOLOGICAL ASPECTS OF VISION LOSS

Vision loss affects all aspects of life. Individuals who have experienced vision loss fear that they will lose their jobs and the ability to support themselves; that they will be unable to take care of themselves; and that they will become the object of pity. Vision loss threatens independence, which in turn diminishes self-esteem. When self-esteem is low, it is often difficult to accept assistance offered by others, including services from professionals.

Individuals with vision loss often need time to adjust psychologically before they are able to begin the rehabilitation process. The amount of time that individuals need before they accept their vision loss and are able to benefit from rehabilitation is a personal matter and may be a matter of days, months, or even years. In many cases, individuals who are slow to accept their prognosis will benefit from speaking to others who have gone through similar experiences or from discussing the situation with a professional counselor.

Progressive vision loss often affects the individual's educational and career plans. An explanation of the likely progression of an individual's eye condition or disease and early referrals for services will facilitate the adjustment process. It will also help individuals make career choices. For example, young people with retinitis pigmentosa or juvenile macular degeneration must be made aware that careers as airplane pilots or surgeons are unrealistic. However, people with these conditions may succeed in a wide variety of demanding professional careers, often with the use of assistive devices.

Some forms of visual impairment or blindness are hereditary, such as albinism, some retinitis pigmentosa syndromes, congenital cataracts, aniridia, and congenital glaucoma. Parents often feel guilty when their children are diagnosed with a hereditary condition that

288

causes visual impairment or blindness. It is often helpful for parents to attend support groups, where they can talk about their feelings and about methods that their family can use to cope with the child's visual impairment or blindness. Genetic counselors may be able to provide information that will help parents decide whether or not to have more children. Learning about the many services, educational programs, and products that enable individuals who are visually impaired or blind to function independently will help alleviate parents' anxieties about their child's future.

PROFESSIONAL SERVICE PROVIDERS

Individuals are often unaware of the causes of visual impairment or blindness or the services provided by health and rehabilitation professionals in the field of vision loss. Individuals with vision loss are an underserved group within the general population, and even more dramatically, in the older population. Not only do elders tend to view loss of vision as an inevitable part of aging and therefore fail to seek support services, but professionals working with elders also tend to have this attitude (Branch et al.: 1989). The role of professional service providers may be crucial in determining individual and family responses to the diagnosis of visual impairment or blindness.

Ophthalmologists (M.D.) are physicians who specialize in diseases of the eye and systemic diseases that affect the eye's functioning. *Optometrists* (O.D.) are trained to conduct refractions and prescribe corrective lenses. In some states, optometrists are also licensed to administer drugs. *Opticians* are trained to make and dispense corrective lenses. All of these practitioners should refer patients for rehabilitation services when medical or surgical treatment and the prescription of corrective lenses do not result in normal visual acuity.

Low vision specialists may be ophthalmologists, optometrists, opticians, or other professionals who are trained to help individuals with vision loss make use of their remaining vision to the greatest extent possible through the use of optical and nonoptical aids.

Rehabilitation counselors serve as case coordinators for individuals who are visually impaired or blind and require rehabilitation services. The rehabilitation counselor establishes a one-to-one relationship in the initial interview. In succeeding contacts, the rehabilitation counselor and the individual jointly develop an Individual Written Rehabilitation Program that is appropriate and realistic. Rehabilitation guidelines have been revised to include the role of "homemaker" as a justifiable rehabilitation goal.

Rehabilitation teachers provide individualized instruction in activities of daily living. This instruction may include adapting the home through the use of large print telephone dials and markers for stoves, thermostats, and medications. Methods to increase home safety are also taught. The rehabilitation teacher provides information about community resources and services.

Orientation and mobility (O and M) instructors orient the individual to his or her home and the immediate areas outside the home; they also teach safe travel skills using the long white cane.

Vision teachers work with the parents of a child who is visually impaired or blind to develop an Individualized Education Program (IEP) which outlines specific instruction, special equipment, and other services to be provided to the child. Vision teachers may provide instruction in typing, braille, and orientation and mobility, while serving as a resource to classroom teachers on methods of working with the child in a regular classroom.

Other health professionals who may be involved in the care of individuals with visual impairment or blindness are *occupational therapists*, *geriatricians*, *diabetologists*, and mental health professionals, such as *psychologists*, *psychiatrists*, and *social workers*.

WHERE TO FIND SERVICES

Services for people who are visually impaired or blind are often offered in ophthalmologists' or optometrists' offices, hospitals, and private or public rehabilitation agencies. These services include the prescription of optical and nonoptical aids which enable individuals to make maximum use of their remaining vision or provide an alternative to visual tasks.

In many states, ophthalmologists and optometrists are required to register individuals who are legally blind with a state agency such as a "Commission for the Blind" or a division of the state vocational rehabilitation agency. Most public agencies require that clients be legally blind in order to receive services. If individuals do not know if they are legally blind, they should ask an ophthalmologist or optometrist. Some agencies that have the word "blind" in their names serve individuals with varying degrees of visual impairment, including low vision. Many private agencies also serve individuals with vision loss; they are usually listed in the "Social Service Organizations" section of the Yellow Pages or in the "Community Services" section of the white pages of local telephone directories.

Children who are visually impaired or blind are eligible for services mandated by the Individuals with Disabilities Education Act (formerly called the Education of the Handicapped Act) and early intervention programs which are available to all children with disabilities (see Chapter 3, "Children and Youths"). Elders who have experienced vision loss but who are not legally blind may be eligible for services from a state department on aging or elder affairs or an area agency on aging. Veterans with vision loss are eligible for services from VA Medical Centers throughout the country, whether or not their vision loss is service related.

ENVIRONMENTAL ADAPTATIONS

The following adaptations are recommended to help people who are visually impaired but who retain some useful vision to function in their homes, schools, and community centers as well as in health and rehabilitation service providers' offices.

Enlarge images and objects. Increasing the size of an object projects it on to a larger part of the retina. Large print labels for telephone dials or push-buttons are two simple examples. Hand-held and stand magnifiers are useful for reading mail, menus, price tags, telephone numbers, newspapers, and books. Closed circuit televisions systems (CCTVs), which enlarge print on a screen, and large print books also make reading easier.

Move closer to the object. Individuals may need to sit closer to the television or hold a book or newspaper closer to their eyes. Children in school may need to sit closer to the chalkboard.

Increase the amount of light. Many individuals with vision loss may find that two to three times more light than usual is necessary. Fluorescent lights diffuse evenly and are inexpensive, but they produce less contrast, may flicker, and are harsh. Diffusing filters may solve these problems. The incandescent light found in a standard bulb offers more contrast and can be directed, but it produces shadows and glare. Halogen bulbs emit a whiter light than incandescent bulbs, making reading easier; last longer; and produce more light per watt. Diffusers and additional lighting spread the light around and reduce shadows. A combination is often the best choice. Sunlight is natural and bright but not easily controlled. Magnifiers with light bulbs in their handles both enlarge and illuminate print.

Control glare. Dimmer switches are useful in controlling glare. Sunglasses worn indoors are helpful in controlling the glare from overhead lights. Many individuals find that an amber tint controls glare without sacrificing clarity. Night lights may help with accommodation problems, avoiding the need to turn on a bright light when rising in a dark room or walking down a dark hall. Even individuals who have very little functional vision complain of problems with glare and may benefit from these suggestions.

Change or improve contrast. The use of light/dark color combinations is important because color perception is often reduced in individuals who are visually impaired. It is a good idea to paint or carpet stairs in a color that contrasts with the floor above and below; to use white or light colored dishes on colored tablecloths; and to pour liquids against contrasting backgrounds. Other practical adaptations are painting stripes or placing tape in contrasting colors on the edges of steps and marking stove and thermostat dials.

The following adaptations are recommended for people who have severe visual impairments or no useful vision. People with less severe visual impairments often utilize these techniques as well.

Use other senses. An individual who becomes visually impaired or blind does not develop a "sixth sense," as is commonly believed. However, individuals learn to use their remaining senses more effectively. Talking calculators, talking watches, and talking clocks provide information aurally; tape recorders are used to take messages; recorded publications played on special tape players provide hours of enjoyment. Items such as canned or frozen foods, spools of thread, or articles of clothing may be marked with tactile labels. Raised large print letters, braille, or special glues which leave a raised "dot" may be used for identification.

Braille uses the sense of touch as an alternative method of reading and writing. Raised dots in various combinations represent the letters of the alphabet, numbers, and punctuation. Most individuals who read and write braille use Grade II braille, which employs the use of contractions, special combinations of letters used in place of an actual word or part of a word. For example, contractions substitute for prepositions such as "with" and "through." Word endings such as "ing" or "ed" use a single symbol, rather than writing each letter of the word ending. Most individuals use a slate and stylus or a braillewriter to produce braille text. The individual using a slate and stylus punches each letter into a cell which accommodates up to six dots (all braille letters, numbers, and contractions, are combinations of one to six dots). Braille is written from right to left so that when the paper is removed from the slate and turned over, the raised dots may be read from left to right. A braillewriter uses six keys, one key for each dot in the braille cell. The user taps various combinations of keys to produce letters, numbers, and punctuation. Braille text may also be produced using a computer and a braille printer.

Most individuals who are congenitally blind use braille as their major reading and writing technique. Children who are blind should also learn to use a regular keyboard at an early age, so that they can communicate in writing with sighted people. Braille literacy has decreased in recent years. The factors that have contributed to this decrease include a decrease in the number of professionals who teach braille; the development and use of low vision aids; and inclusion of children who are visually impaired or blind in regular classes. Individuals who lose vision as adults are less likely to learn braille, especially those whose vision loss is due to the complications of diabetes. These individuals often lose sensitivity in their fingertips and cannot read braille's raised dots. People of any age who are motivated may learn braille from a rehabilitation teacher or teacher of the visually impaired; through correspondence courses; or in braille classes offered in rehabilitation programs. Some individuals with a diminished sense of touch use "jumbo" braille, written with a slate or braillewriter which produces larger dots. Braille users also use recorded materials and computers with speech or braille output.

Special closed-channel radio receivers are used to provide *radio reading services* to individuals whose visual or physical (inability to hold a book or turn pages) disabilities prevent them from reading. Newspapers, books, and local information are read in a recording studio and broadcast over a network of radio reading services. Audio description or *Descriptive Video Service* (see "ORGANIZATIONS" section below) makes television programs or theatrical performances accessible to audiences who are visually impaired or blind. A description is provided of the action taking place, the setting, the actors' clothing, and other visual details. Viewers receive Descriptive Video Services through a stereo television, a videocassette recorder which has a Separate Audio Program (SAP) channel, or a stereo television adapter. Section 713 of the Telecommunications Act of 1996 (P.L. 104-104) requires that video services be accessible to individuals with visual impairments via descriptive video services. The Federal Communications Commission (FCC) is authorized to establish regulations and time tables for implementing this Act.

Family members and professionals may find the following guidelines helpful when living or working with individuals who are visually impaired or blind:

• Always be certain that the individual knows that you are talking to him or her. Use a normal speaking voice unless you know that the individual has a hearing loss. Always look the individual in the eye when speaking.

• Use sighted guide technique: the person who is visually impaired or blind holds the arm of the sighted person just above the elbow and follows a step behind. (An orientation and mobility instructor or a rehabilitation teacher can provide instruction in this simple technique.)

• Tell the individual when you are entering or leaving the room.

• If in doubt about whether individuals need help, simply ask if they need assistance.

There are many useful aids and devices which help individuals who are visually impaired or blind to live independently. One of the simplest aids is the bold pen, available in stationery stores. Other simple writing aids include bold line paper and signature guides.

Banking is easier with large print checks, deposit slips, and check registers. A check writing guide fits over a standard check and provides window guides for filling out the check. Some banks offer special services to customers who are visually impaired or blind, including audiocassette bank statements. Automated teller machines are accessible through the use of braille labels or step-by-step telephone instructions.

Large print reading materials are very popular with individuals who are visually impaired. In addition to popular fiction works, reference books, cookbooks, bibles, and other religious materials are available in large print. Most public libraries have large print collections. Many publications are recorded on audiocassette or flexible discs (thin plastic records) by organizations such as the National Library Service for the Blind and Physically Handicapped (NLS) and Recording for the Blind and Dyslexic (RFB&D). Although RFB&D requires that individuals be legally blind in order to use its services, anyone who is unable to read due to a disability is eligible for NLS services (see "ORGANIZATIONS" section below). Full-length and abridged books are available on audiocassette from local bookstores and libraries. Newsline for the Blind, available in many states, offers an electronic synthetic speech newspaper service, accessed by touchtone telephone.

Telephones are available with high contrast numbers on large buttons, or conventional telephones may be adapted with large print or braille dials or push-button labels. Self-threading needles and large print, audiocassette, or braille instruction books allow individuals who are visually impaired or blind to continue with sewing and other crafts. Large print or braille letters on self-adhesive tape, raised dots, and special glues may be used to label items, such as canned goods, medications, and appliances. Recreational items such as playing cards, bingo cards, or crossword puzzle books are available in large print versions. Braille versions of board games such as Monopoly are available. Watches, thermometers, and blood glucose monitors with speech output and large print or tactile watches and clocks are additional devices that help individuals manage their everyday activities.

Many people with vision loss use "high tech" electronic devices which have been specially adapted to enhance their remaining vision. These aids include closed circuit television systems (CCTVs) and computers with large print, speech, or braille output. Advances in technology have resulted in the proliferation of a wide variety of such devices. These devices enable people to work, keep track of their financial affairs, maintain correspondence, and carry out other activities that require reading and writing (see Chapter 6, High Tech Aids, in "Living with Low Vision: A Resource Guide for People with Sight Loss," listed below under "PUBLICATIONS AND TAPES" to locate manufacturers of these devices)

Many public libraries and universities have established computer access centers where individuals may see the equipment and have "hands-on" experience before making the investment in their own equipment. Some libraries will lend portable equipment to patrons.

References

Age-Related Eye Disease Study Group
2001 "A Randomized, Placebo-controlled, Clinical Trial of High-Dose Supplementation with Vitamins C and E, Beta Carotene, and Zinc for Age-Related Macular Degeneration and Vision Loss: AREDS Report No. 8" Archives of Ophthalmology 119:10(October):1533-1534

Ainlay, Stephen C.
1989 Day Brought Back My Night: Aging and New Vision Loss London and New York, NY: Routledge

Associated Services for the Blind
1988 Volunteers for the Visually Impaired Elderly: A Coordinated Approach to Service Delivery Associated Services for the Blind, 919 Walnut Street, Philadelphia, PA 19107

Branch, Lawrence G., Amy Horowitz, and Cheryl Carr
1989 "The Implications for Everyday Life of Incident Self-Reported Visual Decline Among People Over Age 65 Living in the Community" The Gerontologist 29(March):359-365

Fowles, D.
1991 A Profile of Older Americans Washington, D.C.: American Association of Retired People

Kirchner, Corrinne
1990 "Trends in the Prevalence Rates and Numbers of Blind and Visually Impaired School-Children" Journal of Visual Impairment and Blindness 84:9:478-9

Louis Harris and Associates, Inc.
1995 The Lighthouse National Survey on Vision Loss: The Experience, Attitudes and Knowledge of Middle-Aged and Older Americans New York, NY: The Lighthouse

McNeil, John M.
2001 Americans With Disabilities 1994-95 Washington, DC: U.S. Bureau of the Census Current Population Reports P70-73

Repka, Michael X.
1989 "Update on Retinopathy of Prematurity" Future Reflections 8:3:29-31

Sommer, Alfred et al.
1991 "Racial Differences in the Cause-Specific Prevalence of Blindness in East Baltimore New England Journal of Medicine 325(November 14):1412-7

Tielsch, James M. et al.
1991 "Blindness and Visual Impairment in an American Population" Archives of Ophthalmology 108(February):286-290

Wright, Irving S.
1987 "Keeping an Eye on the Rest of the Body" Ophthalmology 94(September):1196-1198

Zierler, Sally
1988 "Causes of Retinopathy of Prematurity: An Epidemiologic Perspective" pp. 23-33 in John T. Flynn and Dale L. Phelps (eds.) Retinopathy of Prematurity: Problem and Challenge New York, NY: Alan R. Liss, Inc.

AMD Alliance International
1314 Bedford Avenue, Suite 210
Baltimore, MD 21208
(877) 263-7171   e-mail: executivedirector@amdalliance.org
www.amdalliance.org

Offers brochure, toll-free hotline for consumers, and web site.

American Council of the Blind (ACB)
1155 15th Street, NW, Suite 1004
Washington, DC 20005
(800) 424-8666   (202) 467-5081   FAX (202) 467-5085
e-mail: info@acb.org   www.acb.org

National membership organization that provides information and advocates on behalf of individuals who are visually impaired or blind. Has special interest divisions for government employees, students, etc. Makes referrals to local affiliates. Shares parenting information between blind/sighted parents of blind/sighted children. The "Washington Connection," a recorded message about legislation, is available daily, from 5 p.m. to 9 a.m., E.S.T., and weekends by calling the toll-free number. Publishes the "Braille Forum," a monthly newsletter available in alternate formats and on the web site. Membership, $5.00.

American Foundation for the Blind (AFB)
11 Penn Plaza, Suite 300
New York, NY 10001
(800) 232-5463   (212) 502-7600   FAX (212) 502-7774
e-mail: afbinfo@afb.org   www.afb.org

An information clearinghouse on blindness and visual impairment. "AFB Press Catalog of Publications," free. Also available on the web site. "Services Center" is a searchable database, available on the web site, where users may find service providers by name, state, country, or service category.

American Printing House for the Blind (APH)
1839 Frankfort Avenue
PO Box 6085
Louisville, KY 40206-0085
(800) 223-1839   (502) 895-2405   FAX (502) 899-2274
e-mail: info@aph.org   www.aph.org

A major resource for educational materials in large print and braille. Manufactures equipment and assistive devices. Also sells braille children's books.

Association for the Education and Rehabilitation of the Blind and Visually Impaired (AER)
4600 Duke Street, Suite 430
PO Box 22397
Alexandria, VA 22304
(703) 823-9690   FAX (703) 823-9695   www.aerbvi.org

Membership organization of rehabilitation counselors and teachers, orientation and mobility instructors, special educators, and other professionals with an interest in visual impairment and blindness. Holds regional and international meetings; sets standards for certification. Membership, $115.00, includes, "Journal of Visual Impairment and Blindness," published monthly by the American Foundation for the Blind; newsletter, "AER Report;" "RE:view," a quarterly journal; and a monthly publication, "Job Exchange."

Blinded Veterans Association (BVA)
477 H Street, NW
Washington, DC 20001
(800) 669-7079   (202) 371-8880   e-mail: bva@bva.org
www.bva.org

The BVA's field service and outreach employment programs help veterans find rehabilitation services, training, and employment. Offers scholarships to spouses and dependent children of blinded veterans. Membership, $8.00, includes the "BVA Bulletin" in large print and on computer disc. Newsletter also available on the web site.

Council for Exceptional Children (CEC)
1110 North Glebe Road, Suite 300
Arlington, VA 22201
(888) 232-7733   (703) 620-3660   (703) 264-9446
FAX (703) 264-9494   www.cec.sped.org

A professional membership organization that works toward improving the quality of education for children with disabilities. Holds annual conference. Membership dues vary by geographic location. Special division on visual impairments; membership, $20.00.

Descriptive Video Service (DVS)
WGBH
125 Western Avenue
Boston, MA 02134
Information line, (800) 333-1203   (617) 300-3600   e-mail: dvs@wgbh.org
www.dvs.wgbh.org

This organization provides descriptive video services for television programs broadcast on the Public Broadcasting System. Many local Public Broadcasting System affiliates across the country subscribe to this service; a list of these stations is available from DVS. Publishes quarterly newsletter, "DVS Guide," available in large print and braille; on audio through the DVS toll-free information line, (800) 333-1203; and on the Internet at the address above; free. For a biweekly broadcast schedule on PBS and Turner Classic Movies cable, call (800) 333-1203. Sells DVS videotapes of popular movies; call (888) 818-1999 for free catalogue. Special equipment is not required to hear the narration.

Diabetes-Sight.org
www.diabetes-sight.org

Sponsored by Prevent Blindness America, this web site provides information for individuals and professionals about prevention of vision loss due to diabetes. Includes interactive tools such as a quiz, vision loss simulation, and tour of the eye's anatomy as well as research summaries and preferred practice guidelines for clinicians.

Diabetic Retinopathy Foundation
350 North LaSalle, Suite 800
Chicago, IL 60610
www.retinopathy.org

Supports research and public awareness in an effort to prevent diabetic retinopathy. Web site offers information about diabetic retinopathy and links to other web sites.

Federal Communications Commission (FCC)
445 12th Street, SW
Washington, DC 20554
(888) 225-5322   (888) 835-5322 (TTY)   (202) 418-0190
(202) 418-2555 (TTY)   e-mail: fccinfo@fcc.gov   www.fcc.gov

Responsible for developing regulations for telecommunication issues related to federal laws, including the ADA and the Telecommunications Act of 1996.

Foundation Fighting Blindness
11435 Cronhill Drive
Owings Mills, MD 21117
(888) 394-3937   (800) 683-5551 (TTY)   (410) 568-0150
www.blindness.org

Self-help organization and information clearinghouse for individuals with retinal disorders. Local affiliates throughout the country. Supports research, retina donor program, and national retinitis pigmentosa registry. Publishes bimonthly newsletter, "Fighting Blindness News," (three full issues and three "Update" supplements) available in alternate formats and on the web site. Free

Glaucoma Foundation
116 John Street, Suite 1605
New York, NY 10038
(800) 452-8266   (212) 285-0080
e-mail: info@glaucoma-foundation.org
www.glaucoma-foundation.org

Supports research into the causes and treatment of glaucoma. Operates a direct response hot-line. Offers Youth Under Pressure (YUP) and YUP Parents discussion groups on the web site. Publishes "Doctor, I Have a Question: A Guide for Patients and Their Families" and "Eye to Eye," a quarterly newsletter; both in large print. Single copies, free. Also available on the web site.

Glaucoma Research Foundation
200 Pine Street, Suite 200
San Francisco, CA 94104
(800) 826-6693   (415) 986-3162   FAX (415) 986-3763
e-mail: info@glaucoma.org   www.glaucoma.org

Offers public education programs and telephone support network. Quarterly newsletter, "Gleams," free; available in standard print and cassette. Also available on the web site. Operates an eye donor network, which enables researchers to study the eyes donated by individuals with glaucoma and their families.

Helen Keller National Center for Deaf-Blind Youths and Adults   (HKNC)
111 Middle Neck Road
Sands Point, NY 11050
(516) 944-8900   (516) 944-8637 (TTY)   FAX (516) 944-7302
www.helenkeller.org/national

Offers evaluation, vocational rehabilitation training, counseling, job preparation, placement, and related services through ten regional offices. Sponsors a national network of parents and state and local parent organizations. Newsletter, "NAT-CENT NEWS," free to individuals who are deaf-blind and libraries; $10.00 for all others.

Institute for Families of Blind Children
PO Box 54700, Mail Stop #111
Los Angeles, CA 90054
(323) 669-4649   FAX (323) 665-7869
www.instituteforfamilies.org

Provides support to families of children who are blind or visually impaired due to retinoblas-toma, a cancer of the eye. Publishes two quarterly newsletters, "Retinoblastoma Support

News," for parents of children with retinoblastoma, and "Parent to Parent," for parents of children who are blind or visually impaired due to any condition; both free.

Lighthouse International
111 East 59th Street
New York, NY 10022
(800) 334-5497 (V/TTY)   (212) 821-9200   (212) 821-9713 (TTY)
FAX (212) 821-9705   e-mail: info@lighthouse.org
www.lighthouse.org

This organization provides information on vision problems faced by older people and how these problems can be treated. It also promotes understanding of vision loss in children and adolescents, child development, special education, and parent-teacher-professional cooperation. Sells community education materials. Also available on the web site.

Macular Degeneration Foundation (MDF)
PO Box 9752
San Jose, CA 95157
(888) 633-3937   (408) 996-7989
e-mail: info@eyesight.org   www.eyesight.org

Web site provides information and support for individuals with macular degeneration. Produces e-mail newsletter, "The Magnifier."

Macular Degeneration International
6700 North Oracle Road, #505
Tucson, AZ 85704
(800) 393-7634   (520) 797-2525   FAX (520) 797-8018
e-mail: info@maculardegeneration.org
www.maculardegeneration.org

Support network for individuals with early or late onset macular degeneration. Membership, $25.00, includes semi-annual large print newsletter, a large print resource guide, and an audiocassette with "Information and Inspiration."

MEDLINEplus: Vision Disorders and Blindness
www.nlm.nih.gov/medlineplus/visiondisordersblindness.html

This web site provides links to sites for general information about vision disorders and blindness, symptoms and diagnosis, treatment, specific aspects of the condition, clinical trials, statistics, organizations, directories, and research. Includes eye disease simulations and information for children and seniors. Some information is available in Spanish. Provides links to MEDLINE research articles and related MEDLINEplus pages.

National Association for Parents of Children with Visual Impairments (NAPVI)
PO Box 317
Watertown, MA 02471
(800) 562-6265   FAX (617) 972-7444   www.napvi.org

Promotes development of parent groups and provides information through conferences and publications. Local chapters in some states. Free information packet. Membership, parents, $25.00; organizations, $50.00; includes quarterly newsletter, "Awareness."

National Association for Visually Handicapped (NAVH)
22 West 21st Street
New York, NY 10010
(212) 889-3141   FAX (212) 727-2931
e-mail: staff@navh.org   www.navh.org

Sells large print books and low vision aids. Produces three large print newsletters, "Seeing Clearly," "In Focus" (for youths), and "navh UPDATE;" free. Membership, $50.00, includes discounts on purchases and use of library books by mail; limited membership, $25.00 (no library privileges). Free catalogue ($2.50 donation requested).

National Eye Institute (NEI)
Building 31, Room 6A32
2020 Vision Place
Bethesda, MD 20892
(301) 496-5248   www.nei.nih.gov

This federal agency conducts basic and clinical research on the causes and cures of eye diseases. Distributes brochures on eye diseases and conditions, such as age-related macular degeneration, cataract, diabetic retinopathy, and glaucoma, free. NEI also recruits patients as subjects for a variety of clinical studies. Referrals from ophthalmologists are necessary for enrollment in an appropriate study.

National Federation of the Blind (NFB)
1800 Johnson Street
Baltimore, MD 21230
(410) 659-9314   FAX (410) 685-5653
e-mail: nfb@nfb.org   www.nfb.org

National membership organization with chapters in many states. Provides information about available services, laws, and evaluation of new technology. Special interest groups for students, parents of blind children, etc. Holds state and national annual conventions. Sponsors "Newsline," an electronic, synthetic speech newspaper service, and "America's Jobline," an employment database, accessed by touchtone telephone. Regular membership starts at $10.00.

Publishes the "Braille Monitor," a monthly magazine available in standard print and alternate formats. $25.00 a year contribution requested. Also available on the web site.

<u>National Library Service for the Blind and Physically Handicapped</u> (NLS)
1291 Taylor Street, NW
Washington, DC 20542
(800) 424-8567 or 8572 (Reference Section)
(800) 424-9100 (to receive application)
(202) 707-5100   (202) 707-0744 (TTY)   FAX (202) 707-0712
e-mail: nls@loc.gov   www.loc.gov/nls

National library service that serves individuals in the U.S. and U.S. residents living abroad. Regional libraries in many states. Individuals must be unable to read standard print due to visual impairment or physical disability. "Facts: Books for Blind and Physically Handicapped Individuals" describes NLS programs and eligibility requirements. Order form lists general information brochures, magazines and newsletters, directories, reference circulars, and subject and reference bibliographies. "Talking Book Topics," published bimonthly, in alternate formats and on the web site, lists titles recently added to the national collection which are available through the network of regional libraries. All services and publications from NLS are free.

<u>Prevent Blindness America</u>
500 East Remington Road
Schaumburg, IL 60173
(800) 331-2020   (847) 843-2020   FAX (847) 843-8458
e-mail: info@preventblindness.org www.prevent-blindness.org

This organization sponsors vision screenings. Local and state affiliates. Publications related to diseases and eye injuries, including some in large print and Spanish. Free catalogue. Newsletter, "Prevent Blindness News," $12.00; free sample available on the web site.

<u>Recording for the Blind and Dyslexic</u> (RFB&D)
20 Roszel Road
Princeton, NJ 08540
(800) 221-4792   (609) 452-0606
e-mail: custserv@rfbd.org   www.rfbd.org

Records educational materials on four-track audiocassette for people who are legally blind or have physical or perceptual disabilities. RFB&D is a major source of recorded textbooks for college students. Requires certification of disability by a medical or educational professional. Registration fee, $75.00, plus $25.00 annual membership fee. Sells four-track audiocassette players. Catalogue of books is available on the web site. Newsletter, "RFB&D News" published twice a year. Free

Resources for Rehabilitation
22 Bonad Road
Winchester, MA 01890
(781) 368-9094   FAX (781) 368-9096
e-mail: orders@rfr.org   www.rfr.org

Provides training to professionals and the public about resources that help people with disabilities and chronic conditions, including vision loss. Publishes the "Living with Low Vision Series," described in "PUBLICATIONS AND TAPES" section below. Custom designed training programs available. Call for details.

VISION Community Services (VCS)
23A Elm Street
Watertown, MA 02472
(617) 926-4232   In MA, (800) 852-3029   FAX (617) 926-1412
www.mablind.org

Information center for individuals with sight loss. Publishes materials in large print and on audiocassette, including the "VCS Resource List" and "VCS Resource Update," a bimonthly resource newsletter; free.

Blind Children's Center
4120 Marathon Street
Los Angeles, CA 90029
(800) 222-3566   In CA, (800) 222-3567   (323) 664-2153
FAX (323) 665-3828   e-mail: info@blindcntr.org
www.blindcntr.org/bcc

Provides resources and support to parents. Publications include "First Steps: A Handbook for Teaching Young Children Who Are Visually Impaired," $35.00; "Fathers: A Common Ground," "Talk to Me I," "Talk to Me II," "Heart-to-Heart - Parents of Blind and Partially Sighted Children Talk About Their Feelings," "Move with Me," and "Learning to Play: Common Concerns for the Visually Impaired Preschool Child," "Dancing Cheek to Cheek," and "Reaching, Crawling, Walking: Let's Get Moving," $10.00 each.

Can Do Video Series
Visually Impaired Preschool Services
1229 Garvin Place
Louisville, KY 40203
(502) 636-3207   FAX (502) 636-0024   e-mail: info@vips.org
www.vips.org

A series of 11 videotapes that depict six families with children who are visually impaired, ranging from 14 months to six years. Write for description of tapes. Each tape may be purchased separately (prices vary) or the entire set may be purchased for $475.00.

Children's Braille Book Club
National Braille Press
88 St. Stephen Street
Boston, MA 02115
(800) 548-7323   (617) 266-6160   FAX (617) 437-0456
e-mail: orders@nbp.org   www.nbp.org

Braille pages are inserted into standard print children's books. Free membership provides monthly notices with no obligation to buy; $100.00 annual subscription automatically provides one print-braille book per month.

Children with Visual Impairments: A Parents' Guide
by M. Cay Holbrook (ed.)
Woodbine House
6510 Bells Mill Road
Bethesda, MD 20817
(800) 843-7323   (301) 897-3570   FAX (301) 897-5838
e-mail: info@woodbinehouse.com   www.woodbinehouse.com

Discusses the diagnosis of visual impairment, treatment options, special education and legal rights, and coping strategies for children and their families. $16.95 plus $4.50 shipping and handling

Coping with Low Vision
by Marshall E. Flax, Don J. Golembiewski, and Betty L. McCauley
Thomson Learning
PO Box 6904
Florence, KY 41022
(800) 347-7707   FAX (859) 647-5023
www.thomsonlearning.com

This book discusses low vision, vision rehabilitation services, low vision aids, and community resources. Includes resource list of organizations in the U.S. and Canada. Large print, $22.95. Also available on 4-track audiocassette from National Library Service for the Blind and Physically Handicapped regional libraries, RC 38113.

Diagnosis: Retinoblastoma
Institute for Families of Blind Children
PO Box 54700, Mail Stop #111
Los Angeles, CA 90054-0700
(323) 669-4649   FAX (323) 665-7869
www.instituteforfamilies.org

In this videotape, parents discuss their experiences with a child who has retinoblastoma. $10.00 donation required to cover postage and handling.

Dialogue
Blindskills, Inc.
Box 5181
Salem, OR 97304
(800) 860-4224   (503) 581-4224   FAX (503) 581-1078
e-mail: blindskl@teleport.com   www.blindskills.com

Quarterly magazine with information on technology and other resources, special information on child rearing for parents who are visually impaired or blind, and an announcements section. Published in alternate formats. Legally blind readers, $28.00; others, $40.00.

Do You Remember the Color Blue?
by Sally Hobart Alexander
Penguin Putnam, Inc.
(800) 788-6262   www.penguinputnam.com

The author, who lost her sight at age 26, answers questions that children have asked her about being blind. $16.99 Also available on 4-track audiocassette on loan through regional branches of the National Library Service for the Blind and Physically Handicapped. RC 50319

The Encounter
Carmichael Audio-Video Duplication
1025 South Saddleback Creek Road
Omaha, NE 68106
(402) 556-5677   FAX (402) 556-5416

A videotape about interactions between people with normal vision and those who are blind, produced by the Nebraska Department of Public Institutions. The tape uses humor to show how people who are blind are capable of independent activities; it also addresses education and employment opportunities. Available in English and Spanish. 11 minutes. $8.50

A Guide to Independence for the Visually Impaired and Their Families
by Vivian Younger and Jill Sardegna
Demos Medical Publishing
386 Park Avenue South, Suite 201
New York, NY 10016
(800) 532-8663   (212) 683-0072   FAX (212) 683-0118
e-mail: info@demospub.com   www.demosmedpub.com

Written by a vocational counselor who is visually impaired and a writer on disability issues, this book provides practical information for individuals and their families about living independently with vision loss. $29.95 plus $4.00 shipping and handling. Orders made on the Demos web site receive a 15% discount. Available on 4-track audiocassette from National Library Service for the Blind and Physically Handicapped regional libraries, RC 42674.

Helping the Visually Impaired Child with Developmental Problems
by Sally M. Rogow
Teachers College Press, Williston, VT

This book examines the effects of visual impairment in combination with other disabilities on childhood development in the areas of sensorimotor, communication, language, and independence skills. Out of print

If Blindness Strikes: Don't Strike Out
by Margaret Smith
Charles C. Thomas Publisher
2600 South First Street
Springfield, IL 62704
(800) 258-8980   (217) 789-8980   FAX (217) 789-9130
e-mail: books@ccthomas.com   www.ccthomas.com

Written by a rehabilitation counselor who is visually impaired, this book describes many adaptations and strategies for living with vision loss. Hardcover, $54.95; softcover, $38.95; plus $5.95 shipping and handling. Also available on 4-track audiocassette on loan from the National Library Service for the Blind and Physically Handicapped regional libraries, RC 21060. To purchase two-track ($18.00) or 4-track ($6.00) audiocassettes, contact Readings for the Blind, 29451 Greenfield Road, Suite 216, Southfield, MI 48076; (248) 557-7776.

Just Enough to Know Better
by Eileen Curran
National Braille Press
88 St. Stephen Street
Boston, MA 02115
(800) 548-7323   (617) 266-6160   FAX (617) 437-0456
e-mail: orders@nbp.org   www.nbp.org

This self-paced workbook teaches beginning braille skills to sighted parents. $15.00

Living Well with Macular Degeneration
by Bruce P. Rosenthal and Kate Kelley
Penguin Putnam, Inc.
(800) 788-6262   www.penguinputnam.com

This book discusses the symptoms and causes of macular degeneration, describes vision rehabilitation, and provides information about simple and complex assistive devices. Includes chapter on driving and other options. $12.95

Living with Low Vision Series
Resources for Rehabilitation
22 Bonad Road
Winchester, MA 01890
(781) 368-9094   FAX (781) 368-9096
e-mail: orders@rfr.org   www.rfr.org

"Large Print Publications Designed for Distribution by Professionals to People with Vision Loss." Titles include "Living with Low Vision," "How to Keep Reading with Vision Loss," "Aids for Everyday Living with Vision Loss," and disease specific titles. (See order form on last page of this book.)

"Living with Low Vision: A Resource Guide for People with Sight Loss"
A large print (18 point bold type) comprehensive directory that helps people with sight loss locate the services that they need to remain independent. Chapters describe products that enable people to keep reading, working, and carrying out their daily activities. Information about computer bulletin boards and resources on the Internet. $46.95 plus $5.00 shipping and handling

"Meeting the Needs of People with Vision Loss: A Multidisciplinary Perspective"
Susan L. Greenblatt (ed.)
Written by physicians, special educators, counselors, and rehabilitation professionals, this book includes chapters on What People with Vision Loss Need to Know; The Special Needs of Individuals with Diabetes and Vision Loss; Older Adults with Vision and Hearing Losses; Providing Services to Visually Impaired Elders in Long Term Care Facilities; Children with Vision Loss; and The Role of the Family. Available in standard print and on audiocassette. $24.95 plus $5.00 shipping and handling

"Providing Services for People with Vision Loss: A Multidisciplinary Perspective"
Susan L. Greenblatt (ed.)
Written by ophthalmologists and rehabilitation professionals, this book discusses the need to provide coordinated care for people with vision loss. Chapters include Vision Loss: A Patient's Perspective; Operating a Low Vision Aids Service; Vision Loss: An Ophthalmologist's Perspective; The Need for Coordinated Care; Making Referrals for Rehabilitation Services; Mental Health Services: The Missing Link; Self-Help Groups for People with Sight Loss; and Aids and Techniques that Help People with Vision Loss plus a Glossary. Available in standard print and on audiocassette. $19.95 plus $5.00 shipping and handling

Making Life More Livable: Simple Adaptations for Living at Home After Vision Loss
American Foundation for the Blind
AFB Press
PO Box 1020
Sewickley, PA 15143
(800) 232-3044   FAX (412) 741-0609   www.afb.org

Offers simple adaptations to make the home safer for people with visual impairment. Large print. Also available on computer disk. $24.95 plus $10.90 shipping and handling

Meeting the Needs of Employees with Disabilities
Resources for Rehabilitation
22 Bonad Road
Winchester, MA 01890
(781) 368-9094   FAX (781) 368-9096
e-mail: orders@rfr.org   www.rfr.org

This resource guide provides information to help people with disabilities retain or obtain employment. Information on government programs, environmental adaptations, and the transition from school to work is included. Chapters on mobility, vision, and hearing and speech impairments include information on organizations, products, and services that enable employers to accommodate the needs of employees with disabilities. $44.95 plus $5.00 shipping and handling. (See order form on last page of this book.)

My Fake Eye, The Story of My Prosthesis
Institute for Families of Blind Children
PO Box 54700, Mail Stop #111
Los Angeles, CA 90054-0700
(323) 669-4649   FAX (323) 665-7869
www.instituteforfamilies.org

This booklet offers information and support to children, parents, and siblings of children who have had or will have an eye enucleated. $5.00

The New What Do You Do When You See a Blind Person?
AFB Press
PO Box 1020
Sewickley, PA 15143
(800) 232-3044   FAX (412) 741-0609   www.afb.org

This videotape offers tips on interacting with individuals who are blind or visually impaired. 16 minutes. Also available with open captioning or audio description. $39.95 plus $10.90 shipping and handling

On My Own: The Journey Continues
by Sally Hobart Alexander
Von Holtzbrinck Publishing Services, Ortonsville, VA 22942

This book, a sequel to her book listed below, describes the author's additional sight loss and hearing impairment, adjustment, career change, and return to work. Out of print. Also available on 4-track audiocassette on loan through regional branches of the National Library Service for the Blind and Physically Handicapped. RC 45189

Out of the Corner of My Eye: Living with Vision Loss in Later Life
by Nicolette Pernod Ringgold
AFB Press
PO Box 1020
Sewickley, PA 15143
(800) 232-3044   FAX (412) 741-0609   www.afb.org

Written by a woman who became legally blind due to macular degeneration in her late 70s, this book offers practical advice and encouragement for elders with vision loss. Large print and audiocassette. $24.95 plus $10.90 shipping and handling

Pathways to Independence: Orientation and Mobility Skills for Your Infant and Toddler
Lighthouse International
111 East 59th Street
New York, NY 10022
(800) 334-5497 (V/TTY)   (212) 821-9200   (212) 821-9713 (TTY)
FAX (212) 821-9705   www.lighthouse.org

This booklet discusses basic orientation and mobility skills and suggests games and activities for the child with vision loss. Available in English and Spanish. $2.50 plus $2.00 shipping and handling

Planet of the Blind: A Memoir
by Stephen Kuusisto
Random House, Order Department
400 Hahn Road, PO Box 100
Westminster, MD 21157
(800) 733-3000   (410) 848-1900   FAX (410) 386-7013
www.randomhouse.com

Written by a man who was legally blind at birth and encouraged to deny his blindness, this book recounts his experiences at various stages of life, interactions with peers and teachers, and his eventual acceptance of his blindness. $11.95 plus $2.95 shipping and handling

Questions Kids Ask About Blindness
National Federation of the Blind (NFB)
1800 Johnson Street
Baltimore, MD 21230
(410) 659-9314   FAX (410) 685-5653   www.nfb.org

This booklet answers general questions about blindness, braille, canes, guide dogs, and the abilities of individuals who are visually impaired or blind. Describes a typical day in the life of a blind sixth grader attending public school. $5.00 plus $5.00 shipping and handling. Also available on the web site.

Resources for Elders with Disabilities
Resources for Rehabilitation
22 Bonad Road
Winchester, MA 01890
(781) 368-9094   FAX (781) 368-9096
e-mail: orders@rfr.org   www.rfr.org

This large print resource directory meets the needs of elders, family members, and other caregivers. The book provides information about rehabilitation, laws that affect elders with disabilities, and self-help groups. Describes services and products that help elders with disabilities to function independently. Includes chapters on vision loss, hearing loss, stroke, arthritis, Parkinson's disease, diabetes, and osteoporosis. $49.95 plus $5.00 shipping and handling. (See order form on last page of this book.)

Seedlings
PO Box 51924
Livonia, MI 48151-5924
(800) 777-8552   (734) 427-8552
e-mail: seedlink@aol.com   www.seedlings.org

Publishes children's storybooks in braille. Free catalogue. Also available on the web site.

Social Security: If You Are Blind or Have Low Vision - How We Can Help
Social Security Administration
(800) 772-1213   (800) 325-0778 (TTY)   www.ssa.gov

This publication provides information about obtaining Social Security benefits. The Social Security Administration distributes many other titles, including those that are available in standard print, alternate formats, and on the web site. Also available at local Social Security offices. (See Chapter 2, "PUBLICATIONS AND TAPES" section, for other titles available from the Social Security Administration.)

Taking Hold: My Journey into Blindness
by Sally Hobart Alexander
Simon & Schuster
100 Front Street
Riverside, NJ 08075
(888) 866-6631   FAX (800) 943-9831   www.simonsays.com

This book chronicles the author's initial sight loss, adjustment, rehabilitation training, and return to work. $14.95 plus $7.50 shipping and handling. Also available on 4-track audiocassette on loan through regional branches of the National Library Service for the Blind and Physically Handicapped. RC 40247

<u>TJ's Story</u>
by Arlene Schulman
Lerner Publishing Group
1251 Washington Avenue North
Minneapolis, MN 55401
(800) 328-4929   (612) 332-3344   FAX (612) 204-9208
www.lernerbooks.com

In this book, a nine year old boy who is blind describes his everyday activities, reading braille, attending public school, using assistive technology, and playing with his friends. $21.27 plus $5.00 shipping and handling

<u>Understanding and Living with Glaucoma: A Reference Guide for Patients and Their Families</u>
Glaucoma Research Foundation
200 Pine Street, Suite 200
San Francisco, CA 94104
(800) 826-6693   (415) 986-3162   FAX (415) 986-3763
e-mail: info@glaucoma.org   www.glaucoma.org

Written by an individual with glaucoma, this booklet describes living with a chronic health condition. Single copy, free.

RESOURCES FOR ASSISTIVE DEVICES

Listed below are catalogues that specialize in devices for people who are visually impaired or blind. Unless otherwise noted, these vendors sell a variety of products, and their catalogues are free.

<u>Ann Morris Enterprises</u>
551 Hosner Mountain Road
Stormville, NY 12582
(800) 454-3175   (845) 227-9659   FAX (845) 226-2793
e-mail: annmor@webspan.net   www.annmorris.com

Catalogue available in alternate formats; free. Braille catalogue, $10.00; $6.00 with an order.

<u>Exceptional Teaching Aids</u>
20102 Woodbine Avenue
Castro Valley, CA 94546
(800) 549-6999   FAX (510) 582-5911
www.exceptionalteaching.com

Braille and low vision aids; adapted computer software; art, science, and mathematical aids.

<u>Florida New Concepts Marketing</u>
PO Box 261
Port Richey, FL 34673
(800) 456-7097   (727) 842-3231 (V/FAX)
e-mail: compulenz@gte.net   gulfside.com/compulenz

Sells Compulenz, which fits on most computer monitors, and enlarges character size while eliminating distortion and light reflection. Prices vary with monitor size.

<u>Independent Living Aids, Inc.</u> (ILA)
200 Robbins Lane
Jericho, NY 11753
(800) 537-2118   FAX (516) 752-3135
e-mail: can-do@independentliving.com
www.independentliving.com

Catalogue is available in standard print and audiocassette.

Lighthouse Consumer Products
36-20 Northern Boulevard
Long Island City, NY 11101
(800) 829-0500   FAX (718) 786-0437
www.lighthouse.org

Large print catalogue.

LS & S Group Inc. Catalogue
PO Box 673
Northbrook, IL 60065
(800) 468-4789   (800) 317-8533 (TTY)   FAX (847) 498-1482
e-mail: vision@lssgrp.com   www.lssgroup.com

Catalogue in standard print, free, and audiocassette, $3.00, applied to purchase.

Mons International
6595 Roswell NE, #224
Atlanta, GA 30328
(800) 541-7903   e-mail: mons@negia.net   www.magnifiers.com

Large print catalogue.

National Federation of the Blind
Materials Center
1800 Johnson Street
Baltimore, MD 21230
(410) 659-9314   FAX (410) 685-5653   www.nfb.org

Catalogue available in standard print and alternate formats.

Visual Aids and Informational Material
National Association for the Visually Handicapped (NAVH)
22 West 21st Street
New York, NY 10010
(212) 889-3141   FAX (212) 727-2931
e-mail: staff@navh.org   www.navh.org

Large print catalogue; members, free; nonmembers, $2.50 donation requested.

INDEX TO ORGANIZATIONS

This index contains only those organizations listed under sections titled "ORGANIZA-TIONS." These organizations may also be listed as vendors of publications, tapes, and other products.

ABLEDATA 102
Access-Able Travel Service 98
Access Outdoors 102
Achilles Track Club 102
ADED - Association for Driver Rehabilitation Specialists 98
Administration on Developmental Disabilities 71
Agency for Healthcare Research and Quality 19
Air Travel Consumer Report 98
Alexander Graham Bell Association for the Deaf 126
AMD Alliance International 295
American Academy of Orthopaedic Surgeons 227
American Association of Diabetes Educators 176
American Association of Kidney Patients 176
American Association of Spinal Cord Injury Nurses 271
American Autoimmune Related Diseases Association 245
American Back Society 227
American Canoe Association 102
American Chronic Pain Association 227
American Cleft Palate-Craniofacial Association 151
American Council of the Blind 295
American Council on Rural Special Education 71
American Diabetes Association 176
American Dietetic Association 177
American Disabled for Attendant Programs Today 19
American Foundation for the Blind 295
American Indian Rehabilitation Research and Training Center 19
American Kidney Fund 177
American Pain Foundation 227
American Pain Society 228
American Paraplegia Society 271
American Printing House for the Blind 295
American Self-Help Clearinghouse 20
American Society for Deaf Children 126
American Speech-Language-Hearing Association 126, 151
American Spinal Injury Association 271
American Tinnitus Association 126
Amputee Coalition of America 177
Amtrak 98

Antiepileptic Drug Pregnancy Registry 205

Architectural and Transportation Barriers Compliance Board 50, 91, 98

Arthritis Foundation 228

Association for the Education and Rehabilitation of the Blind 296

Association of Late-Deafened Adults 127

Association on Higher Education and Disability 71

Auto Channel 99

Automobility Program 99

Avonex Alliance 245

Avonex Start Assistance Program 245

Barrier Free Education, Center for Assistive Technology and Environmental
        Access 72

Beach Center on Disability 20, 72

Betaseron Foundation 245

Blinded Veterans Association 296

Brain Injury Association 205

Brain Resources and Information Network 245, 271

Breckenridge Outdoor Education Center 102

Canine Companions for Independence 127

Captioned Media Program 134

CDC Division of Diabetes Translation 177

Center for Hereditary Hearing Loss, Boys Town National Research Hospital 127

Center for Universal Design 91

Challenged Athletes Foundation 102

Christopher Reeve Paralysis Foundation 272

Clearinghouse on Disability Information 50, 72

Client Assistance Program, U.S. Department of Education, Rehabilitation
        Services Administration 50

ClinicalTrials.gov 20, 228

Cochlear Implant Association, Inc. 127

Combined Health Information Database 20

Commission on Accreditation of Rehabilitation Facilities 21, 228, 272

Commission on Mental and Physical Disability Law 51

Commission on Rehabilitation Counselor Certification 21·

Consortium of Multiple Sclerosis Centers/North American Research Committee
        on Multiple Sclerosis 246

Council for Exceptional Children 73, 128, 151, 296

Craig Hospital Aging with Spinal Cord Injury 272

Descriptive Video Service 296

Diabetes Action Network, National Federation of the Blind 178

Diabetes Exercise and Sports Association 178

Diabetes-Sight.org 178, 297

Diabetic Retinopathy Foundation 297

Disability.gov 21, 51

DisabilityResources.org 21
Disability Rights Education and Defense Fund 51
Disability Rights Section, U.S. Department of Justice, Civil Rights Division 51
Disability Statistics Center 21
Disabled Sports, U.S.A. 103
Disabled Sports U.S.A. Volleyball 103
Dogs for the Deaf 128
EDLAW Center 73
Educational Equity Concepts 73
Epilepsy Foundation 205
Epilepsy-L 205
Equal Employment Opportunity Commission 52
ERIC Clearinghouse on Disabilities and Gifted Education 73
Fannie Mae 52
Federal Communications Commission 52, 128, 297
Fishing Has No Boundaries 103
Ford Mobility Motoring Program 99
Foundation Fighting Blindness 297
Foundation for Spinal Cord Injury Prevention, Care and Cure 272
Functional Electrical Stimulation Information Center 246, 273
Gallaudet Research Institute 128
Gallaudet University 129
GE Answer Center 91
General Motors Mobility Assistance Center 99
Genetic Alliance 22
Glaucoma Foundation 298
Glaucoma Research Foundation 298
Greyhound Lines, Inc. 100
Handicapped Scuba Association 103
Healthfinder 22
Healthpages 22
HealthWeb 22
Hear Now 129
Helen Keller National Center for Deaf-Blind Youths and Adults 129, 298
Independent Living Research Utilization 22
Institute for Families of Blind Children 298
Insure Kids Now 74
Internal Revenue Service 52
International Association of Laryngectomees 151
International Association of Rehabilitation Professionals 23
Juvenile Diabetes Research Foundation International 178
Ketogenic Diet 205
Kids on the Block 74
Laurent Clerc National Deaf Education Network and Clearinghouse 129

Lekotek Toy Resource Helpline 74
Lexington School and Center for the Deaf, Inc. 130
Librarians' Index to the Internet 23
Lighthouse International 299
Macular Degeneration Foundation 299
Macular Degeneration International 299
Medicinenet 23
MEDLINEplus: Back Pain 229
MEDLINEplus: Diabetes 179
MEDLINEplus: Epilepsy 206
MEDLINEplus: Hearing Disorders and Deafness 130
MEDLINEplus: Multiple Sclerosis 246
MEDLINEplus: Speech and Communication Disorders 152
MEDLINEplus: Spinal Cord Injuries 273
MEDLINEplus: Vision Disorders and Blindness 299
Miami Project to Cure Paralysis 273
Mobility International USA 100
MossRehab ResourceNet 100
MSActiveSource.com 246
MS Pathways 247
MSWatch 247
National Ability Center 104
National Aphasia Association 152
National Association for Continence 247, 273
National Association for Parents of Children with Visual Impairment 300
National Association for the Education of Young Children 74
National Association for Visually Handicapped 300
National Association of Epilepsy Centers 206
National Association of Home Builders 92
National Association of the Deaf 130
National Association on Alcohol, Drugs, and Disability, Inc. 23, 274
National Center for Medical Rehabilitation Research 23
National Center for Stuttering 152
National Center for the Dissemination of Disability Research 24
National Chronic Pain Outreach Association 229
National Council of State Housing Agencies 53, 92
National Council on Disability 24, 53
National Craniofacial Association 152
National Diabetes Education Program 179
National Diabetes Information Clearinghouse 179
National Easter Seal Society 104, 153, 247, 274
National Epilepsy Library 206
National Eye Institute 300
National Family Caregivers Association 24

National Federation of the Blind 300
National Health Information Center 25
National Home of Your Own Alliance 53
National Information Center for Children and Youth with Disabilities 74
National Institute of Arthritis and Musculoskeletal and Skin Diseases 229
National Institute of Arthritis and Musculoskeletal and Skin Diseases Information
    Clearinghouse 229
National Institute of Diabetes and Digestive and Kidney Diseases 179
National Institute of Neurological Disorders and Stroke 153, 206, 247
National Institute on Deafness and Other Communication Disorders 130, 153
National Institute on Deafness and Other Communication Disorders Information
    Clearinghouse 131, 153
National Institute on Disability and Rehabilitation Research
U.S. Department of Education 25, 274
National Institutes of Health Information 25
National Kidney and Urologic Diseases Information Clearinghouse 180
National Kidney Foundation 180
National Library of Medicine 25
National Library Service for the Blind and Physically Handicap 75, 301
National Mobility Equipment Dealers Association 100
National Multiple Sclerosis Society 248
National Organization for Rare Disorders 26
National Organization on Disability 26
National Parent Network on Disabilities 75
National Park Service 100
National Rehabilitation Association 26
National Rehabilitation Information Center 27
National Resource Center for Parents with Disabilities 27
National Self-Help Clearinghouse 27
National Spinal Cord Injury Association 274
National Sports Center for the Disabled 104
National Stroke Association 154, 207
National Stuttering Association 154
National Technical Institute for the Deaf 131
National Wheelchair Basketball Association 104
Native American Research and Training Center 27
Neuropathy Association 180
Nolo Law for All 53
North American Riding for the Handicapped Association 104
Office for Civil Rights, U.S. Department of Health and Human Services 54
Office of Civil Rights, Federal Transit Administration 54
Office of Civil Rights, U.S. Department of Education 54
Office of Fair Housing and Equal Opportunity, U.S. Department of Housing and
    Urban Development 54

Office of Federal Contract Compliance Programs, U.S. Department of Labor, Employment Standards Administration 55

Office of General Counsel, U.S. Department of Transportation 55

PACER Center 75

Paralyzed Veterans of America 275

Parent Education and Assistance for Kids 75

Prevent Blindness America 301

Project ACTION Accessible Traveler's Database 101

Recording for the Blind and Dyslexic 301

Registry of Interpreters of the Deaf 131

Rehabilitation Engineering and Assistive Technology Society of North America 28

Rehabilitation Research and Training Center for Persons Who Are Deaf or Hard of Hearing 131

Rehabilitation Research & Training Center for Persons Who Are Hard of Hearing or Late Deafened 132

Rehabilitation Research and Training Center on Secondary Complications of Spinal Cord Injury 275

Research and Training Center on Independent Living 28

Research and Training Center on Rural Rehabilitation 28

Resources for Rehabilitation 29, 302

Rural Housing Service National Office, U.S. Department of Agriculture 55, 92

Sailors with Special Needs 105

Self Help for Hard of Hearing People 132

Shared Solutions 248

Sibling Support Project, Children's Hospital and Medical Center 29, 76

Simon Foundation for Continence 248, 275

Social Security Administration 55

Society for Accessible Travel and Hospitality 101

Society for Disability Studies 29

Spine-health.com 230

Stroke Connection 154

Stuttering Foundation of America 154

Substance Abuse Resources & Disability Issues 29, 276

TASH: The Association for Persons with Severe Handicaps 30, 76

TDI 132

The Technical Assistance Alliance for Parent Centers, PACER Center 76

Thomas 56

Toys for Special Children & Enabling Devices 77

United Cerebral Palsy Association 155

United States Golf Association 105

United Way of America 30

Universal Wheelchair Football Association 105

University of California San Francisco Center on Deafness 132

Untangling the Web 30
U.S. Department of Housing and Urban Development 56, 92
U.S. Department of Veterans Affairs 30, 133
U.S. Society for Augmentative and Alternative Communication 155
VSA Arts 105
Vestibular Disorders Association 133
VISION Community Services 302
Vocational Rehabilitation and Employment, Veterans Benefits
        Administration 30, 276
Well Spouse Foundation 31
WheelchairNet 276
Wheelers Accessible Van Rental 101
Wilderness Inquiry 106
World Institute on Disability 31
Wright's Law 77

PUBLICATIONS FROM RESOURCES FOR REHABILITATION

Resources for People with Disabilities and Chronic Conditions

This comprehensive resource guide has chapters on spinal cord injury, low back pain, diabetes, multiple sclerosis, hearing and speech impairments, visual impairment and blindness, and epilepsy. Each chapter includes information about the disease or condition; psychological aspects of the condition; professional service providers; environmental adaptations; assistive devices; and descriptions of organizations, publications, and products. Chapters on rehabilitation services, independent living, self-help, laws that affect people with disabilities (including the ADA), and making everyday living easier. Special information for children is also included. Includes Internet resources.

Fifth edition, 2002   ISBN 0-929718-30-5 $56.95

"...wide coverage and excellent organization of this encyclopedic guide...recommended..." Choice
"...an excellent guide" Reference Books Bulletin/Booklist
"Sensitive to the tremendous variety of needs and circumstances of living with a disability" American Libraries
"...improves the chances of library patrons finding needed services..." American Reference Books Annual

Making Wise Medical Decisions
How to Get the Information You Need

This book includes a wealth of information about where to go and what to read in order to make informed, rational, medical decisions. It describes a plan for obtaining relevant health information and evaluating the quality of medical tests and procedures, health care providers, and health facilities. Each chapter includes extensive resources to help the reader get started. Chapters include Getting the Information You Need to Make Wise Medical Decisions; Locating Appropriate Health Care; Asking the Right Questions About Medical Tests and Procedures; Protecting Yourself in the Hospital; Medical Benefits and Legal Rights; Drugs; Protecting the Health of Children Who Are Ill; Special Issues Facing Elders; People with Chronic Illnesses and Disabilities and the Health Care System; Making Decisions About Current Medical Controversies; Terminal Illness. Includes Internet resources.

Second edition, 2001   ISBN 0-929718-29-1 $42.95

"It is refreshing to find a source of practical information on how to proceed through the medical maze...this should become a popular resource in any public, hospital, or academic library's consumer health collection."
Library Journal
"The book is very, very good. There's so much information, it's definitely worth buying." A health care consumer

The Mental Health Resource Guide

In a landmark report, the Surgeon General declared that mental illness is a public health problem of great magnitude. Both the public and professionals hold misconceptions about mental disorders. **The Mental Health Resource Guide** is designed to help individuals who are mentally ill, family members, and health professionals understand the issues surrounding mental illness and find services. The book provides information on treatments in current use, medications, laws that affect individuals who are mentally ill, employment, and the needs of children and elders. The effects of mental illness on the family and caregivers are also addressed. Chapters on anxiety disorders, eating disorders, depressive disorders, schizophrenia, and substance abuse include information about causes, diagnoses, and treatments as well as descriptions of helpful organizations, publications, and tapes. Includes Internet resources.

2001   ISBN 0-929718-27-5 $39.95

"...authoritative...will add value to professional health care collections and public libraries." Library Journal
"packed full of information...in crisp, clear prose."   American Reference Books Annual

Resources for Elders with Disabilities

This book provides information that enables elders, family members and other caregivers, and service providers to locate appropriate services. Published in LARGE PRINT (18 point bold type), the book provides information about rehabilitation, laws that affect elders with disabilities, and self-help groups. Each chapter that deals with a specific disability or condition has information on the causes and treatments for the condition; psychological aspects; professional service providers; where to find services; environmental adaptations; and suggestions for making everyday living safer and easier. Chapters on hearing loss, vision loss, Parkinson's disease, stroke, arthritis, osteoporosis, and diabetes also provide information on organizations, publications and tapes, and assistive devices. Throughout the book are practical suggestions to prevent accidents and to facilitate interactions with family members, friends, and service providers. Includes Internet resources.

Fourth edition, 1999　　　　　　　ISBN 0-929718-24-0　　　　　　　　　$49.95

"...especially useful for older readers. Highly recommended."　　　*Library Journal*
"...a valuable, well organized, easy-to-read reference source."　*American Reference Books Annual*

LARGE PRINT PUBLICATIONS

Designed for distribution by professionals, these publications serve as self-help guides for people with disabilities and chronic conditions. They include information on the condition, rehabilitation services, professional service providers, products, and resources that help people with disabilities and chronic conditions to live independently. Titles include "Living with Low Vision," "How to Keep Reading with Vision Loss," and "Living with Diabetic Retinopathy." Printed in 18 point bold type on ivory paper with black ink for maximum contrast. 8 1/2" by 11" Sold in minimum quantities of 25 copies per title. See order form on last page of this book for complete list of titles.

"These are exciting products. We look forward to doing business with you again."
A rehabilitation professional

Living with Low Vision
A Resource Guide for People with Sight Loss

This LARGE PRINT (18 point bold type) comprehensive directory helps people with sight loss locate the services, products, and publications that they need to keep reading, working, and enjoying life. Chapters for children and elders plus information on self-help groups, how to keep reading and working with vision loss, and making everyday living easier. Information on laws that affect people with vision loss, including the ADA, and high tech equipment that promotes independence and employment. Includes Internet resources.

Sixth edition 2001　　　　　　　ISBN 0-929718-28-3　　　　　　　　　$46.95

"no other complete resource guide exists..an invaluable tool for locating services.. for public and academic libraries."
　　　　Library Journal
"This volume is a treasure chest of concise, useful information."　*OT Week*

A Woman's Guide to Coping with Disability

This **unique** book addresses the special needs of women with disabilities and chronic conditions, such as social relationships, sexual functioning, pregnancy, childrearing, caregiving, and employment. Special attention is paid to ways in which women can advocate for their rights with the health care and rehabilitation systems. Written for women in all age categories, the book has chapters on the disabilities that are most prevalent in women or likely to affect the roles and physical functions unique to women. Included are arthritis, diabetes, epilepsy, lupus, multiple sclerosis, osteoporosis, and spinal cord injury. Each chapter also includes information about the condition, service providers, and psychological aspects plus descriptions of organizations, publications and tapes, and special assistive devices. Includes Internet resources.

Third edition 2000   ISBN 0-929718-26-7 $44.95

"...this excellent, empowering resource belongs in all collections." *Library Journal*
"...crucial information women need to be informed, empowered, and in control of their lives. *Excellent* self-help information... *Highly recommended* for public and academic libraries." *Choice*
"...a *marvelous* publication...will help women feel more in control of their lives."
                                        A nurse who became disabled

A Man's Guide to Coping with Disability

Written to fill the void in the literature regarding the special needs of men with disabilities, this book includes information about men's responses to disability, with a special emphasis on the values men place on independence, occupational achievement, and physical activity. Information on finding local services, self-help groups, laws that affect men with disabilities, sports and recreation, and employment is applicable to men with any type of disability or chronic condition. The disabilities that are most prevalent in men or that affect men's special roles in society are included. Chapters on coronary heart disease, diabetes, HIV/AIDS, multiple sclerosis, prostate conditions, spinal cord injury, and stroke include information about the disease or condition, psychological aspects, sexual functioning, where to find services, environmental adaptations, and annotated entries of organizations, publications and tapes, and resources for assistive devices. Includes Internet resources.

Second edition 1999   ISBN 0-929718-23-2 $44.95

"a unique reference source." *Library Journal*
"a unique purchase for public libraries" *Booklist/Reference Books Bulletin*
"...Thank you for the **high quality** books you provide."   *A nurse's aide*

Meeting the Needs of Employees with Disabilities

A comprehensive resource guide that provides employers and counselors with the information they need to help people with disabilities retain or obtain employment. Includes information on government programs and laws, such as the Americans with Disabilities Act, training programs, supported employment, transition from school to work, and environmental adaptations. Chapters on hearing and speech impairments, mobility impairments, visual impairment and blindness describe organizations, adaptive equipment, and services plus suggestions for a safe and friendly workplace. Individuals with disabilities also will find this to be a valuable resource guide. Includes Internet resources.

Third edition 1999   ISBN 0-929718-25-9 $44.95

"...recommended for public libraries and for academic libraries..." Choice
"...a valuable resource...an informative reference for professionals and the public...a good reference for human resources personnel..." Journal of Applied Rehabilitation Counseling

Providing Services for People with Vision Loss
A Multidisciplinary Perspective
Susan L. Greenblatt, Editor

Written by ophthalmologists, rehabilitation professionals, a physician who has experienced - vision loss, and a sociologist, this book discusses how various professionals can work together to provide coordinated care for people with vision loss. Chapters include Vision Loss: A Patient's Perspective; Vision Loss: An Ophthalmologist's Perspective; Operating a Low Vision Aids Service; The Need for Coordinated Care; Making Referrals for Rehabilitation Services; Mental Health Services: The Missing Link; Self-Help Groups for People with Sight Loss; and Aids and Techniques that Help People with Vision Loss plus a Glossary. Available in standard print and on audiocassette.

1989   ISBN 0-929718-02-X $19.95

"an excellent overview of the perspectives and clinical services that facilitate rehabilitation."
Archives of Ophthalmology
"...an excellent guide for professionals" Journal of Rehabilitation

Meeting the Needs of People with Vision Loss
A Multidisciplinary Perspective
Susan L. Greenblatt, Editor

Written by rehabilitation professionals, physicians, and a sociologist, this book discusses how to provide appropriate information and how to serve special populations. Chapters include What People with Vision Loss Need to Know; Information and Referral Services for People with Vision Loss; The Role of the Family in the Adjustment to Blindness or Visual Impairment; Diabetes and Vision Loss - Special Considerations; Special Needs of Children and Adolescents; Older Adults with Vision and Hearing Losses; Providing Services to Visually Impaired Elders in Long Term Care Facilities; plus a series of Multidisciplinary Case Studies. Available in standard print and on audiocassette.

1991   ISBN 0-929718-07-0 $24.95

"...of use to anyone concerned with improving service delivery to the growing population of people who are visually impaired." American Journal of Occupational Therapy

RESOURCES for REHABILITATION →

22 Bonad Road • Winchester, MA 01890 • (781) 368-9094 • FAX (781) 368-9096
e-mail: orders@rfr.org • www.rfr.org
Our Federal Employer Identification Number is 04-2975-007

NAME _____

ORGANIZATION _____

ADDRESS _____

PHONE _____

[ ] Check or signed institutional purchase order enclosed for full amount of order. Purchase orders accepted fr
government agencies, hospitals, and universities <u>only</u>.

[ ] Mastercard/VISA Card number: _____

Signature: _____ Expiration date: _____

ALL ORDERS OF $100.00 OR LESS <u>MUST</u> BE PREPAID.

TITLE	QUANTITY		PRICE	TOTAL
Resources for people with disabilities and chronic conditions	____	X	$ 56.95	_____
Resources for elders with disabilities	____	X	49.95	_____
Making wise medical decisions	____	X	42.95	_____
Living with low vision: A resource guide	____	X	46.95	_____
A woman's guide to coping with disability	____	X	44.95	_____
A man's guide to coping with disability	____	X	44.95	_____
The mental health resource guide	____	X	39.95	_____
Providing services for people with vision loss	____	X	19.95	_____
[ ] Check here for audiocassette edition				
Meeting the needs of people with vision loss	____	X	24.95	_____
[ ] Check here for audiocassette edition				
Meeting the needs of employees with disabilities	____	X	44.95	_____

<u>MINIMUM PURCHASE OF 25 COPIES PER TITLE FOR THE FOLLOWING PUBLICATIONS</u>
Call for discount on purchases of 100 or more copies of any single title.

Living with diabetes	____	X	1.75	_____
Living with low vision	____	X	2.00	_____
How to keep reading with vision loss	____	X	1.75	_____
Living with diabetic retinopathy	____	X	1.75	_____
Living with age-related macular degeneration	____	X	1.25	_____
Aids for everyday living with vision loss	____	X	1.25	_____
High tech aids for people with vision loss	____	X	1.75	_____
	SUB-TOTAL			_____

SHIPPING & HANDLING: $50.00 or less, add $5.00; $50.01 to 100.00, add $8.00;
add $4.00 for each additional $100.00 or fraction of $100.00. Alaska, Hawaii,
U.S. territories, and Canada, add $3.00 to shipping and handling charges
Foreign orders must be prepaid in U.S. currency.
Please write for shipping charges.

SHIPPING/HANDLING _____

<u>Prices are subject to change.</u>

TOTAL $_____